Susan Curtis has worked with natural remedies since 1979. She originally trained as a homoeopath, and has since studied and used other forms of natural healing including herbs, essential oils and flower remedies. For several years, Susan practised professionally at a clinic of natural medicine in London, but recently she has committed herself to helping people to treat themselves using natural remedies. She is a co-author, with Romy Fraser, of *Neal's Yard Natural Remedies*. Susan is married and lives in South London.

Romy Fraser founded the innovative and highly successful Neal's Yard Remedies, specialising in alternative medicines and natural cosmetics, in 1981. Its franchises are being set up all over Britain, and the range of Neal's Yard Remedies products is available in Australia and the United States. Romy has two children and lives in London.

Natural Healing
for Women

Caring for yourself with herbs,
homoeopathy & essential oils

Susan Curtis & Romy Fraser

An Imprint of HarperCollins*Publishers*

Pandora
An Imprint of HarperCollins *Publishers*
77–85 Fulham Palace Road,
Hammersmith, London W6 8JB

First published by Pandora in 1991
10 9 8 7 6

British Library Cataloguing in Publication Data
can be obtained from the British Library.

ISBN 0 04 440645 2

Printed in Great Britain by
HarperCollinsManufacturing Glasgow

This book is presented as a collection of natural remedies
and as an aid in understanding the various theories and
practices underlying their use. The book does not
represent an endorsement or guarantee as to the efficacy
of any remedy, or of its preparation. The remedies are not
intended to replace or supersede medical consultation
and treatment.

Contents

Acknowledgements

Grateful thanks for their valuable contributions to this book are extended to David Loxley, Rachel Packer and Cathy Roguski, and to Ginny Iliff and Candida Lacey at Pandora Press.

Introduction

The most interesting thing about natural medicines is what lies behind them, what the way of life is that incorporates them. The reawakening of interest in natural medicine in the western world is part of the process of re-evaluation of technology and materialism that has been occurring in the past few decades. As our respect for the earth as an infinitely complex living organism grows, so we can begin to trust her more to provide what we need. To trust and respect nature is to trust and respect your body, and your body's own healing potential.

The same attitude that has allowed us to exploit resources and pollute the earth has led us to filling our body's with chemicals from drugs and in our food. The ecosystems of the earth are suffering from pollution, destruction of natural habitats and depletion of resources. Our health is suffering from diets which are nutrient deficient and affected by chemical toxicity and the stress of living in inhospitable environments. These problems are of a chronic nature; they did not arrive overnight, and they will not disappear without a lot of effort and re-education.

Using natural remedies is one of the ways in which we can make a positive step towards improving the quality of our life and health. What is exciting about natural remedies is that they can be used by everyone, on themselves. This is very empowering. Once we have access to our own healing we can take fuller responsibility for our lives as a whole.

The first step towards natural healing may well be visiting a practitioner. A good practitioner will encourage you to become involved in your own healing whilst using their knowledge and skill to help you overcome your present symptoms. Later, by learning yourself about natural remedies, through courses, reading books like this one and, above all, by trying out the remedies, you can begin to make your own decisions about what you need.

If at any time you feel stuck in an uncomfortable frame of mind, or with a particular set of symptoms, despite attempts to treat yourself, then it is probably time to accept that you may need to consult a practitioner. Being healthy is not about cutting yourself off from other people, avoiding difficulties, or even setting yourself up in an ideal environment on an organic farm in the middle of the countryside. It is about being prepared to change and grow as a person, and developing a greater contact with your purpose for living – your spirit, if you like.

Ultimately, it may well be that we no longer need even natural remedies because we become so in tune with our needs that we are able to stay in balance without recourse to anything external. But natural remedies are there to help us, they are safe when used sensibly and they are an exciting part of the learning process; so use them.

The Body's Systems and Their Diseases

Introduction

Our body, with all its idiosyncracies and symptoms, is a perfect reflection of whom we are. We are each a unity made up of myriad components. You cannot look at your stomach in isolation from the rest of your body, your eating habits and lifestyle, any more than you can look at your physical body without considering the feeling and thinking person that inhabits it.

Modern science has taught us to become accustomed to isolating parts of our body, and its symptoms and illnesses, without considering the interconnected nature of all life. This has led us to develop drugs and surgical techniques that are effective in a particular way, but do not support the organism as a whole. Looking for causes of disease within an individual's life has become neglected, as has a genuine consideration for the overall well-being of the patient.

Natural healing methods should always consider the person as a whole being. The remedies are generally gentler in action than drugs, and support the energy of the body, and not override it. We can often treat ourselves with natural medicine, thus taking a greater responsibility for our own lives as opposed to placing them in the hands of doctors and experts.

We can look at the different systems of the body just as we contemplate the rivers, mountains and clouds of the earth. This is not to forget that each is part of a whole. The different systems of the body display particular types of symptoms and we can use these to help us trace the cause and the cure of illness. Certain natural remedies have an affinity for particular parts of the body. This was understood in medieval times and used by herbalists to develop the 'doctrine of signatures'. They recognised that certain plants which looked like parts of the body could be used to cure disease in that area. For example, the pansy flower has petals shaped like a heart, and was used to treat diseases of that organ; hence its other name, heartsease.

The remedies that are mentioned here under a particular disease heading are merely suggestions. They should not be used without first looking them up in the Materia Medica section and considering their appropriateness in your own case. They are suggested because they do have an affinity for a particular disease, but each disease and each symptom is unique to you as an individual. When we have a disease we have the opportunity to learn something about ourselves. Taking a remedy should be part of that learning process.

Accidents and Injuries

Taking full responsibility for our lives as a whole means taking on board all the experiences that come to us, even the unexpected or painful ones. Many of us find it particularly difficult to accept that we create a need for the experience of an accident, and that we cannot simply blame the outside world. However, Freud and many psychologists since, have developed the concept that accidents, like slips of the tongue and forgetting things, are actually products of our unconscious intentions. It is actually very empowering to see that we create our own experiences in life, and that we are never simply the victims of it.

To gain an understanding of the role of an accident in your life requires investigating the circumstances and its effects in detail, and applying what you discovered to your current situation. The underlying causes of an accident can be immensely varied, although amongst the most common is the idea that we are resisting or avoiding a change that needs to be made.

By discussing and questioning what might be behind the experience of an accident with trusted friends, or a therapist, it is nearly always possible to come to understand it; and it is remarkable how a person always seems to be able to recognise one explanation that seems particularly appropriate when the various possibilities are explored. A book that throws more light on the role of accidents in our lives is *The Healing Power of Illness* by T. Dethlefsen and R. Dahlke (Element Books).

See also the First Aid Kit on pages 389–91.

Bites and Stings

Some people are more sensitive to insect stings and bites than others. If symptoms of collapse or breathing difficulties develop then seek emergency medical advice. The remedies mentioned here will help you to deal with any pain or minor reaction, but it is also important to use methods that prevent infection from developing.

Herbs that will help to relieve pain and inflammation resulting from a bite or sting include: CHAMOMILE, MARSHMALLOW and WITCHAZEL. These should be infused and applied locally. Those that prevent infection and promote healing include: MARIGOLD and ST JOHN'S WORT. These should also be infused or used as tinctures to apply locally. GARLIC and ECHINACEA may be taken internally to prevent infection. Herbs may also be used to repel insects – try an infusion or the tinctures of the following: LAVENDER, PENNYROYAL, PYRETHRUM and WORMWOOD. Apply these to the skin, or spray them in a room.

The essential oils of EUCALYPTUS, LAVENDER or MELISSA may be dabbed onto the site of a sting or insect bite to relieve inflammation. BERGAMOT or TEA TREE essential oils may be used to prevent infection. The essential oils that repel insects, include: CITRONELLA, LAVENDER, LEMON GRASS and PEPPERMINT. These may be diluted in vegetable oil and applied to exposed skin, or burnt in a room.

Homoeopathic remedies can be very effective at treating the symptoms of insect bites and stings, and animal bites. Consider the following remedies by looking them up in the Materia Medica section: APIS, ARNICA, CALADIUM, HYPERICUM, LACHESIS, LEDUM and STAPHYSAGRIA.

Bruises

A bruise is the result of a blow or fall that causes damage to the soft tissue beneath the skin, and breaks the skin capillaries. The skin becomes discoloured where the blood clots in the bruised area.

The two most effective remedies to treat bruising are ARNICA and WITCHAZEL. These may be applied locally in the form of a lotion or ointment. Other anti-inflammatory herbs that may be used as a compress to relieve bruising, include: COMFREY, MARIGOLD and YARROW.

Essential oils may also bring relief to the discomfort of bruising. The most effective are LAVENDER and MARJORAM, and are best applied as a compress.

For more severe cases of bruising, homoeopathic remedies can treat shock, relieve pain, and reduce inflammation. The first remedy to consider is ARNICA, although HYPERICUM, LEDUM or RUTA may also be appropriate.

Burns

The correct treatment for a burn depends on how severe it is. Minor burns and scalds can be dealt with safely at home, but the emergency services should be called for more serious burns. In a serious case, do not attempt to remove clothing before getting to casualty, as this may damage the skin further. Burns resulting from exposure to chemicals should be treated first by bathing the affected area with cold running water for at least five minutes.

When you treat minor or severe burns one of the most important things is to prevent an infection developing. Use only clean gauze and sterile utensils, if these are not available then leave the burns exposed to the air and take great pains to keep them clean. If blisters form, do not puncture or interfere with them, as they form a protective cushion for the damaged skin.

Internal treatment for shock, for example homoeopathic ARNICA or the Healing Herbs of Dr Bach FIRST-AID REMEDY, may safely be given in any case where a burn is involved. Other homoeopathic remedies that may be used in the treatment of burns include: CANTHARIS, CAUSTICUM, KALI BICH and URTICA URENS.

The most effective emergency treatment for burns that we know is to pour the essential oil of LAVENDER over the area: this is soothing, prevents infection, and promotes new tissue growth. Herbal or homoeopathic tinctures that you may use in the same way are: HYPERICUM and URTICA URENS. The juice of the ALOE VERA plant is also effective; grow the plant in your kitchen so that you can break a piece of the leaf off and squeeze the gel onto a burn whenever necessary.

An antiseptic and healing wash can be made by infusing the herbs COMFREY, MARIGOLD and ST JOHN'S WORT, and bathing the affected part.

COMFREY ointment may be used once the burn has healed over, to reduce scarring.

Eye Injuries

Because the eyes are so delicate, any eye injury should be examined by a physician to assess the damage.

Loose foreign bodies or splashes of chemical substances in the eye should be flushed out with plenty of cool, clean water.

Anti-inflammatory herbs may be used to bathe the eye by cooling down an infusion, or diluting the tinctures; consider especially: CHAMOMILE, EYEBRIGHT and WITCHAZEL. Homoeopathic remedies to consider, depending upon the nature of the injury, include: ARNICA, LEDUM, SILICA and SYMPHYTUM. Consult the Materia Medica section to find the most appropriate remedy.

Fractures

It can be difficult to tell if a bone is broken – an X-ray may be needed. Then the bone has to be set in plaster to keep it rigid and allow it to heal. Take the homoeopathic remedy ARNICA immediately to treat any shock, reduce bruising and promote healing from the beginning.

The most common sites of fractures are the wrist, ankle and collar bone. Elderly people are more prone to fractures as their bones tend to be more brittle.

The most effective way to promote the healing of broken bones externally is to apply a compress. Make an infusion of the herbs COMFREY, HORSETAIL and MOUSEAR to apply locally (obviously this will not be possible until any plaster cast has been removed). COMFREY ROOT may also be taken internally to encourage the healing of the bone. Essential oils may be applied as a compress, or diluted in vegetable oil to massage into the area: LAVENDER, MARJORAM, ROSEMARY and THYME will soothe any aching and promote healing.

Homoeopathic remedies to consider to promote healing, and ease any symptoms of discomfort include: ARNICA, BRYONIA, EUPATORIUM PERF, HYPERICUM, RUTA and SYMPHYTUM. Consult the Materia Medica section to see which is most appropriate.

Head Injuries

For any injury to the head that involves a loss of consciousness, however brief, professional medical advice should be sought immediately. Following a head injury the person should be treated as for Shock (see below).

If the person is unconscious, check that their air passages are clear, and place them in the 'recovery position': lying on their front or side, with their head turned to the side so that any vomit or secretions drain out of the mouth instead of down into their lungs. The Healing Herbs of Dr Bach FIRST-AID REMEDY may be placed on exposed pulse points while awaiting the emergency services.

If the person is conscious, give them some homoeopathic ARNICA while awaiting medical advice. ARNICA should also be given when concussion follows a blow to the head. The homoeopathic remedy NATRUM SULPH should also be considered after a head injury.

Shock

Physical shock is a reaction that occurs when the blood flow is reduced to below its normal levels. Some degree of shock can occur after any injury, burn or illness that involves the loss of blood or other body fluids. Shock can also occur following coronary thrombosis, allergic reaction, severe infection or malfunction of the nervous system. The characteristics of shock are: general weakness; cold, clammy, pale skin; a rapid, weak pulse; reduced alertness; and shallow breathing. Nausea may also be present. Hot sweetened tea will help for minor shock.

You should suspect shock following any accident or injury, and apply first-aid measures, then call the emergency services if the injury is severe. The first-aid treatment of shock is to reassure the patient; keep them lying down, with their legs higher than their head if they feel faint (except in the case of a head or chest injury where the head should be higher than the feet); and keep them warm.

A herbal infusion that will help with minor cases of shock, or may be administered while you are awaiting emergency medical treatment, can be made from: BALM, CHAMOMILE, PEPPERMINT and SCULLCAP. This infusion can be sweetened with honey. Do not give

11

the patient anything to drink before medical investigations in the case of an abdominal injury.

The first homoeopathic remedy to administer for shock is ARNICA. If available, the following homoeopathic remedies can also be useful: ACONITE, CHAMOMILLA, CHINA and IGNATIA.

The essential oils of LAVENDER, MELISSA, NEROLI or PEPPERMINT will alleviate the symptoms of shock. Place a few drops on a tissue so the patient can inhale the vapours, or massage a couple of drops onto their temple.

Sprains and Strains

Sprains and strains are caused by an injury that tears or stretches the supporting tissue of a joint. The most common sites of such damage are the ankles, wrists and knees.

Cold water compressess will offer some relief as a first-aid measure. If symptoms appear at all severe, seek medical advice to rule out the possibility of a fracture. A supporting bandage may be helpful to take the strain off the affected joint while it heals.

An anti-inflammatory and healing compress can be made by using an infusion, or the diluted tinctures, of the herbs ARNICA, COMFREY or WITCHAZEL. ARNICA, COMFREY and RHUS TOX are all available as ointments to massage into the site of a sprain, strain or pulled muscle. A compress may be made using the essential oils of EUCALYPTUS, LAVENDER, MARJORAM or ROSEMARY, or add a few drops of one to a warm bath.

Immediately after the injury treat the patient with the homoeopathic remedy ARNICA. Then consult the Materia Medica section to see which of the following homoeopathic remedies is best indicated for your particular symptoms: BELLIS PERENNIS, BRYONIA, RHUS TOX and RUTA.

Sunburn

Prolonged exposure to the sun causes dehydration of the skin. To prevent painful burning or blistering occuring, keep the skin protected with a sunscreen lotion, and only expose yourself to the sun for short periods of time until you become accustomed to it.

If you do become sunburned treat it in the same way as a burn (see page 9). Bathe the area with a cooled herbal infusion, or diluted tinctures, of CHAMOMILE, ST JOHN'S WORT or WITCHAZEL. Apply the infused herbal oils of MARIGOLD or ST JOHN'S WORT; or add some CALENDULA tincture to OLIVE OIL and apply that to the burned skin. ALOE VERA gel will have a cooling and healing effect. The essential oils of BERGAMOT or LAVENDER may be diluted in vegetable oil and applied locally.

If the person becomes severely overheated, and the cooling mechanism of the skin fails, then sunstroke will occur. The skin becomes hot and dry with sunstroke, and the body temperature rises; this can be dangerous and you should get medical advice. Other symptoms of sunstroke are feelings of dizziness, nausea or feverishness, and a severe headache. The first-aid treatment for sunstroke is to cool the person off by bathing them in cool water, and give a glass of cool water with half a teaspoon of salt in it to promote perspiration.

The most important homoeopathic remedies that may be indicated after too much sun or sunstroke are BELLADONNA and GLONOINE.

Wounds

Wounds may be classified as contused, incised, lacerated, perforated or punctured, and each one needs to be dealt with individually:

CONTUSED: Severe contusions or bruises, for example following a car accident, may indicate serious underlying injury, and the emergency services must be called. Treat for Shock (pages 11–12) as a first-aid measure. For minor contusions see Bruises (pages 8–9).

INCISED: Wounds made by cutting, for example with a knife, tend to bleed a good deal and the edges gape. If blood loss is severe, hold a clean cloth tightly against the wound and call the emergency services. After it has been cleaned the edges may need to be stitched together. The wound should heal within a week or two providing there is no infection.

To clean an incised wound bathe the area with the diluted tincture of HYPERICUM. To promote rapid healing apply the diluted tincture of CALENDULA. The antiseptic essential oils of BERGAMOT, LAVENDER or TEA TREE may be applied on clean gauze to prevent infection. If

13

the wound becomes weepy then apply the essential oil of MYRRH in the same way. Immediately after sustaining the wound give the homoeopathic remedy ARNICA; to promote rapid healing give the homoeopathic remedy CALENDULA.

LACERATED: Torn wounds are the most likely wounds to become infected. These are the most likely to be sustained in a car accident. A severe, lacerated wound should be treated by a surgeon, who will clean them thoroughly. Minor, lacerated wounds may be treated at home in the same way as incised wounds.

PERFORATING: Wounds that pass through part of the body, for example caused by bullets or fragments of metal, are called perforating. These wounds will need to be treated by a surgeon. As a first-aid measure treat as for Shock (see pages 11–12).

PUNCTURED: Punctured wounds are caused by a sharp object, for example a nail or needle, perforating the skin. Punctures can be dangerous because it may be impossible to tell how far the puncturing object has penetrated: if there is any question of deep penetration call the emergency services. The homoeopathic remedy ARNICA may be given to relieve shock. If the wound is very painful administer the homoeopathic remedy HYPERICUM. The homoeopathic remedy LEDUM may be used as a prophylactic for tetanus.

Breasts and Breastfeeding

Breasts have developed in certain female mammals, including humans, as a method of producing milk to feed their young. Their growth and development are regulated by hormones, first during puberty and then for milk production during pregnancy and childbirth.

Each breast is divided into about twenty compartments containing systems of branching tubes lined by cells that secrete milk. In each compartment, the tubes join together to form a single duct that opens out on the surface of the nipple, making about twenty openings in total. The tissue between the tubes is filled with muscle fibres, fibrous strands and fat.

Traditionally breasts are a symbol of fertility, fecundity and motherhood; they connect humanity with the abundance of nature. However, in western society breasts have become estranged from this symbolism so that they have more to do with sexuality, stimulation and titillation; women have become objects of fantasy and breasts fashion accessories.

Breast Disease

Many women find that their breasts swell and become tender before a period. This process is regulated by our hormones and in the second half of the menstrual cycle, the breast builds up fluid and glandular tissue to prepare for pregnancy. If conception does not occur, the body reabsorbs all this extra substance via the lymph system, which acts as a drain for the breasts.

If the process of fluid and tissue build-up followed by drainage becomes inefficient, congestion will develop, and this may become

Cross Section of the Breast

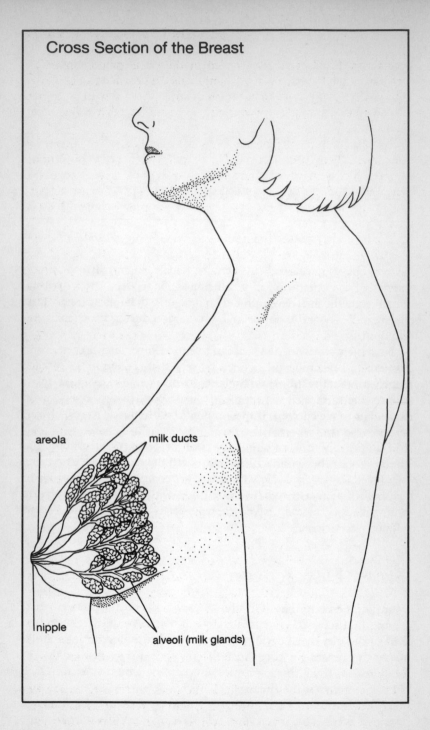

areola

milk ducts

nipple

alveoli (milk glands)

permanent. Fluids can get trapped in the ducts of the breast to form sacs called cysts, or solid lumps called fibroadenomas. When a generally lumpy and swollen condition results then it is either fibroadenosis (multiple tiny nodules) or cystic mastitis (fibrocystic disease).

Over 80 per cent of reported cases of breast lumps are caused by one of these 'benign' conditions. Cancer of the breast can also exist as a lump, which is usually hard and may be tender or painless. Symptoms may also include a discharge of bloody or clear fluid from the nipple, flaking or puckering of the skin over the lump or enlarged lymph glands in the armpit.

Around 95 per cent of breast cancers are discovered by the women themselves, and all Family Planning and Health Clinics now have leaflets explaining how to do a breast self-examination. This involves examining the breasts visually and by touch for any unusual lumps or skin changes that remain for more than one menstrual cycle. The examination is best carried out at the same time each month, just after your period has finished, and when the breasts are no longer swollen.

Orthodox treatment of breast cancer includes surgery, radiation and chemotherapy. Some women prefer to consider alternative systems of medicine such as herbalism, homoeopathy, acupuncture and nutritional or psychological approaches. Many will try a combination of orthodox and alternative treatments. Whichever approach you chose, dealing with the cancer in its early stages is likely to be more successful than when it is well advanced.

Since initial stages of breast disease lie in the lymphatic system's inability to drain and reabsorb waste matter which accumulates during the menstrual cycle, and by an imbalance of the hormones oestrogen and progesterone, it is very important that this system is healthy in order to avoid or treat breast disease. See Lymphatic System beginning on page 89 for suggestions on improving its function.

Caffeine presents a problem for the lymphatic system because it is difficult to eliminate; it is also known to aggravate any tendency you may have to develop fibroids and cysts. Both of these are good reasons to avoid caffeine, whether it is in coffee, cola drinks or chocolate. Try dandelion coffee or herb teas instead. Fresh fruit and fresh green vegetables, preferably organically grown, are good things to eat.

The herbs that are most useful in the treatment of breast disease are those that assist the lymphatic system in its task of drainage. Consider especially: CLEAVERS, GOLDEN SEAL, MARIGOLD, MARSHMALLOW,

NETTLES, RED CLOVER, SLIPPERY ELM, and YELLOW DOCK. The herb VITEX should also be considered when there is a hormonal imbalance contributing to breast disease.

There is a specialist form of massage known as 'Lymphatic drainage'; this is particularly good when it is combined with the right essential oils. Essential oils that encourage lymph drainage, help to regulate any hormone imbalance and relieve symptoms of breast disease include: FENNEL, GERANIUM, LAVENDER, JUNIPER and ROSEMARY. These oils can be added to the bath too. **Important**: None of the lymphatic drainage methods should be used if you have cancer as it tends to spread via the lymphatic system, and speeding up the flow of lymph fluid may encourage secondary sites of the cancer to develop.

EVENING PRIMROSE OIL has been found to be effective for treating symptoms of breast disease, such as swelling and tenderness, that are markedly worse before a period. You can take it in capsule form throughout the cycle or for ten days before each period.

Homoeopathic treatment can be very successful in treating breast disease, but you will probably need constitutional treatment by a qualified practitioner to find the right remedy or remedies that take all the contributory factors into account. Among those homoeopathic remedies to be considered are: BRYONIA, LACHESIS, PHYTOLACCA, PULSATILLA and SILICA. All the remedies mentioned here should be cross-referenced in the Materia Medica section of this book.

See also the information on pre-menstrual tension on page 147 in the Reproductive System.

Breastfeeding

The evidence for the benefits of breastfeeding compared to bottle feeding is so overwhelming that it is a good example of the need that existed to return to a way of life that has more respect for what is natural. Bottle feeding became increasingly popular in the decades immediately following the 1939–45 War. It represented the success of technology over the primitive and natural. Food and drug companies soon invested huge amounts of money in promoting their baby feeds as the best. In more recent years, increased interest in natural health combined with the realisation that breastfed babies are healthier, has led to the recognition that 'breast is best'.

Bottle-fed babies are more prone to suffer from allergies,

gastrointestinal, ear, respiratory, viral and yeast infections, and from being overweight, than their breastfed counterparts. Breast milk is full of antibodies and anti-allergens that protect the baby from disease and infection. It is also easily digestible, as well as warm, fresh, sterile and conveniently available.

Breastfeeding also has benefits for the mother. Suckling after child-birth stimulates the pituitary gland to release oxytocin, the hormone that makes the uterus contract and helps it return to its normal size and shape. Any extra weight gained during pregnancy will be more easily lost at a slow and steady pace while breastfeeding, without the need for dieting. Breastfeeding usually delays the resumption of ovulation and menstruation for some months, although birth control methods should still be used to avoid pregnancy, as you can never be sure when ovulation resumes until after the event (i.e. with menstruation or another pregnancy!).

Breastfeeding should not have any effect on the size or shape of the breasts, as long as a well-made maternity bra is worn to support the extra weight. There is some suggestion that women who have breastfed are at less risk of developing breast cancer, although there are other factors that are more important here (such as family tendency and previous breast disease).

It is possible for nearly all women to breastfeed their babies. The only contra-indications are if the mother has some serious infectious illness, e.g. tuberculosis, or needs to take drugs that will pass through the breast milk to the baby. Inverted nipples will often become more prominent during pregnancy, and this process can be assisted by regularly pulling the nipple out with the fingers and gently squeezing and rolling it around. If the nipple remains inverted you can use a special plastic shield to assist breastfeeding.

It is best to start breastfeeding immediately after the birth, even before the umbilical cord is cut, when the baby's sucking reflex is strongest. Often babies are put to the breast far too late in hospitals, so try to make it clear to the staff that you would like the baby to suckle on the delivery table beforehand. Breastfeeding this early is an important part of the bonding process, it makes use of the baby's early sucking reflex, it stimulates the process of expelling the placenta and uterine readjustment for the mother, and it prevents the breasts from becoming too full and hard which would make feeding more difficult later on.

If the baby has to be put in an incubator, or has a feeding difficulty (such as a cleft palate), then it is still possible to give breast milk by expressing the milk and giving it to him in a bottle. A breast pump should be supplied by the hospital or midwife to help you do this. You can sterilize an ice-cube tray and fill it with breast milk, then freeze it and store in a plastic bag (e.g. bottle liner).

For the first few weeks of breastfeeding a new baby, feeding on demand is virtually essential. This means feeding the baby when he wants to be fed, instead of trying to impose a regime on feeding times. Most babies thrive on being fed little and often during the first few weeks. Feeding regimes (such as four-hourly feeds) were designed for bottle-fed babies who need to have their feeds carefully measured and timed. Most hospitals these days will allow feeding on demand, but if you come up against a member of staff who does not approve of it, you may need to be quite insistent and determined if this is what you want.

During the last few months of pregnancy your breasts will be making colostrum, and this is what you feed your baby for the first couple of days after the birth. Colostrum is rich in protein, minerals, vitamin A and nitrogen. It also contains antibodies that will help to protect the newborn against infections and diseases such as polio, colds, gastro-enteritis, bronchitis, pneumonia, asthma, eczema, colic and measles. It is impossible to manufacture a complex substance such as colostrum synthetically, and this is one reason why it is so important to breastfeed your baby, even if only for one or two weeks. After two or three days of suckling your baby, the milk proper will come in.

Breasts quite naturally produce milk according to the baby's demands: more frequent suckling at the breast stimulates an increase in the milk produced. If you are advised that your baby is not gaining enough weight, simply let her suckle more often. Breastfed babies usually either stay the same weight in the first week after birth, or lose weight: this is quite normal. If your baby loses weight after the first week you should seek medical advice.

After the first few weeks you can try to establish a more regular breastfeeding pattern if you find it helpful, such as feeding every 3–4 hours. After the first month or two, you could try letting someone else give your baby an occasional bottle, but try not to miss two consecutive feeds. If this is successful, it should be possible when the baby is two or three months old, to miss one feed during the day regularly and replace it with a bottle. Missing the same feed every day is the key to successful part-time breastfeeding, if this is what you need to establish. The substitute bottles can contain either formula milk or, preferably, pumped breast milk.

Breastfeeding can supply the total nutritional needs of your baby for up to six months, and can supply three-quarters of their needs for up to a year. However, formula milk, correctly prepared, is perfectly adequate to give occasionally after the first couple of months, and solids or cereals can be introduced slowly after about four months. All these suggestions are very general, and one baby will vary very much from another as to his or her feeding wants and needs. Great flexibility is required to establish feeding patterns that are acceptable for the parents and appropriate for the baby.

If you cannot breastfeed, it can be difficult not to feel guilty about it, but instead put your energy into finding out about the best feeds available, and creating a pleasant and relaxed feeding environment. Cow's milk is best avoided by babies because it is a common cause of allergies, mucous congestion and colic. Goat's milk is much more similar than cow's milk to human breast milk and is much less likely to cause digestive upsets. Soya milk is not rich enough in iron and calcium to be given on its own, but the unsweetened variety can be mixed with goat's or sheep's milk.

Nursing mothers require plenty of protein, vitamins and iron in their diet. You do not need to eat any one thing in particular, but ensure that your diet contains plenty of fresh fruit and vegetables, whole grains and protein-rich foods (such as soya beans, cheese, lentils, lean meat, fish, eggs and nuts). If you suspect at any time that you may be anaemic, have a blood test, and then follow the advice in this book under Anaemia in the section on the Circulatory System (see pages 55–6). Dieting can quickly result in a reduction in the milk supply, so do not try any crash diets, but avoid refined sugar and refined carbohydrates (e.g. white flour), and remember that breastfeeding will slowly use up the stores of fat that were laid down during pregnancy for that purpose.

It is important to drink plenty of liquids whilst breastfeeding: try to drink at least 2 litres (4 pints) of liquid a day.

BREAST ENGORGEMENT

On the third day after giving birth a reflex occurs that stimulates the breasts to produce milk in place of the colostrum that the breasts have been producing during pregnancy. If the milk comes in suddenly the breasts can feel full, heavy, lumpy and tender. The milk needs to be cleared from the breasts regularly, either by the baby suckling or manually, until things have settled down. If the baby has been encouraged to suckle immediately after labour, and on demand following that, painful engorgement is much less likely to occur.

If the breasts do become engorged and painful try placing flannels that have been immersed in very cold water onto the breasts. Consider taking the homoeopathic remedy BRYONIA if the breasts are very hard and painful. A compress made using a few drops of the anti-inflammatory essential oils of CHAMOMILE, GERANIUM, LAVENDER or ROSE in warm water can be applied to the breasts at regular intervals to relieve engorgement. Remember to wash any residue of the oils off before feeding the baby again. A compress of herbs made up of MARSHMALLOW and SLIPPERY ELM can be very helpful, or take POKE ROOT and MARSHMALLOW internally.

Engorgement will also occur if you have to stop breastfeeding the baby suddenly for any reason. If you are only stopping temporarily you can keep the breasts clear and still produce milk by using a pump to express the milk. If you want to stop producing milk altogether then taking the homoeopathic remedy LAC CANINUM will help you. Try taking just one dose of 200C and only repeat after a couple of days if necessary. You can also drink an infusion of the herb RED SAGE, or GARDEN SAGE if only this is available. Drink a cupful three times a day for several days.

CRACKED NIPPLES

Sore and cracked nipples can be quite agonising and need to be dealt with promptly if the mother is to be able to continue breastfeeding. Cracks in the nipples can be an entrance point for bacteria, so the nipples should be carefully washed and dried after every feed to prevent any infection developing. Special nipple shields can be worn inside the bra to allow air to circulate around the nipple so that it can dry out between feeds.

If you have delicate skin, or your nipples are sore, try massaging an oil made by adding a few drops of essential oil of ROSE to a vegetable oil base onto the nipple and surrounding area after each feed. If you get cracked nipples, look up the homoeopathic remedies of CAUSTICUM, GRAPHITES and SILICA in the Materia Medica section of this book to see which one is the most suitable. Also, dilute the tinctures of MARIGOLD and ST JOHN'S WORT in a little boiled water and dap onto the cracked nipples after each feed. COMFREY ointment can also be applied to cracked nipples for a soothing and healing effect. Any substance applied to the nipple should be rinsed off thoroughly using clean water before attempting to feed the baby again. Breast milk is good and healing.

MASTITIS

Mastitis means inflammation of the mammaries (the breasts).

Inflammation may occur due to engorgement, a blocked milk duct or if an infection develops (usually by bacteria entering through a cracked nipple). The symptoms of mastitis are a feeling of heaviness and fullness in the breast, combined with tenderness, pain, heat and possibly redness.

To avoid mastitis developing it is important to regularly empty each breast of milk, and also to wash and dry the nipples carefully after each feed. Mastitis can lead to 'milk fever', which was a common cause of death amongst women in the past. Thus it is important to act quickly to reduce the local symptoms of inflammation, and if the symptoms are persistent, and particularly if the general temperature of the mother continues to rise after a few hours, seek immediate professional advice.

As soon as any symptoms of mastitis develop immerse flannels in very cold water and then apply them to the breast. Take the most appropriate homoeopathic remedy after looking the following up in the Materia Medica section of this book to see which is most suitable: BELLADONNA, BRYONIA and PHYTOLACCA. A paste can be made by mixing MARIGOLD, POKE ROOT and SLIPPERY ELM powder with water; this can be spread over the breast and left on for a couple of hours to reduce the inflammation. Alternatively, add a few drops of the essential oils of CHAMOMILE, LAVENDER or ROSE to some warm water, immerse a clean cloth in the water, and apply to the breast as a compress. Anything applied externally near the nipple should be rinsed off before attempting to feed the baby again. BORAGE or FENNEL will encourage the milk to flow. Also, take ECHINACEA for infection.

POOR MILK SUPPLY

Breast milk should smell good, be pure white (almost bluish-white) in colour, flow easily and taste sweet. It is unusual not to produce enough milk for the baby's demands because generally a hungry baby will stimulate the breasts to produce more milk when allowed to suckle more. However, if the quality or supply of milk does need to be improved, a combination of the herbs and seeds of ANISEED, BORAGE, FENNEL and HOLY THISTLE can be made into an infusion. Drink a cupful two or three times a day for a few weeks. If the breast milk seems to cause your baby to have colic then try drinking an infusion made from the seeds of DILL before each feed.

WEANING

The least traumatic way of weaning your baby is to do it gradually.

You can try replacing one feed at the same time each day with a bottle feed once the baby is a few months old. Solids can be introduced slowly and made a regular part of the diet once your baby seems able to digest them easily (this time will vary from baby to baby but you can try after four months or so).

Eventually you will probably get breastfeeding down to an evening feed, and probably the odd 'comfort' feed during the night or on a difficult day. Some babies seem quite willing to make the step to not being breastfed from this part-time feeding, whilst for other babies this step will seem impossible without causing great trauma to both mother and baby. Some mothers have found that taking the Healing Herbs of Dr Bach remedy WALNUT, and giving it to the baby, helps them both to make the transition go more smoothly.

When you have determined that it is the right time to wean your baby, you can dry up your breast milk by drinking an infusion of the herb RED SAGE three times a day. Alternatively, take one dose of the homoeopathic remedy LAC CANINUM 200C, and only repeat this after a few days if necessary.

Cancer

Cancer is the name given to a group of diseases all characterised by abnormal cell division. Normal cells reproduce in an orderly fashion to carry on their work of tissue growth and repair; cancer cells begin to divide in an uncontrolled way, creating a mass of extra cells or tissue. When the mass of cancerous cells takes on a solid form it is called a tumour.

Cancer may be invasive, that is when it infiltrates and destroys surrounding healthy tissue. It may also metastasize, when it spreads to other parts of the body and forms new growths called metastases. Untreated cancer is often fatal because it displaces healthy tissue and causes organs to cease functioning until the patient dies. However, the disease may go into spontaneous remission, and the symptoms then decrease or disappear altogether.

Cancer can attack nearly all of the body's organs, and the disease is often named after the organ where it originated – breast cancer, stomach cancer and so on. In women, nearly half of all cases of cancer affect the reproductive system: of these breast cancer accounts for about one quarter of cases, and cancers of the pelvic area account for the rest.

The causes of cancer appear to be very complex. Some substances are known to be carcinogens and can trigger the disease, for example radiation or cigarette smoke. However, even when we are exposed to carcinogens there is an element of individual susceptibility, because not every heavy smoker will develop lung cancer. There are some indications that certain viruses have a role to play in developing cancer, and there are also indications that there may be a hereditary component. Diet is considered to be another significant factor. A diet high in refined and processed foods, and low in fresh vegetables and fibre, is considered to be more likely to lead to certain types of cancer.

Psychological factors also have a role to play, probably by increasing an individual's susceptibility to the disease. It is known, for example, that the incidence of cancer rises considerably for an individual in the two years following the death of a close member of the family. Studies indicate that unassertive people who have difficulty expressing their emotions and forming close personal relationships, are more likely to develop cancer and are also less likely to respond well to treatment.

With cancer what is happening is that a group of cells is dividing itself off from the rest of the organism and developing without regard for the whole. The cancer cells exploit and eventually threaten the life of the rest of the organism, and thereby of course destroy their own source of existence. The exploitation of the well-being of the whole, and the alienation from the essential purpose of the organism, that occurs with cancer, is a revealing metaphor for the problems that are occuring in our society. The increasing incidence of cancer may well be a reflection of the central issues that we need to sort out in order to become a healthier society. For example, many pollutants are known to be carcinogens. Our western diet of refined, low-fibre foods is known to contribute to cancer. We live in a society that does not always encourage the expression of emotion and the development of a sense of purpose. A cure for cancer is not going to come about by finding a wonder-drug, or more sophisticated surgical procedure. Cancer can only be cured by readdressing the factors that contribute to it on every level – physical, emotional and spiritual.

On an individual basis, the fight against cancer is also more likely to be successful if we reassess all the contributive factors and the patient's whole lifestyle. Whatever approach you take to deal with the physical symptoms of cancer, whether it is orthodox chemotherapy or radiotherapy, or by using natural remedies such as herbs, homoeopathy or dietary supplements, your chances of recovery will be improved if you also cultivate a positive, 'fighting' attitude to your disease, and a sense of purpose for your life.

There are many therapies that can help fight the disease and enhance the quality of your life while doing so. A professional herbalist or homoeopath will be able to select the remedies that are most appropriate to your individual case from those that are known to be effective in the treatment of cancer. Specialised forms of diet have been developed specifically to help eliminate chronic diseases such as cancer, so you might consider consulting a naturopath or dietary therapist for advice. Psychotherapists and counsellors have evolved techniques that are particularly appropriate for cancer sufferers. One of the most widely used is known as 'creative visualisation', whereby people are taught to use their imagination, to see themselves fighting off the disease and building a positive image of health.

It is unfortunate that there is so much fear surrounding everything to do with cancer because this tends to undermine our ability to fight the disease successfully. It is partly a reflection of our society's attitude to death as something to be afraid of, to hide away from, ignore and avoid, whatever the cost to our quality of life. Any therapist who has treated people with cancer will recognise the profound personal growth and self-learning that they experience. Indeed, like any other disease, cancer can be an exceptional opportunity to reassess what is valuable in life, to develop a less obsessive attitude towards end results, and concentrate on the quality and purpose of our existence.

See also Stress (page 109), Shock (page 11), Addiction (page 100–2) and Depression (page 103).

Childbirth

The act of giving birth is for many women one of their most powerful life experiences. During childbirth the most amazing physical, emotional and spiritual processes occur in unison – they require a tremendous output of energy and effort by the mother. The overwhelming experience of delivery heralds the arrival of a new person who will affect the inter-relationship of a whole family and the total life of the mother.

The preparation for birth means creating a context in which a new human can thrive physically, emotionally and spiritually. It is no wonder that so many of those involved in the birthing process today place more and more emphasis on improving the quality of the whole experience for all concerned, while at the same time doing everything possible to assist the mother and baby through it safely.

Interest in natural medicine has developed alongside an increasing awareness of the benefits of natural childbirth: a movement towards childbirth that is mother and baby-oriented, and not doctor and technology centred. There are a growing number of midwives today who are reclaiming their traditional role of assisting at home births; there is a growing awareness of the benefits of active birth; and for those who choose or need a hospital environment for childbirth, there is an increasing tendency towards allowing the mother more choice about such things as who attends the birth, what position she adopts during labour and maintaining physical contact with the baby following delivery. However, there are still doctors who believe that all deliveries should be obstetrically controlled, and the rate of caesarean sections is still alarmingly high, so it can require great determination and forward-planning on the part of the mother if she wants to be able to choose the course her labour will follow.

There are some excellent books on childbirth, and it is well worth reading several in advance to learn what options are available, and to read about other women's experiences. Three particularly useful books are: *New Active Birth* by Janet Balaskas (Unwin Paperbacks), *Spiritual Midwifery* by Ina May Gaskin (The Book Publishing Company), and *Freedom and Choice in Childbirth* by Sheila Kitzinger (Penguin). For details on other relevant reading see page 405.

Preparation for the Birth

Many women have benefitted from yoga classes or active birth classes during pregnancy. It is ideal if you can find a yoga class specifically for pregnant women, if not do make sure that your yoga teacher knows that you are pregnant. Your teacher should concentrate on exercises that tone the pelvic floor muscles. The exercises strengthen the muscles that support the weight of the uterus and baby, prepare the muscles for the delivery, and make the muscles more elastic so that they spring back into shape more readily after the birth.

A good yoga or active birth class will also work on breathing techniques and special exercises and positions that can be used during labour. Ask at your local natural health centre or contact the Active Birth Centre (see page 398) for details about classes in your area.

Thinking ahead and making plans for your labour can mean that you have a lot more choice about how it will be. The basic things to consider well in advance are: whether to employ an independent midwife (addresses on page 398) or use the NHS, whether to have a home or a hospital birth, who your birth companions will be, and whether or not you intend to have an active birth.

If you choose to have a home birth you will have a lot more control over such things as who your companions will be, soft lighting, music, your freedom to move around, the amount of contact with the baby following the birth, and soon. Hospitals do vary a lot in their approaches to childbirth these days: some have special rooms with soft lighting, facilities for a companion to stay and an attitude which welcomes natural childbirth where possible. Others are very much stuck on the need for total obstetric control and it can end up like being in a ward for acutely sick people. If you are going to have your baby in hospital, do try and visit it beforehand, and if you are not happy with it ask your doctor or midwife to suggest another.

There are a relatively small number of women who are in one of the categories that make it advisable for them to have a hospital birth for health and safety reasons. Otherwise it really should be your choice, based on where you feel happiest and most relaxed. A hospital birth is advisable for those women who are under 16 or over 40, if the baby engages in a particularly difficult presentation, if there has been bleeding during the third trimester, and for those women who suffer with toxaemia or epilepsy or who have experienced severe postpartum haemorrhage previously.

One thing that many women find particularly important to establish in advance is their hospital's policy on allowing the mother to keep the baby with her. It should be possible to explain that you want to maintain physical contact with the baby immediately after the birth, and to allow the baby to suckle as soon as he or she wishes. Following the birth, some hospitals remove the baby to another room for several hours, and only bring him in at set intervals to be fed. However, others have 'rooming in' facilities so that you can keep the baby with you and feed on demand. The first few days following the birth are now known to be crucial for the bonding of a loving relationship between mother and baby, and this can only develop with plenty of contact. Mothers who do have the chance to bond well with their babies are known to be less likely to suffer from postnatal depression.

It can be helpful to draw up a birth plan that covers all eventualities, when labour and birth go well and what you will choose if things get difficult. This means that you need to work out, ahead of time, whether you want the freedom to move around during labour, what, if any, forms of pain relief you find acceptable, under what circumstances you would opt for induction or a caesarean, whether you want to deliver the placenta naturally or with Syntometrine, when you want to be discharged from hospital, and so on. You can give copies of the birth plan to your companion, midwife and doctor. For a detailed explanation on how to draw up a birth plan, the book *Freedom and Choice in Childbirth* by Sheila Kitzinger (Penguin) is very helpful.

It is worth bearing in mind that while planning and preparation are helpful and useful, no two births are ever the same, and that you cannot really know how your birth is going to be. Indeed, birth is about letting yourself go in the experience of bringing a new person into the world, and no amount of forward-planning can really prepare you for the reality of that experience. Many women who carefully plan and organise a totally natural birth, end up receiving a lot of obstetric assistance, and we should all be grateful that such technology is there when it is needed. If a birth does not go the way it was planned it is certainly not something that any woman should feel guilty about.

In addition to eating well, taking regular exercise and getting enough rest and relaxation during pregnancy, there are several natural remedies that have been used over the ages to facilitate an easier delivery. An herbal infusion taken traditionally to tone the uterus and help to make the labour easier is RASPBERRY LEAF: make an infusion with a teaspoon of herb to a cupful of boiling water, and drink two or three times a day throughout the last three months of pregnancy. SQUAW VINE is a Native American herb used for the same purpose: make a decoction and drink a cupful once a day throughout the last two months of pregnancy. Many women find that taking the homoeopathic remedy CAULOPHYLLUM helps them to have an easier birth. Ask your homoeopath what she recommends, or try taking one dose of 30C a week during the last month of pregnancy. All these remedies may be looked up in the Materia Medica section of this book.

Massaging the perineum during the last couple of months of your pregnancy will help it to become more elastic and reduce the likelihood of a tear or the need for an episiotomy. Use either ALMOND OIL or WHEATGERM OIL and massage the area twice a day.

During Labour

Labour begins when contractions of the uterine muscles, aided by hormonal changes, cause the cervix to soften, thin out and dilate in order to allow the baby through. For medical purposes labour is divided into three stages: the first is the dilatation of the cervix, the second the expulsion of the baby and the third the delivery of the placenta. However, you may experience several different phases of mood and activity during each of these stages.

The average length of the first stage of labour with a first baby is about twelve hours, and with subsequent children about seven hours. However, this stage may take anywhere from two to twenty-four hours, or more, depending on the size of the baby, her position, the size of the mother's pelvic area and the behaviour of the uterus. First-stage labour is itself split into two categories: early and late.

During early first-stage labour, the cervix is drawn up and thinned out and dilates to 5–6 centimetres (2½ inches). There is no single sign that heralds the onset of labour, but occasional contractions become longer and stronger and more regular until they occur about every four or five minutes. You may have a 'show' if you have not already had one: this is the appearance of some blood-stained mucus, like the beginning of a period. The show is the mucous plug that was in the cervix to protect the uterus from any germs travelling up from the vagina. The waters of the amniotic sac may burst either with a slow leak, or so that water streams out. Once the bag of waters have burst there is usually an increase in contractions and your midwife or hospital should be contacted.

If labour starts fairly slowly this can be a useful time to have a light meal – perhaps soup and fruit. You should also be able to get some rest or sleep at this time, if you need it.

By the late-first stage the contractions will be getting stronger, longer and closer together until they come every two or three minutes and last sixty seconds or more. You can use breathing techniques – welcoming a contraction by a slow breath out, then breathing more lightly over the peak of the contraction, and giving another long breath out as the contraction finishes. The cervix be dilating to 5–8 centimetres.

You may find it good to sip iced water, grape juice or honeyed water at this stage. If a mother becomes tense or anxious then sipping a glass of water with a few drops of the Healing Herbs of Dr Bach remedy RESCUE REMEDY added to it can be very calming.

During this stage, the birth companion can be a great help: massaging, breathing with the mother, helping her into a more comfortable position when required, and encouraging her to relax between contractions. A helpful massage oil can be made by blending the essential oils of CLARY SAGE, JASMINE and ROSE into a vegetable-oil base: this feels wonderful when it is massaged firmly into the lower back by your companion. Alternatively, a few drops of essential oil of BERGAMOT or LAVENDER added to some water in a plant spray, can be sprayed around the birth room to freshen and disinfect the atmosphere.

The herb BLUE COHOSH may be taken throughout labour to tone the uterus and keep the contractions strong and regular. Make a decoction and drink a cupful every hour, or use the tincture. If labour becomes protracted and the strength of the contractions seems to be waning, then the herb BLUE COHOSH may be safely used to strengthen and support the action of the uterus. The dosage should be one size 'O' capsule every half-hour.

There are many homoeopathic remedies that can be invaluable during labour. It is ideal if you can have a homoeopath present at the birth to prescribe for you when needed, so if you have previously consulted one, ask her if she will attend your labour. We can mention a few remedies that will be useful for you, your companion and preferably your midwife to know about here. If the mother becomes very fearful and anxious for any reason during labour, try ACONITE 30 or 200; if she becomes totally exhausted during a long labour then try CARBO VEG 30 or 200. When contractions are weak and irregular, or stop altogether, try CAULOPHYLLUM 30 or 200. If the mother becomes anxious and trembles, and the contractions are not productive, try GELSEMIUM 30 or 200. If she becomes irritable and weepy, and the labour pains are weak, try PULSATILLA 30 or 200.

Towards the end of the first stage of labour, just before the cervix dilates to its full 10 centimetres, the contractions become much more painful, longer and with less time to relax between them. This period is called transition and may be accompanied by nausea, vomiting, trembling and feelings of irritability. Fortunately, transition only lasts a short time – from between one contraction to half an hour, or, rarely, a couple of hours – and some women do not experience it at all. With positive encouragement all women who have made it this far can get through transition without pain-relieving drugs. This is important because drugs at this late stage in labour are likely to have a detrimental effect on the newborn baby's breathing. If the mother complains that the pain is unbearable, and becomes very irritable, then the homoeopathic remedy CHAMOMILLA can be given in 30C or 200C to give some relief.

The second stage of labour begins with the complete dilatation of the cervix and ends with the delivery of the baby. During this stage, the baby descends as it is pushed downwards by the uterine muscles with the help of the abdominal muscles and the diaphragm. The amniotic membranes usually rupture during this stage if they have not done so already.

The urge to push gets stronger as the baby gets lower. The contractions may be further apart, and the degree and timing of the pushing urge may vary with each contraction. Advocates of natural childbirth now believe that once the cervix is fully dilated, the right time to push is when you want to, and that it is not helpful to encourage a mother to push when the urge is not there. The most helpful image at this stage is of opening up and breathing out the baby, not becoming tense by straining to push too hurriedly. Try MOTHERWORT and BLACK COHOSH after RASPBERRY LEAF and SQUAW VINE.

Different positions may be tried during this stage. Some women prefer squatting, kneeling or being supported from behind, and standing. The old-fashioned idea of making a women lie flat on her back during second-stage labour was based on making it easier for the doctor to intervene, not on helping the mother to give birth.

Towards the end of the second stage you may begin to feel a hot, tingling sensation around the vagina; this occurs as the baby's head begins to press against and stretch the perineum. It means that his head is about to crown and that the birth is imminent. At this stage it is important to try and relax, not push too hard, and ease or breathe the baby out, otherwise you may tear the perineum before it has a chance to stretch fully. Trying to keep your mouth and lips loose can have a relaxing influence on the muscles of the vagina.

Your baby's head will emerge following a contraction; then the baby's whole body will slip out. The mother can reach out her arms and embrace and welcome the baby.

The third stage of labour is the delivery of the placenta. The placenta begins to separate naturally from the inner lining of the uterus as soon as the baby is born. Within about forty five minutes the placenta is expelled by the final contractions. If you want to deliver the placenta naturally it is important not to have the umbilical cord clamped until it has stopped pulsating, to remain in a squatting or kneeling position if necessary to allow gravity to assist the expulsion, and to push down if the midwife suggests you should.

In western countries, it has become the habit to clamp the umbilical cord as soon as the baby has been born, and to give the mother an injection of Ergometrine or Syntometrine, which contracts the uterus and expels the placenta rapidly. However, this speeding up of the third stage tends to increase the incidence of retained placenta and maternal blood loss. It should be possible to reserve the use of Ergometrine or Syntometrine for those cases where the women is bleeding excessively and things need to be hurried up.

Clamping the umbilical cord before it stops pulsating has the disadvantages of depriving the baby of blood which is rightly its own, of cutting off the oxygen supply to the baby and throwing it onto its own resources, and prolonging the length of the third stage. However, if an injection of Ergometrine is given, it is important to have the umbilical cord clamped to prevent the baby receiving too much blood too quickly and then developing jaundice.

If you are hoping to deliver the placenta naturally and things do not seem to be happening fast enough, there are some herbs that can help the process. ANGELICA ROOT, RASPBERRY LEAF and SHEPHERD'S PURSE may be taken as a decoction; one cup is usually enough, although another may be taken after half an hour if necessary. You can also try BLACK or BLUE COHOSH: drink a cupful of the decoction, or take ten drops of the tincture.

Haemorrhage

A postpartum haemorrhage is defined as blood loss of more than 500ml (just less than 1 pint) within twenty-four hours of delivery. The bleeding may come on very suddenly by gushing out or, more usually, it may be constant but moderate over a period of hours. The causes of postpartum haemorrhage may be: when the uterus does not contract sufficiently after delivery of the placenta; failure to expel all of the placenta from the uterus; bleeding from lacerations in the cervix or lower segment of the uterus (for example, following the use of forceps); or a clotting disorder of the blood.

Postpartum haemorrhage is a very serious situation and can be life threatening if it is severe. The orthodox management of a haemorrhage like this is an injection of Syntometrine, and if it is severe a blood transfusion.

There are natural remedies that have been used over the years to deal with postpartum haemorrhage, but you will probably need a midwife who is confident about the properties of natural medicine, or a practitioner such as a herbalist or homoeopath present, in order to be given the chance to try these first. One effective herbal treatment that has been used to stop uterine haemorrhage is a combination of SHEPHERD'S PURSE, RASPBERRY LEAF and GOLDEN SEAL: a decoction of these should be made in advance to drink if necessary, or take the tinctures.

Homoeopathic remedies that have been used successfully to treat postpartum haemorrhage include: ARNICA, if the haemorrhage is due to lacerations or trauma; CAULOPHYLLUM, if the labour has been long and exhausting and the uterus is too weak to contract; IPECAC, if the bleeding is sudden and profuse, and especially if the mother feels nauseous; and SABINA, if the blood is dark and there are severe pains in the uterine area. These homoeopathic remedies need to be given in a fairly high potency, say 200C potency, to work quickly and effectively.

Caesarean Birth

During a caesarean section, the act of delivery is taken over from the mother by the surgeon. An opening is cut into the abdomen of the mother and the baby is lifted out.

Despite many drawbacks to the mother and infant, the rate of caesarean sections has risen dramatically in western countries since the 1970s. As with most methods of obstetric control, this intervention can be the wonderful use of life-saving technology but only too often it is performed routinely, for reasons such as the doctor's desire to control nature, fear and for the convenience of medical staff.

The most frequent situation that leads to a caesarean section is when labour is slow (dystocia). Planning your labour ahead and thinking about such things as how you would cope with a long, tiring labour, whether you have the freedom to move about, have a bath or rest, and if you will be with a companion and midwife committed to natural birth, can be really important in avoiding an unnecessary caesarean delivery.

Other common reasons for caesarean births are repeat caesareans, breech births and foetal distress. A repeat caesarean section is often performed because it is feared that the scar from the previous operation may rupture. If the labour is managed carefully, and oxytocin is avoided, many women can in fact go on to have a perfectly normal vaginal delivery. If you want to have a go at a normal birth following a caesarean, you will have to press your doctor and midwife for a 'trial of labour'.

Caesarean sections are given for breech births on the basis that when the baby is born bottom-first there is a chance of a hold-up with the delivery of the head and then the baby will be starved of oxygen. However, studies have shown that the risk to the baby from a vaginal breech delivery is no greater than that from a caesarean section. Certainly you should be able to opt for a trial of labour if you have a normal-sized pelvis, the baby is not very large, and if the baby is curled up with its head forward onto its chest (frank breech).

Try to be well-nourished, and rested when labour starts to avoid the likelihood of foetal distress. Decline induction, oxytocin stimulation and drugs during labour. Move about when you want to, lie down on your side rather than your back, rest and relax when possible, breathe deeply between contractions, and avoid prolonged breath-holding and over-straining.

The main disadvantages of a caesarean section are: that the risk of mortality to the mother increases by 400 per cent; it is more likely to result in an infection in the mother; and it is more likely to result in breathing difficulties for the baby after delivery.

If it is necessary for you to have a caesarean there are lots of natural remedies that you can use afterwards to lessen the impact of such a major operation. Herbs to take internally to promote healing and reduce the chance of an infection developing include: COMFREY, DAISY, ECHINACEA, MARIGOLD, RASPBERRY LEAF and MARSHMALLOW. These may be combined and taken as a decoction (or as tinctures) three times a day for up to a month after the birth. Taking homoeopathic ARNICA immediately after the caesarean will help to prevent infection and promote healing: take either a couple of doses of 200C or one 30C dose a day for five days. The homoeopathic remedy BELLIS PERENNIS is also very useful after a caesarean to relieve discomfort and promote tissue healing: try taking 30C each day for five days following the ARNICA. If, after two or three weeks, there is still a lot of abdominal discomfort, or the wound is slow to heal, try taking the homoeopathic remedy STAPHYSAGRIA: one dose of 200C should be sufficient.

Externally, compresses can be used to promote healing, soothe inflammation and prevent an infection developing (but not on raw stitches). A suitable compress can be made from an infusion of the herbs COMFREY, MARIGOLD and ST JOHN'S WORT. This should be applied using clean lint when the infusion has cooled to blood temperature. Alternatively, a compress can be made using a few drops of the essential oils of LAVENDER, TEA TREE and MYRRH added to warm water. Once the wound has closed over then COMFREY ointment can be massaged in daily to reduce scarring.

After the Birth

Once the baby has been born, we begin the time of physical readjustment and healing, getting to know the baby, and adjusting to our new role of being a mother. A few hours after the birth, your body will start to return to its normal, non-pregnant condition.

If this is your second or subsequent baby, you may feel afterpains, which occur as the uterus contracts back to its normal size (involution). Afterpains are not usually experienced with first babies because the uterus has not been stretched so much. These cramps may last several days, and can be quite strong, especially when breastfeeding. The homoeopathic tissue salt MAG PHOS 6X may be taken every few hours for up to five days to relieve the pain of the spasms. If they are very severe, and particularly if they make you feel irritable, then try the homoeopathic remedy CHAMOMILLA. A herbal combination that will relieve afterpains at the same time as helping the uterus to readjust can be made from BLACK COHOSH, BLUE COHOSH, CRAMP BARK and RASPBERRY LEAF. Make a decoction to drink three times a day for a few days, or use the tinctures. Alternatively, try adding a few drops of the anti-spasmodic essential oils of CHAMOMILE, LAVENDER or MARJORAM to a warm bath, or apply to the abdomen as a warm compress.

For a few weeks following the birth you can expect to have a vaginal discharge. It will change during this time from being bloody to pinkish-brown to yellowish-white. This discharge, called lochia, should not smell bad; if it does begin to smell bad at any time, seek urgent medical advice because this is a sign of infection. Also, seek advice if the lochia is still bloody after a few days because this may indicate that some placental tissue remains in the uterus. Other symptoms that should lead you to take urgent medical advice, are: persistent abdominal pain, the inability to urinate, or any feelings of feverishness or a temperature that rises above 38°C.

If you have been unfortunate enough to tear or have had an episiotomy during labour, there are several remedies that you can use to relieve the discomfort and promote healing. Internally, the homoeopathic remedies to compare are: firstly, ARNICA; if the stitches are very painful HYPERICUM; if the wound is slow to heal, CALENDULA. Externally, take sitz baths containing an infusion of the healing herbs COMFREY, MARIGOLD and ST JOHN'S WORT. A poultice made of MARIGOLD LEAF, GOLDEN SEAL, SLIPPERY ELM, CHAMOMILE and MARSHMALLOW LEAF in gauze and held against the perineum by a sanitary towel is very good. Alternatively, add a few drops of the essential oils of CHAMOMILE, CYPRESS and/or LAVENDER to the warm water in a sitz bath. Use a clean washing-up bowl or a baby bath (if you are small) for a sitz bath. Pour warm water into the bowl, then add the infusion of herbs or the essential oils and lower yourself into the water for several minutes. Dry yourself carefully when you get out. Ideally, you should take a sitz bath two or three times a day at first, and less frequently as you begin to heal up.

Feeling tired after the birth of a child is very common, and most women feel exhausted for a while at some point in the weeks after delivery. This is not surprising when you consider the tremendous hard work and emotional intensity of the birth, the sweeping hormonal changes that are occuring at this time, and the irregular sleeping pattern that having a new baby involves. Having help around the house and with other children, and getting plenty of rest after the birth, are the first requirements in dealing with this.

There is an excellent combination of Chinese herbs that has been used by thousands of women over the centuries in China, to restore energy and tonify the blood and generative organs following childbirth, made from: CHINESE ANGELICA (DANG GUI) and REHMANIA ROOT (SHU DI HUANG). These are available as tinctures (take 5ml in water three times a day), or as herbs, so you will need to make a decoction (see page 182 for details). Other herbs you can try at this time are: ANGELICA, ELDERBERRY and LIQUORICE. If you are exhausted after losing a large amount of blood during labour, consider the homoeopathic remedy CHINA. If you are anaemic following childbirth, check the suggestions under Anaemia in the Circulatory System on page 55.

If your tiredness seems to be directly related to having your sleeping pattern disturbed, try taking the homoeopathic tissue salt KALI PHOS 6X three times a day for up to ten days. If you just feel generally weary and exhausted, then the Healing Herbs of Dr Bach remedy OLIVE can help you to keep going. All these remedies should be compared in the Materia Medica section of this book to check that they are suitable.

Immediately after the birth you may feel excited and relieved about the arrival of your baby. It is not unusual for this to be followed after a couple of days by a sudden feeling of deflation when you feel exhausted and achy. The breast milk comes in around the third day and this is a common time for the 'baby blues', when you may feel depressed and tearful. This feeling of depression only lasts a day or two for most women, but if it becomes severe, or persists for more than a couple of days, then do talk to your doctor or natural therapist urgently, because postnatal depression can become a serious and ongoing problem if it is not dealt with properly in its early stages.

For mild postnatal blues, a herbal tonic to balance the hormones and nervous system may be made from BALM, BLACK COHOSH, BORAGE, LADY'S SLIPPER and OATS. Make a decoction to drink three times a day or take the tinctures. Essential oils that will have a good uplifting and antidepressant effect include GERANIUM, LAVENDER, MELISSA, NEROLI and ROSE. Choose one or two of these to be diluted in vegetable oil for a massage, or add a couple of drops of one to a warm bath.

If the Baby Dies

A baby may die in the womb during the last few months of pregnancy. The mother will still need to give birth to the dead baby because this is the least hazardous way of delivery. Sadly, some babies also die during labour. While allowing yourself to experience the grief is the only way to emerge from such a life-trauma, there are several things that can be done to assist the grieving process.

Other mothers who have lived through the experience of their new babies dying say how helpful they found it to hold their dead baby for a few moments. Holding, or at least seeing the baby, gave them someone to remember, rather than an intangible, nightmarish experience. Be firm and build this requirement into your birth plan if you think it would help you in the same situation. Hospitals vary greatly in their ability to deal with a grieving mother sensitively, but you should have the right to insist on a room away from other mothers and babies, and to have your companion with you as much as possible, if that helps.

Your body will have to make all the physical and hormonal readjustments following any pregnancy. These can be particularly painful reminders of your loss. To help stop your breasts producing unneeded milk, you can drink an infusion of the herb SAGE three times a day. The homoeopathic remedy LAC CANINUM will have a similar effect: try taking one dose of 200C and repeat after a couple of days only if necessary.

If you find it increasingly difficult to cope with your feelings of grief, or if you feel very depressed, then do seek professional counselling to help you at this time. It is better to avoid taking tranquillizers and sedatives if you can, because these only tend to delay the natural grieving process. Natural remedies can help you to feel stronger and calmer without the numbing and heavily-sedating effect of drugs.

The Healing Herbs of Dr Bach RESCUE REMEDY is a useful natural remedy that may be taken several times a day during an emotional crisis. The homoeopathic remedy IGNATIA is also likely to be helpful. Herbs that can be taken during this stressful time include: BALM, CHAMOMILE, OATS, SCULLCAP and VERVAIN. These may be combined and an infusion drunk up to three times a day. Essential oils with a mildly sedative and antidepressant action include: CLARY

SAGE, LAVENDER, MELISSA, MYRRH and NEROLI. Choose one or two of these to burn in your room, add to a bath, or use in a massage. All these remedies may be looked up in the Materia Medica section of this book to help you find the most useful one for yourself.

Children's Illnesses

The vitality of a normally healthy child is exceptionally strong and children have remarkable powers of recovery. A child can have a high temperature and look very poorly one minute and be running around full of energy, looking completely well again, within the hour. At least, this was the picture until fairly recently. Nowadays, more and more children have begun to suffer from chronic complaints, and most notably from allergies.

All practitioners of alternative medicine have numerous cases on their books of children brought by parents who feel that they are not as healthy as they should be. They may have specific complaints, most commonly asthma, eczema or digestive problems, or their parents may have noticed that they do not throw off colds and viruses as quickly as they should.

The main reason for this decline in our children's health is the onslaught that their developing immune systems have to deal with in the modern world. Just as improved hygiene and nutrition began to make a real impact on reducing acute infections and deficiency diseases, other conditions have become worse to the extent that a whole new range of chronic illness is becoming increasingly widespread.

A child's vital organs and immune system is developing and growing all the time. For the first few months of her life, a baby relies on antibodies inherited from her mother to protect her from disease. This immunity is further enhanced if the baby is breastfed because there are antibodies and nutrients present in breast milk. This is why being breastfed is such an important factor in a child's health (see also the entry on breastfeeding on page 18).

A growing child will be less likely to develop a properly functioning immune system and good health if he or she is affected by such things as: a poor physical inheritance (that is, unhealthy parents); a poor diet (for example, a diet of refined, additive-laden processed foods); a polluted environment (perhaps living or going to school near a main road or polluted industrial site); polluted drinking water (containing toxic metals or an excess of chemicals such as nitrates); too much medication (most commonly in the form of antibiotics); and over-vaccination.

The damage done to a developing immune system by vaccination, in particular, is often underestimated. Viral elements injected into a child's body as vaccinations may persist and sometimes mutate in the system for years. Because of this, many people working in health care now believe that vaccinations may actually suppress and damage the immune response mechanism. Studies indicate that there is a direct link between the increased incidence of auto-immune diseases in recent decades and the increase in vaccination.

Furthermore, as a result of injecting a vaccine directly into the body, only the antibody response is stimulated, as opposed to the general immune response that occurs during the normal process of illness and recovery. The inflammatory response to an infectious illness (for example a fever, rash or cough) represents the body's natural efforts to clear the virus from the system. In this way the entire immune system is profoundly stimulated, and not only will the child who recovers from the illness have a natural immunity to it, but he will be able to respond rapidly and effectively to other infections. In fact, infectious diseases are necessary for the maturation of a healthy immune system (this is particularly true of the 'common' childhood illnesses such as chickenpox, measles and mumps).

Many medical professionals recommend vaccines, arguing that immunisation has been responsible for the decline in infectious illnesses like diptheria. In fact, because of better sanitation and hygiene, most of these diseases – including diptheria, cholera and typhoid – were in rapid and continuous decline well before the introduction of immunisation procedures.

It is not irresponsible to decide against vaccination for our children. As the World Health Organisation maintains, 'the best vaccine against common infectious diseases is an adequate diet'. A healthy diet – one sufficient in nutrients, based on unrefined foods and containing plenty of fresh fruit and vegetables – will help a child to resist disease, and when illness does occur her body will be in good shape to deal with it rapidly and effectively. Natural remedies will help a child to recover from an infectious illness by supporting his immune system, and not suppressing it. It is a good idea to register your child with a practitioner of natural medicine, such as a homoeopath, so that if he does become ill, you can get professional advice quickly.

If you do opt to have your child vaccinated be selective about it. If she goes swimming in public baths, this is a good reason for having the polio vaccine. If she gets a deep punctured wound, then consider the tetanus vaccine. If you must travel to an area where there is an outbreak of yellow fever, or other tropical diseases, then it may be necessary to consider some other immunisations. If you keep vaccination to a minimum you will greatly increase your child's chances of becoming a healthy adult with a well-functioning immune system.

See also the section on the Immune System beginning on page 79.

Bedwetting

Bedwetting is not usually considered a problem until a child reaches school age. Many children go through a phase of bedwetting and there is nearly always a psychological factor to take into account. Prolonged bedwetting often causes considerable stress to both child and parents, and great care and understanding are necessary to solve the problem.

It may be caused by an organic problem, such as a kidney defect, so if the problem persists, it is advisable to take the child to a physician for an examination.

A child's tendency to wet her bed will be aggravated by fizzy drinks, refined sugar and food additives (especially food colourings), so these should be avoided. It sometimes helps if you avoid giving her a drink too late in the evening, and to wake her up to urinate when you go to bed.

If the problem persists, try consulting a practitioner of natural medicine. Homoeopathy is often particularly good at treating bedwetting. Homoeopathic remedies to consider include: CALC CARB, CAUSTICUM, EQUISETUM and KREOSOTUM. A herbal infusion that may be given to strengthen the urinary system, and gently help to relieve any stress, can be made from: CATNIP, CHAMOMILE, HORSETAIL and ST JOHN'S WORT. This infusion may be sweetened with buckwheat honey and drunk twice a day.

Chickenpox

Chickenpox is one of the most contagious of all the childhood illnesses and it provides a great opportunity for the vitality of the child to assert itself and throw off inherited or acquired toxicity. Any distressing or uncomfortable symptoms can be effectively treated using natural remedies, but seek professional advice if the symptoms seem particularly severe, or if the spots become seriously infected.

The contagious period for chickenpox lasts from twenty-four hours before the rash starts to the time the spots scab over. A rash is often the first sign of chickenpox, but it may begin with a temperature or general malaise. The rash will appear on different parts of the body and will be extremely itchy. At first, the spots are like dark red pimples, and within a few hours these will develop a small blister on top; this will eventually form a scab and drop off.

A herbal infusion may be drunk every few hours to soothe the child and encourage a rapid recovery. Consider the herbs BALM, CHAMOMILE, BURDOCK, ELDERFLOWER and HEARTSEASE. Also, sponge the child down with a soothing lotion made by infusing the herbs CHICKWEED, LAVENDER, MARIGOLD and ST JOHN'S WORT and then waiting for the infusion to cool. Diluted WITCHAZEL also has a pleasantly cooling and soothing effect.

Consult the Materia Medica section of this book to see which of the following homoeopathic remedies are best for your child's particular symptoms: ANT CRUD, ARS ALB, BELLADONNA, PULSATILLA and RHUS TOX. Of these, the most commonly indicated homoeopathic remedy for chickenpox symptoms is RHUS TOX.

Essential oils may be diluted into a vegetable-base oil and then gently rubbed onto the skin for a soothing and healing effect. Try a combination of CHAMOMILE, LAVENDER and TEA TREE. COMFREY ointment may be massaged into the skin once the scabs have fallen off to prevent scarring.

Colic

Colic is experienced as a spasmodic pain in the abdomen. It usually comes on after feeding in a baby and causes the infant to cry in pain and pass wind. Most babies outgrow colic at around three to four months, but it can be very distressing to deal with at the time. If the symptoms are very severe or persistent, or if there is any doubt about the diagnosis, then professional advice should be sought. For older children, a warm hot-water bottle hugged to the stomach will often bring relief. An infusion of the herbs CHAMOMILE and DILL SEEDS will be soothing and ease griping pains in children or babies. This infusion may be given in a bottle or beaker while it is still warm.

The homoeopathic remedies that are most often used to relieve colic are CHAMOMILLA, COLOCYNTH, LYCOPODIUM, MAG PHOS and NUX VOMICA. You can blend a couple of drops of the essential oils of CHAMOMILE or MELISSA with almond oil to gently massage into the abdomen to relieve colic in children. Do not use essential oils to treat very young babies.

Croup

Croup is a harsh cough accompanied by loud, laboured breathing. It generally occurs at night. You need to seek emergency care if the symptoms persist for more than half an hour, or in any case where the child appears to have severe breathing difficulties.

A traditional remedy is to make a steamy atmosphere by boiling a kettle in a room and this helps the child to breathe. EUCALYPTUS leaves, or a few drops of the essential oil, can be added to a basin of boiling water and placed near the child so that he can inhale the vapours. CHAMOMILE essential oil also relaxes the respiratory system. LAVENDER essential oil may be applied to the child's head and chest as a soothing compress.

A mixture of herbs to drink as an infusion to relieve croup can be made from ANISEED, CATNIP, CHAMOMILE and WHITE HOREHOUND. Homoeopathic remedies to treat croup include ACONITE, HEPAR SULPH and SPONGIA. Compare these in the Materia Medica to see which is the best for your child.

Earache

Ear infection is one of the most common childhood illnesses and almost every child will experience at least one before he or she is

7 years old. Unfortunately, for many children, ear infections are a frequently recurring problem.

Not all earaches are due to infection – catarrh and inflammation during a cold will often cause ear pains or impaired hearing. These symptoms are generally less dramatic than when there is infection.

Ear infections develop when germ-laden fluids from the nose and throat enter the middle ear. This may happen as a result of a cold or allergy, or because the Eustachian tube is so small and short in young children. As the infection develops, white blood cells and antibodies are secreted into the tissues of the middle ear area where they attack and kill infecting bacteria. As dead bacteria and white blood cells accumulate, pus forms and puts pressure on the ear drum; as the thin membrane bulges outward from the pressure the pain increases. Sometimes the membrane bursts, allowing pus to drain out of the ear; this is the body's way of expelling the pus. The torn eardrum will usually heal rapidly in children, although take care to prevent water, soap or shampoo getting into the ear until the membrane is fully healed.

The orthodox treatment for an ear infection is with antibiotics. However, recent studies have revealed that children who were given antibiotics were significantly more likely to have recurrent ear infections than children who did without.

If your child develops an ear infection, you could consider treating her yourself with natural remedies. But if the symptoms are severe or persistent contact a practitioner, such as a homoeopath, for advice. And if the child has other symptoms, such as a severe headache, a stiff neck or swelling or tenderness of the bony area around the ear, then seek medical advice immediately.

If ear infections keep coming back, you should also seek constitutional treatment by a qualified practitioner of natural medicine, such as a homoeopath, in order to prevent or treat any hearing loss, and to improve the child's health and resistance.

Anti-inflammatory and anti-microbial herbs can be used to treat a child suffering from an ear infection. Consider especially: CHAMOMILE, ECHINACEA, GOLDEN ROD, PLANTAIN and GOLDEN SEAL. An oil macerated with the herb MULLEIN is a traditional herbal treatment for earache: place a few drops of the oil on a piece of cotton wool and gently place it inside the outer ear. Earache can be greatly relieved by making a bag from clean cotton, filling it with salt, and heating it in a pan until it is thoroughly warm but not too hot. Then hold it against the ear. This method is useful if you do not have any other remedies to hand.

The essential oils of CHAMOMILE and LAVENDER can both be effective in treating an ear infection; put a few drops on a piece of cotton wool and place gently inside the outer ear. Alternatively, use as a compress over the ear area.

Homoeopathic remedies can work quickly and effectively if you find the right remedy. Consider the following by looking them up in the Materia Medica: ACONITE, BELLADONNA, CHAMOMILLA, HEPAR SULPH, KALI MUR, MERC SOL, PULSATILLA and SILICA.

German Measles (Rubella)

German measles is a harmless disease in children. It is shorter and less severe than regular measles and usually lasts three days or less. An infected child will often be slightly feverish, have a nasal discharge and develop a rash of small, lightly raised spots that tends to move down the body. If any uncomfortable symptoms do arise, use the remedies suggested for the treatment of measles on pages 49–50.

German measles is a potential threat to pregnant women, since those who contract it during the first three months of pregnancy are at risk of having a baby with birth defects, including blindness, deafness, a heart condition, cleft palate and mental problems. The natural immunity from having had German measles offers more protection than a vaccination, so try to ensure that your daughter catches it as a child.

It makes more sense to restrict vaccinations to those young women who have not managed to contract German measles by the time they get to childbearing age rather than vaccinating all children against it. There is a test that can be carried out to test for a natural immunity to the disease if there is any doubt. This would prevent unnecessarily vaccinating entire generations of children.

Measles

Measles is another classic childhood illness. The early symptoms of measles are a sore throat, cold symptoms, inflamed eyes, a cough and feverishness. It may be possible to observe Koplik's spots – small white spots on the inside of the cheeks – at the beginning of the illness. On about the fourth day a rash appears on the child's neck and behind his ears, which gradually moves downwards to cover the rest of the body. Most children will recover without treatment after seven to ten days.

The incubation period for measles is ten to twelve days, and the most infectious period is the few days before the rash appears.

Measles is not usually a dangerous disease, and like scarlet fever, it has tended to become milder in the last twenty years or so. Complications do develop very occasionally. These are usually caused by dehydration from a high fever or breathing difficulties because of a secondary chest infection. Contrary to the popular myth, there is no danger of permanent eye damage resulting from measles, although if the child is sensitive to bright light during the illness you should keep her in a darkened room to help her rest and heal quickly.

A more serious complication involving inflammation of the brain tissues (encephalitis) may develop very rarely. Look out for any unusual drowsiness, a severe headache or marked irritability, and seek urgent treatment if any of these symptoms becomes apparent. Encephalitis is most likely to result from 'atypical measles', which is in fact more common in those children who have received the measles vaccine.

A recent Danish study has shown also that the measles vaccine leads to a predisposition to arthritis, dermatitis and bone diseases later in life. Chinese medicine believes that measles is a chance for the child to eliminate those poisons that accumulated during pregnancy. If the child is immunised, they cannot be eliminated and this will make the child vulnerable to other disorders later in life.

The measles rash can be very itchy and this is the most likely cause of your child's discomfort. Antibiotics do not have any effect on the measles virus, so they should not be considered unless a secondary infection has developed. General home care should involve bed rest, sponging down with tepid water during the fever, and responding to any uncomfortable symptoms as they arise with natural remedies.

You can give an infusion made from the herbs BURDOCK LEAVES, BONESET, CHAMOMILE and ELDERFLOWER to soothe the child, bring down the fever and promote healing. If her eyes are sore and inflamed then add the herb EYEBRIGHT to the mixture (this may also be bought in tincture form to dilute and bathe the eyes). An infusion made from the herbs CHAMOMILE, CHICKWEED, MARIGOLD and MARSHMALLOW and used when cool to sponge down the child, will help to relieve feverishness and itching. Alternatively, add a few drops of the essential oils of CHAMOMILE, EUCALYPTUS or LAVENDER to tepid water and use this to sponge the child.

The most commonly indicated homoeopathic remedy for measles symptoms is PULSATILLA. Other homoeopathic remedies to consider include: ACONITE, BELLADONNA, BRYONIA, EUPHRASIA, KALI BICH and RHUS TOX.

Mumps

Mumps is a highly infectious but usually harmless childhood disease. The virus causes one or both salivary glands (parotids), located just below and in front of the ears, to swell. Other symptoms of mumps include feverishness and a sore throat. The gland-swelling usually begins to diminish after two or three days, although one gland may become affected first and the other several days later.

These days many infants are immunised against mumps along with measles and rubella, in the MMR vaccine. This vaccination is promoted on the basis that although mumps is not a serious childhood disease, it may lead to orchitis (a complication affecting the testicles) in the adult male. Orchitis can cause sterility, although this is rare because usually only one testicle is affected.

If you have mumps as a child it nearly always leads to a life-long immunity. It is not known whether the mumps vaccination confers an immunity that lasts into the adult years. Consequently, there is the possibility that if a child is immunised against mumps in childhood he or she may suffer more serious consequences if they catch it as an adult. The side-effects of the mumps vaccine can be severe, ranging from allergic reactions to, more rarely, febrile seizures, nerve deafness and encephalitis.

A child who has mumps needs plenty of rest and lots of fluids. Try a soothing drink made from an infusion of BALM, BORAGE and CHAMOMILE. If the illness lasts for more than a couple of days add ECHINACEA, POKE ROOT and YARROW to the mixture.

A compress can be very pleasant and will have a soothing and healing effect. Add a couple of drops of the essential oils of CHAMOMILE and LAVENDER to water and apply to the child's forehead and neck. The essential oils of EUCALYPTUS or THYME, added to a steam inhalation, will act as a decongestant and help the body fight the infection. You can also dilute these oils in water and spray them around the child's room with a plant spray.

The homoeopathic remedies that are most frequently indicated for treating the symptoms of mumps include: ACONITE, APIS, BELLADONNA, MERC SOL, PHYTOLACCA and PULSATILLA.

Whooping Cough

Whooping cough (pertussis) is an infectious disease that affects the mucous membranes of the air passages, and usually occurs in children. The initial symptoms are like those of a common cold but after about a week a violent, convulsive cough, often accompanied by vomiting, follows. At first the cough occurs only at night, but as the illness progresses it may appear during the day as well.

Whooping cough can be a very distressing and exhausting experience for the parents and the child. The child may cough a dozen times with each breath, and his face may darken to a bluish or purple hue. During a coughing bout you may hear the characteristic 'whoop' as the child struggles to inhale. This may not happen during a mild attack but you should always seek careful treatment and professional help with a case of whooping cough, especially in babies, in case they contract pneumonia or damage their lungs.

Although the vaccine against whooping cough has been used for decades, it is one of the most controversial of the immunisations. Doubts persist about its effectiveness, and many health care professionals are concerned that the potentially damaging side-effects of the vaccine, which include skin conditions and convulsions (in rare cases leading to permanent brain damage), may outweigh the alleged benefits.

Using natural remedies to treat whooping cough can reduce the risk of complications setting in and help to shorten the illness. However, the following suggestions should be used in addition to professional supervision, and not as an alternative to it.

A herbal infusion to reduce the spasms, fight the infection and strengthen the lungs can be made from ANISEED, COLTSFOOT, HOREHOUND, HYSSOP, LIQUORICE and THYME. Add two teaspoons of herbs to a cup of boiling water (it may be sweetened with honey). The dosage for babies is one teaspoon of infusion every four hours; for children of 6 months to 5 years two teaspoons every four hours; and for children over 5 years one tablespoon every four hours.

Essential oils may be added to steaming water so that the child can inhale the vapours, or add a few drops to a vegetable-oil base and massage onto the chest. Those oils to consider are CYPRESS, LAVENDER, ROSEMARY, TEA TREE and THYME. They may be used in a combination.

51

You can get excellent results by treating whooping cough with homoeopathic remedies. However, finding the right remedy is not always easy and it is advisable to consult a qualified homoeopath for advice. The most frequently indicated homoeopathic remedies for whooping cough include: BELLADONNA, BRYONIA, COCCUS CACTI, DROSERA and IPECAC.

The Circulatory System

The blood circulatory system is the transport system of the body. It carries oxygen from the lungs to the tissues, and carbon dioxide in the opposite direction. It transfers absorbed food substances from the gut to the liver and then throughout the body. It carries waste products from the tissues to the liver and kidneys for detoxication and excretion. The heart is the pump in this system, the blood vessels provide the route and the blood is the carrier.

Blood is the prime symbol of life and vitality for many cultures. Its ability to flow throughout the body and distribute nutrients is a symbol of the free circulation and sharing of resources throughout any system, personal or planetary. Diseases of the circulatory system are caused by and result in congestion, stagnation and decay; an appropriate image for this is a polluted river. Rivers should flow freely, carrying great life in their waters, but when they are polluted they become stagnant, poisonous and unable to support life.

Cardiovascular diseases are on the increase and are already the major cause of death among adults in the developed world. Considerable changes in attitude and lifestyle are necessary to revert this trend. The dictum 'Prevention is better than cure' is never more true than in the case of circulatory system diseases. Once the symptoms of heart disease are established, natural medicines have a lot to offer, but an individual case should be assessed by a suitably qualified practitioner.

Diet is a major factor to consider in the prevention of heart disease. It is well known that those people who eat foods that are high in animal fats are more prone to heart disease: food containing animal fats is slowly digested and is more likely to cause excessive cholesterol levels in the body. Cholesterol is a waxy substance that is produced naturally by the liver and adrenal glands, any excess

The Circulatory System

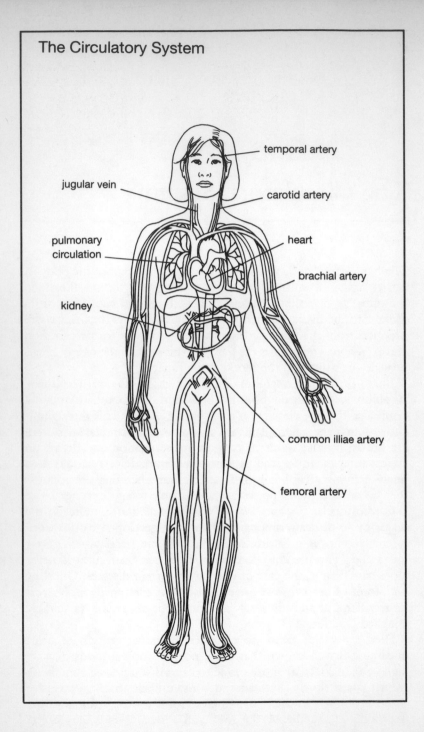

temporal artery

jugular vein

carotid artery

pulmonary circulation

heart

brachial artery

kidney

common illiae artery

femoral artery

can be considered a waste product. Its build-up in the bloodstream contributes to hardened arteries, and strokes and coronary disease are likely to result. Foods that are particularly high in cholesterol and should be kept to a minimum are: butter, cream, cheese, eggs and meat. Conversely, natural foods such as unprocessed fruits, vegetables, grains, legumes, nuts and seeds, contribute towards the liver's production of lecithin, which acts as a fat-dissolving agent and protects the body from excess accumulations of fats within the arteries. Heat and other processes of extraction will destroy lecithin in foods. This shows how much better it is to use cold pressed vegetable oils, whole grains and unprocessed and unrefined foods.

It is advisable to stick to a low-salt diet to keep the risk of heart disease to a minimum. Smoking should definitely be avoided, and keep your alcohol intake to a moderate amount.

Exercise is important to keep the tone of the circulatory system in good order. Regular daily exercise which makes you feel warmed up and slightly short of breath, is preferable to infrequent but excessive exertion.

Stress is widely acknowledged to be a major contributory factor to heart disease. Stress can become such a part of your lifestyle that it may be necessary to seek advice about trying to reduce it. There are many kinds of relaxation therapies available if you are aware that you do not relax easily. If you have been under a lot of emotional stress, some form of personal counselling can be a great help.

Anaemia

Anaemia may be the result of either a reduction in the number of red blood cells, or a lack of haemoglobin (the red pigment in blood that carries iron). Red blood cells carry oxygen from the lungs to the rest of the body, the oxygen combining with iron to form haemoglobin. Symptoms of anaemia include general weariness, debility, dizziness and headaches; a simple blood test will establish whether you are anaemic or not.

A common cause of anaemia is loss of blood, which may be sudden, as after an operation, an accident or childbirth, or sustained over some time, as with a heavy menstrual flow, bleeding from a peptic ulcer or haemorrhoids. Other causes are defective blood formation after or during severe or chronic infections, lack of iron in the diet, or inadequate absorption of iron from the digestive tract in disorders of the intestine. Pregnant women are more susceptible to anaemia due to the increased nutritional demands on the body. There are also a group of hereditary blood disorders, including sickle cell disease, that cause anaemia. Its cure must include the treatment of the condition causing it as well as increasing the intake of iron.

Calcium and copper, Vitamin C and the B group vitamins must also be present for the body to be able to assimilate iron. A balanced diet of natural foods should supply sufficient quantities of these vitamins and minerals, otherwise food supplements may be taken; vegetarians in particular may need to take extra Vitamin B12. Foods that are naturally rich in iron include: meat, eggs, lentils, apricots, green-leaf vegetables, molasses and beetroot. The cruder forms of iron supplements, such as those usually recommended during pregnancy, often causes digestive upsets and constipation. FLORADIX is an excellent plant-based iron tonic which may be used to supplement the diet and can be taken during pregnancy.

The herbs ALFALFA, DANDELION ROOT, NETTLES, WATERCRESS and YELLOW DOCK are all rich in iron and may be taken regularly as an infusion. The homoeopathic tissue salt FERRUM PHOS can aid the assimilation of iron from the diet.

Artery Disease

The arteries are responsible for bringing oxygen and nourishment to the vital organs and other parts of the body. Without this they become diseased and die. Therefore the condition of the arteries is of prime importance to the overall health of the body. The most common cause of death in adults in Britain is insufficient circulation to the brain or heart because of disease of the arteries.

The arteries are tubes with muscular walls. When these walls become thickened and lose their elasticity, the condition is called arteriosclerosis. This is usually associated with high blood pressure. When the arteries become thickened by localised accumulations of fatty substances (atheroma), the condition is called atherosclerosis.

Atherosclerosis may begin early in life and often no symptoms are experienced for many years. Gradually the walls of the arteries become thicker and the flow of blood becomes restricted. Eventually atheroma may completely block a major artery with dramatic, maybe fatal, results – a heart attack or stroke. Atheroma also promotes the clotting of blood in arteries, and when these clots create a blockage in an artery supplying either the heart or the brain (a thrombosis), a similar crisis results.

A combination of arteriosclerosis and high blood pressure may result in angina which is caused by a reduction in the blood supply, and therefore oxygen, to the muscle of the heart. Angina pain is of a dull, gripping nature and is characteristically felt across the upper part of the chest, radiating down the left or sometimes right arm. The pain comes on during exertion, often it is most noticeable when going up a slope or climbing stairs. The pain is relieved by rest.

All the general advice about diet and lifestyle in the introductory section to the Circulatory System is relevant to diseases of the arteries (see pages 53–5). The main causes of hardening of and deposits in the arteries are a high cholesterol diet, smoking, high alcohol consumption and a lack of exercise. It is only by changing these habits that this major disease of the modern world can be prevented. Natural medicines have a lot to offer, but obviously they will only be of long-term benefit if they are used alongside changes in diet and lifestyle.

The use of fresh GARLIC in your daily diet will help your body to break down any deposits of cholesterol that have built up. COD LIVER OIL and HALIBUT LIVER OIL also keep the arteries clean – they may be taken as capsules. Specific herbs for artery disease are HAWTHORN TOPS and its berries and LIME BLOSSOM. For the treatment of angina MOTHERWORT should also be considered. A regular massage with the essential oils of JUNIPER and LEMON can also help to break down fatty deposits in the arteries.

Heart Weakness

Conventional medicine divides heart disease up into several different categories, but in natural medicine there are many remedies that can help to strengthen the heart and circulation generally. If there are symptoms of suspected heart disease, such as breathlessness when you exert yourself, pains in the chest or down the arms, or if you are already on medication, a professional therapist should be consulted.

The most important herbal heart and circulation tonic is HAWTHORN TOPS. This may safely be taken as an infusion or a tincture for several months. Other particularly useful herbal heart tonics are BALM, LIME BLOSSOM and MOTHERWORT. Among essential oils the main cardiac

tonics are LAVENDER, MARJORAM, MELISSA, ROSE and ROSEMARY. These
may be used singly or as a combination, and added to the bath or
used for a massage.

High Blood Pressure (Hypertension)

Blood pressure depends on two main factors: first, the strength of
the contraction of the heart; and second, the peripheral resistance to
the blood flow which is determined by the size and condition of the
smaller arteries. The more constricted these tiny arteries the greater
the resistance, and the higher the blood pressure reading. As we get
older, the arteries become thicker and less elastic; this leads to a rise
in blood pressure, and explains why it tends to be higher in older
people.

There are two figures to a blood pressure recording: the higher
number (systolic pressure) is written over the lower number (diastolic pressure). The systolic pressure, produced when the heart
contracts, is more susceptible to changes induced by exercise and
emotion, and more liable to fall when the subject is at rest. The
diastolic pressure, the pressure maintained when the heart relaxes
between beats, depends more on the state of the arteries and is less
likely to be affected by outside events. Below the age of about 50
years, the diastolic pressure is normally less than 85.

There is usually no warning symptom of high blood pressure until
a person suffers from one of its complications – most commonly a
heart attack, stroke or kidney disease. The only way to discover the
disease in advance is to have the blood pressure measured with a
sphygmomanometer.

Some forms of kidney disease and certain gland disorders may lead
to high blood pressure, but no obvious cause is found in the majority
of people. Hypertension is equally common in women and men and
it affects about 15 per cent of British adults. Sometimes the disease
is hereditary. Mild cases of hypertension will often respond quickly to
dietary changes, increased relaxation and natural medicines. Periods
of trauma in people's lives can result in high blood pressure. In most
people this will return to normal once the trauma is resolved. More
severe cases of hypertension will need treatment over an indefinite
period of time, in order to prevent strokes, kidney disease or
heart failure.

Conventionally, hypertension is often treated with both a diuretic and a sympathetic nervous system depressant, which reduces the ability of the nervous system to constrict blood vessels. Increasingly, a type of drug called beta-blockers is prescribed. Sometimes vasodilators are used to relax the walls of the arteries. If you are receiving medication for high blood pressure, you must consult a qualified practitioner before attempting to try any other remedies or cut down on the drugs.

If you have high blood pressure, you must make changes to your diet and reappraise the amount of stress in your lifestyle. Smoking must be avoided. Your diet should be low in animal fats and you should not add any salt to food during or after cooking. Eat plenty of raw garlic.

The recognition and control of stress in your life is vital if you suffer from hypertension; this is probably the single factor that has the greatest effect in the long-term management of high blood pressure. It is often people who drive themselves very hard and have high standards who are most prone to high blood pressure. You need to reassess the amount of stress at work and within your personal relationships, possibly with the help of a professional counsellor. Consider some sort of relaxation therapy or meditation classes, too.

For a mild case of high blood pressure the following herbs may be tried: HAWTHORN BERRIES should be ground, infused and drunk on a regular basis (or use the tincture); CRAMP BARK can be used to encourage the arteries to dilate; and other herbs to consider are LIME BLOSSOM and YARROW. Herbal medicine should not be used by someone already taking drugs for high blood pressure without consulting a professional herbalist as we have already stated.

A regular massage by a skilled aromatherapist can really help to reduce high blood pressure. The oils with a particular role in the treatment of hypertension are LAVENDER, MARJORAM and YLANG YLANG. These may be used in the bath or for a relaxing and therapeutic massage.

There are many examples of cases of hypertension that have responded well to acupuncture treatment, so it may be well worth consulting an acupuncturist from one of the acupuncture registers (see page 397 for addresses).

Low Blood Pressure (Hypotension)

This problem is less common and has less serious implications than high blood pressure, but it can be distressing to the sufferer – causing fainting and weakness. It may be associated with a weak circulation, or with general debility. Some teenagers experience a bout of low blood pressure, associated with periods of fainting, which then clears up of its own accord.

BROOM is one of the most important herbs for treating low blood pressure – it tones the arterial system. Other herbs to consider are GINGER, HAWTHORN TOPS and ROSEMARY. If the low blood pressure is associated with general weakness and debility, you should consider nutritious herbs such as ALFALFA, NETTLES and PARSLEY. An invigorating massage with the stimulating oils of BLACK PEPPER, ROSEMARY or SAGE may also be of benefit.

Palpitations

Palpitations are experienced when the heart beats forcibly or irregularly and the individual becomes aware of its action. Although palpitations do occur with other symptoms of true heart disease, the vast majority of people experience them as a result of anxiety, and not as a direct result of heart disease at all. After a physical examination by your doctor to rule out organic heart disease, these remedies may be tried to relieve palpitations associated with stress or anxiety.

Look up the following herbs in the Materia Medica section to see which are the most suitable for you: BROOM, LIMEFLOWERS, MISTLETOE, MOTHERWORT and VALERIAN. The essential oils which are particularly good for the treatment of palpitations, include: ANISEED, LAVENDER, MELISSA, NEROLI, PEPPERMINT, ROSEMARY and YLANG YLANG. A regular visit to an aromatherapist for a relaxing massage will be of most benefit.

Many people find palpitations very frightening, which of course makes the palpitations worse. In this situation, the Healing Herbs of Dr Bach RESCUE REMEDY can help to calm the feelings of panic and anxiety. If stress and anxiety are known to be the cause of palpitations then deep relaxation, as taught by relaxation therapists, can be a great help.

Poor Circulation and Chilblains

Poor circulation will cause cold extremities, and in a cold winter chilblains may develop. All the general advice at the beginning of this section is appropriate to tonify and improve the circulation. In addition, a mixture of the following herbs may be taken for several weeks: GINGER, HAWTHORN, PRICKLY ASH BARK and ROSEMARY. MUSTARD foot baths can also be very good for cold feet.

The essential oils of BLACK PEPPER, CYPRESS and MARJORAM will all help to stimulate the circulation, so try a regular, invigorating massage of these oils diluted in vegetable oil.

If you are prone to getting chilblains, you should wear warm socks and shoes and gloves when outdoors in cold weather. On returning indoors, you should warm your hands and feet slowly at room temperature, do not expose them to direct heat which will only aggravate the chilblains.

For the treatment of chilblains, compare the homoeopathic remedies of: FERRUM PHOS and PULSATILLA. There is also a homoeopathic ointment made to relieve the itching called TAMUS OINTMENT. If the chilblains have caused the skin to break then use CALENDULA OINTMENT to promote healing. Essential oils that may be used to heal chilblains are CHAMOMILE and LAVENDER – these are both anti-inflammatory.

Varicose Veins

Blood is returned to the heart through the veins of the legs by the contraction of the leg muscles. Within the veins there are one-way valves which keep the blood flowing in the right direction. When the valves fail, the veins swell and the blood stagnates within them; this is the condition described as varicose veins.

Varicose veins are common in adults of both sexes, although they are about twice as common among women. They may be caused by constipation, pregnancy or other causes which partially block the veins in the pelvis, and by jobs which involve a great deal of standing without much movement, for example hairdressing and dentistry. There appears to be a hereditary factor involved as the condition tends to run in families. High levels of oestrogen, such as occur during pregnancy and from some forms of the birth control pill, may also cause varicose veins. During pregnancy, they may appear in the early months but often disappear entirely after the delivery.

Varicose veins are usually just unsightly, but they may cause aching, heaviness of the legs and swelling of the ankles, especially at the end of the day. These symptoms are usually relieved if you rest with your feet up. When a clot occurs in the veins of the legs (the condition is called phlebitis), it causes local inflammation and pain, and must be urgently looked at by a practitioner to make sure that there is no danger of further complications.

Conventional treatment of varicose veins includes injecting them with a substance that will close off the affected part of the vein, or by surgically stripping the affected veins out of the leg. In both instances, the varicose veins often recur because the reasons why they developed in the first place have probably not been tackled.

It is difficult to cure varicose veins once they exist, but it is quite possible to prevent them from getting worse. It is important to avoid becoming constipated, so stick to a whole-food, high-fibre diet. Do not drink strong tea or more than one or two cups of weak tea a day. Avoid becoming overweight. Make sure that you get plenty of regular leg exercise such as walking, cycling or swimming. Avoid wearing tight boots, trousers or pants, and do not sit with your legs crossed. If varicose veins begin during pregnancy then elastic support tights can relieve any aching.

RUTIN helps to keep the vein walls in good shape, so eat plenty of buckwheat (its natural source), or take RUTIN tablets. The homoeopathic tissue salt CALC FLUOR promotes the elasticity of vein walls and may be taken as a course for two or three weeks (this may be taken during pregnancy). HAMAMELIS, in homoeopathic form, will relieve varicose veins that are aching and causing a feeling of fullness in the leg.

Herbs to repair and tone the venous system are HAWTHORN BERRIES, HORSE CHESTNUT, PRICKLY ASH and YARROW; these should be infused and taken internally. An ointment made from MARIGOLD or WITCHAZEL may be used externally if there is any irritation. The essential oils of JUNIPER, LAVENDER or CYPRESS may be diluted and massaged into the area around but not directly on the varicose vein, or add a couple of drops to a bath.

The Digestive System

Our health and energy is determined to a great extent by what we ingest into our bodies. Our digestive system is our prime contact with the produce of the earth. The food that we eat and feed to our families is one of the most important factors involved in caring for the physical body.

There is a great deal written about what we should and should not eat, in fact so much has been said that it can be quite overwhelming. We suggest a very common-sense approach to diet, with a few basic guidelines: eat food that is as fresh as possible; with as few additives and as little processing as possible; try to eat regular meals; eat a variety of foods for a well-balanced diet; and try not to overeat as this will put a strain on all your body's systems.

If the digestive system is already showing symptoms of disease and you suspect that your diet is not very good now, or has not been in the past, then it can be a great help to consult a dietary therapist or a naturopath. He or she should be able to isolate foods that aggravate your condition and guide you through a detoxification programme if that is considered advisable (or try the one on page 395). To help you find a naturopath or dietary therapist consult page 397 of this book. For general information on food and diet see pages 379–83 in the Lifestyle section of this book.

Colitis

Colitis is an inflammation of part of the large intestine (colon); if ulcers develop the condition is called ulcerative colitis. The symptoms

The Digestive System

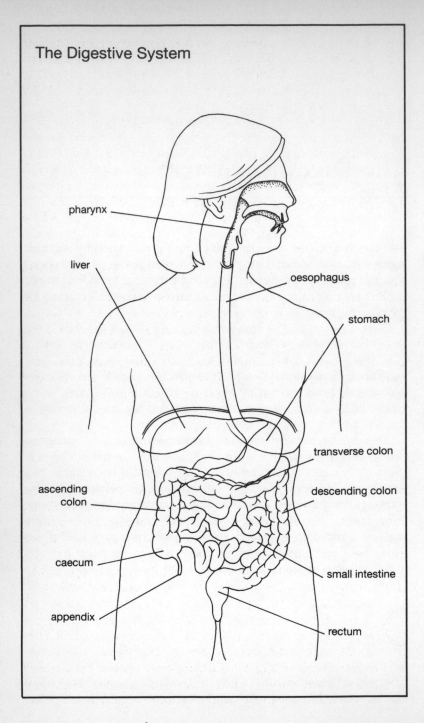

pharynx

liver

oesophagus

stomach

transverse colon

ascending colon

descending colon

caecum

small intestine

appendix

rectum

are colicky pains in the abdomen and diarrhoea which may alternate with constipation and depression. The condition may have phases of active symptoms followed by periods of remission. A medical diagnosis is advisable if you suspect that you have a bowel problem, as these symptoms are also shared by other illnesses.

Colitis will often improve with a change of diet; try bland, easily digested foods, at least during its active bouts. Dairy products, red meat, bran products, rich, fatty foods, highly-spiced food, coffee and excessive alcohol, should be avoided at all times by sufferers of this disease. Colitis is increasingly common in our modern, high-stress lives, and dealing with stress and tension must be taken into account when it is treated. Although the following suggestions may relieve your symptoms if you suffer with this distressing disease, if the problem is longstanding, or it has a hereditary background, only prolonged treatment by a qualified practitioner will be of lasting benefit.

Study the following herbs in the Materia Medica section of this book to see which seem the most appropriate to take as an infusion: AGRIMONY, COMFREY ROOT, FENUGREEK, MARIGOLD, MARSHMALLOW ROOT, MEADOWSWEET and SLIPPERY ELM. Do not use mucilagenous herbs if you have mucus colitis. The essential oils of BERGAMOT, CHAMOMILE, LAVENDER or ROSEMARY may be diluted in vegetable oil and massaged over the abdomen for a soothing and healing effect.

Constipation

There are conflicting ideas about how frequent bowel movements should be. It is considered to be normal to open your bowels twice or more a day, or only two or three times a week; however, most women seem to feel better if they have a regular, daily bowel movement.

While constipation is not a disease itself, there can be uncomfortable symptoms associated with it, such as bloatedness, abdominal pains or headaches. The factors that tend to lead to constipation are a diet that is rich in refined foods, stress, and not putting the time aside for a bowel movement. Chronic constipation – a long-term tendency to infrequent bowel movements – can often only be treated by a radical change in diet. Even adding more fibre to the diet may not help sufficiently, without first going on a cleansing programme to clear out the system and establish a more regular bowel habit.

It may be best to consult a naturopath or dietary therapist to get advice about a detoxification programme, or try the cleansing diet on page 395.

Eat more foods that are high in fibre, fresh fruit and vegetables to help avoid constipation. The recent tendency to add bran to everything doesn't suit everyone; it can be rather drying in the bowel. Plain oats soaked in fruit juice can make a better alternative to bran or toast for breakfast. Linseed can also be a valuable addition to the diet; sprinkle a tablespoon of the seeds onto the oats at breakfast, or stir into a glass of water or juice. It can also be helpful to drink more water.

Avoid the frequent use of laxatives as they can irritate the gut and weaken the tone of the bowel thus making the constipation worse. The following suggestions will be good for the odd bout of constipation, but if you suffer from chronic constipation you should seek constitutional treatment from a practitioner of natural medicine.

For a herbal infusion that has a laxative effect, choose from: BUCKTHORN, CASCARA SAGRADA, FENNEL, LIQUORICE, MARSHMALLOW ROOT, RHUBARB ROOT and SENNA LEAVES. The main homoeopathic remedies to choose from are: ALUMINA, BRYONIA, NAT MUR, NUX VOMICA and SEPIA. A pleasant way to relieve constipation is to massage a few drops of FENNEL, MARJORAM or ROSEMARY essential oils, diluted in vegetable oil, onto the abdomen. Look all these remedies up in the Materia Medica section of this book to help you choose the most appropriate ones for yourself.

Gastro-enteritis

Gastro-enteritis means an inflammation of the stomach, often causing nausea and vomiting, accompanied by inflammation of the small intestine, causing diarrhoea. Abdominal colic and sometimes fever may also be present.

The main causes of gastro-enteritis are food poisoning and any infection or virus that affects the small intestine. Food infected with the Salmonella organism is responsible for many outbreaks of acute gastro-enteritis.

If someone is vomiting or has diarrhoea care must be taken to ensure that the person does not become dehydrated – this is particularly crucial with infants. Failure to hold down clear fluids, drowsiness, disinterest in fluids and decreased urination are all warning signs of the need for urgent medical advice in a young child.

Following the onset of gastro-enteritis, the stomach should be rested for the first eight hours with sips of water; after that plenty of fluids should be taken to prevent dehydration, possibly with a little honey added. After twenty-four hours plain, light food such as soup, plain crackers, ARROWROOT or SLIPPERY ELM may be introduced. If symptoms are not relieved after twenty-four hours of home care, or twelve hours in young children, seek immediate medical assistance.

The main herbs used in the treatment of gastro-enteritis are COMFREY ROOT, HOPS, GOLDEN SEAL, MARSHMALLOW ROOT, MEADOWSWEET, RASPBERRY LEAF, SLIPPERY ELM and THYME. After comparing these herbs in the Materia Medica section, choose one or two of them to make into a drink, and take every four hours until symptoms are relieved. There are many homoeopathic remedies that may be indicated, so you will need to compare: ARS ALB, CHAMOMILLA, COLOCYNTH, IPECAC, MAG PHOS, NUX VOMICA, PHOSPHORUS and PULSATILLA. The essential oils of CHAMOMILE or GERANIUM may be diluted and massaged into the abdomen to bring relief.

Gum Disease

Receding or bleeding gums are symptoms of gum disease. When the gum becomes loosened around the teeth, pockets tend to form and bacteria can accumulate; the gum margin and the underlying tissues can then become inflamed. This is called gingivitis. In more advanced cases, called pyorrhoea, the teeth become loose and may even fall out. One of the main causes of gum disease is a diet of soft, refined foods: the gums are stimulated by chewing crunchy and fibrous foods and this helps to keep them healthy.

The most important herbs to use to treat gum infections and gum disease are CALENDULA, ECHINACEA, HYPERICUM, MYRRH and SAGE; the best way to use them is to buy a selection of the tinctures and make up a mouthwash for regular use. The essential oils of FENNEL, LAVENDER and MYRRH are healing and antiseptic, and a couple of drops of one of them may be added to warm water to rinse around the gums. There are several brands of herbal toothpastes on the market these days that contain some of these herbs and oils.

Haemorrhoids (Piles)

Haemorrhoids are varicose veins that develop either inside or just outside the anus. The main causes are being overweight, chronic constipation, straining during a bowel movement, the use of powerful laxatives, and pregnancy and labour. The symptoms are itching or pain at the anus, and if the pile ruptures, bleeding. Haemorrhoids are a common complaint that can be helped considerably by preventing constipation (see pages 65–6) and correct treatment, but other forms of rectal bleeding may mimic or co-exist with them, and a diagnosis should be established if this particular symptom is persistent.

RUTIN tablets may be taken as a dietary supplement to improve the strength of the capillary walls in the bowel. Internally, a course of the herbs DANDELION ROOT, GOLDEN SEAL, HORSECHESTNUT, HAWTHORN, STONE ROOT and YARROW can be helpful. Externally, an infusion or the diluted tinctures of HORSECHESTNUT, PILEWORT or WITCHAZEL may be applied. Homoeopathically, the main remedies to consider are: ARNICA, CALC FLUOR, HAMAMELIS, NIT AC, NUX VOMICA, SEPIA and SULPHUR. A homoeopathic ointment containing AESCULUS, HAMAMELIS and PAEONIA is available from many health shops for the treatment of haemorrhoids. A local compress of the essential oils of CYPRESS, FRANKINCENSE, LAVENDER or MYRRH will be very soothing and healing; these oils may also be added to a warm bath. Compare all these remedies in the Materia Medica section of this book to see which ones are most suitable for you.

Indigestion

The stomach may be upset by diseases directly affecting the stomach and also by any general illness. In addition, nervous tension or anxiety frequently causes a digestive upset; most people experience loss of appetite, 'queasiness' and tension in the stomach when they are under emotional strain, or before an exam or interview. Other common causes of indigestion are eating rich food, drinking or smoking too much, eating too fast and eating at irregular times.

Symptoms of indigestion include heartburn, nausea, waterbrash, flatulence and general discomfort in the stomach region. Occasional symptoms of indigestion are felt by most people sometimes, but if the problem is more persistent or constitutes a marked change from a previously stable pattern, you should seek professional advice. Recurrent indigestion can be an early symptom of several different digestive diseases.

You can chew the seeds of ANISEED, CARDAMOM or FENNEL after meals as an aid to digestion. An infusion of BALM, CHAMOMILE, ORANGE PEEL or BLOSSOM, MEADOWSWEET, PEPPERMINT or VERVAIN will be soothing and can be drunk in combination or singly as required. Compare the homoeopathic remedies of CARBO VEG, KALI MUR, NUX VOMICA and PULSATILLA to treat indigestion. Alternatively, the essential oils of CARDAMOM, FENNEL or PEPPERMINT may be diluted and massaged into the stomach area. All these suggestions should be looked up in the Materia Medica section of this book before use.

Mouth Abscess

A mouth or tooth abscess is a collection of pus that has gathered under a tooth. If this becomes inflamed the site will became hot, red and you will feel a throbbing pain. The fact that such an infection has developed shows that your gums are not healthy, and that your resistance to infection is probably low. A cleansing diet (try the one on page 399) or constitutional treatment by a natural health practitioner should be considered if your abscesses keep coming back.

The following herbs should be considered for mouth abscesses: BURDOCK ROOT, CLEAVERS, ECHINACEA, GOLDEN SEAL and YELLOW DOCK. Make a decoction of these herbs, or buy them as tinctures, and take three times a day for three weeks. A compress of the essential oils of CHAMOMILE or LAVENDER may be applied externally. The homoeopathic remedies to consider are: APIS, BELLADONNA, HEPAR SULPH and SILICA. Compare all these remedies in the Materia Medica section of this book to see which are most suitable for you. Eat plenty of GARLIC in your diet to help fight the infection.

Mouth Ulcer

Mouth ulcers are small, painful blisters that appear on the tongue, gums or lining of the mouth. They usually indicate a need to improve the general health of the sufferer, and a natural therapist should be consulted for constitutional treatment, especially if they are recurrent. The odd mouth ulcer can be treated at home using natural remedies.

An infusion of the herbs MARIGOLD, RASPBERRY LEAF, RED SAGE and THYME may be used as a mouthwash to heal mouth ulcers quickly. Alternatively you can dab either the tincture or the essential oil of MYRRH on to the ulcer. Compare the homoeopathic remedies BORAX, MERCURIUS and NAT PHOS.

Peptic Ulcer

Peptic ulcers are ulcers of the digestive system, they are usually either gastric (stomach) ulcers, or duodenal (small intestine) ulcers. Part of the mucous membrane of the stomach or duodenum becomes eaten away by the highly acidic digestive juices.

The main things that lead to a peptic ulcer are a faulty diet (too rich in fats and refined carbohydrates), smoking, an excessive intake of stimulants, such as coffee or highly-spiced food, and alcohol. Emotional stress tends to increase the secretion of digestive acids and this can also contribute to the formation of an ulcer.

The first symptom of a peptic ulcer is pain, this may be felt anywhere in the upper abdomen but usually under the sternum. The pain is often relieved for a short time after eating and by vomiting. Heartburn and nausea are other common symptoms. Most bleed at times and this may cause anaemia. Peptic ulcers are a very serious condition and complications include sudden and severe bleeding, perforation of the stomach or duodenum and a narrowing of the outlet of the stomach. Any persistent pain associated with the stomach should be referred to a medical practitioner for diagnosis, as other diseases may show similar symptoms.

The following suggestions will almost certainly bring relief to the painful symptoms of a peptic ulcer, but unless you are prepared to change your lifestyle, and particularly the level of stress in your life and your diet, home remedies will only temporarily alleviate the symptoms without really getting to the cause of the problem. We advise you to seek professional advice from a natural therapist, as this may well be a necessary part of the healing process.

The herbs to consider in the treatment of peptic ulcers are COMFREY, LIQUORICE, MARIGOLD, MARSHMALLOW ROOT, MEADOWSWEET and SLIPPERY ELM. The essential oils of CHAMOMILE, FRANKINCENSE, GERANIUM, MARIGOLD or MARJORAM may be diluted and massaged into the abdomen. Look all these remedies up in the Materia Medica section to see which ones are the best indicated for your particular symptoms.

Threadworms

Threadworms (pinworms) are a very common complaint, especially in children of school age. The worms are passed on by taking the eggs into the mouth, usually after touching the anus, where the worms descend from the rectum to lay their eggs. The lifecycle from the egg to the threadworm is about ten days, so treatment must be aimed at breaking this cycle as well as alleviating the symptoms.

The sorts of symptoms to watch out for with threadworms are irritability, a desire to pick at the nose, and most markedly an itchy anus that will be worse in the evening when the worms come out to lay their eggs. Diagnosis may be confirmed by seeing the worms in the stools or around the anus in the evening.

The elimination of worms requires scrupulous hygiene. The hands should be washed with hot water and soap after every visit to the lavatory. Underwear, towels and bed linen must be changed regularly. Close-fitting underwear should be worn at night so that the anus cannot be scratched inadvertently.

Dietary control of threadworms involves eating plenty of the foods that the worms cannot thrive on, such as: raw carrots, apples, onions, garlic and pumpkin seeds. All foods containing sugar, even natural sweeteners such as malt or honey, should be avoided because the worms live on sugars. ACIDOPHILUS tablets or capsules can be taken for several weeks to improve the general health of the bowel.

One very useful method of treatment is to add a few drops of EUCALYPTUS or LAVENDER essential oil to either CALENDULA OINTMENT or Vaseline and apply it to the anus every evening. This will help to stop the worms laying their eggs as well as relieve the itching. A mixture of the herbs BALMONY, LIQUORICE and WORMWOOD may be taken as an infusion or as an enema. One of the most useful homoeopathic remedies in the treatment of threadworms is CINA. Look all these remedies up in the Materia Medica section to check how suitable they are for you or your children.

Toothache

Persistent or severe toothache should be assessed by a dentist, but there are a few remedies that can be used to relieve the pain and inflammation temporarily, and that will help relieve transient tooth pains.

Biting on a couple of CLOVES will release the analgesic oil that they contain; alternatively, apply a few drops of CLOVE essential oil onto cotton wool and place over the area. A strong infusion of the herbs MARSHMALLOW, SAGE and THYME will have an antiseptic and soothing effect. Make an infusion to rinse around the mouth and then drink. The homoeopathic remedies of ARNICA, KALI PHOS, MAG PHOS and SILICA should be compared in the Materia Medica section to see which is the most appropriate for your toothache symptoms.

The Eyes

Any eye or vision problem should be considered on a psychological level as well as a physical level so that you can understand what the underlying problem really is. The eye enables us to see and build up information about the outside world; also, it tells other people about us. Other people 'look us in the eye' when they want to find out more about us. It is the eyes that break into tears, and they reveal to the outside world what is happening with our emotions inside. They are the 'mirrors of the soul' and they are the outward manifestation of the qualities of vision and insight in our life. If an eye problem arises we should consider what it is in our lives that we do not want to see, and what it is in ourselves that we do not want to look at.

Conjunctivitis

The conjunctiva is the mucous membrane that covers the eyeball and lines the lids. Inflammation of this membrane is known as conjunctivitis, and the affected eye will water and look bloodshot. If the inflammation is a symptom of a cold then there will be a clear and watery discharge; allergic conjunctivitis is accompanied by itching; and bacterial infections result in a thick, yellow-green discharge.

If the symptoms of conjunctivitis persist for more than three days, if they are associated with any loss of vision or pain in the eye, or following an injury or possible exposure to flying fragments of metal or grit, then seek emergency medical advice.

When you treat the eyes take care to wash your hands and utensils carefully, and use only cool, boiled or distilled water on the eye.

The herbs that you can take to help conjunctivitis include: ECHINACEA, ELDERFLOWER, EYEBRIGHT, GOLDEN SEAL and SAGE. Herbs that should be considered for infusions for external use include: CHAMOMILE, ELDERFLOWER, EYEBRIGHT, GOLDEN SEAL and MARIGOLD. Consult the Materia Medica section and make up a mixture of the best herbs for your own use. EYEBRIGHT may be bought as a tincture that can be diluted to make a soothing and healing eyewash.

The homoeopathic remedies that should be considered to treat these symptoms include: APIS, ARS ALB, BELLADONNA, EUPHRASIA, HEPAR SULPH and PULSATILLA.

Eye Strain

Eye strain may develop after a long bout of focusing the eyes on one object or at one particular distance, for example, when you are sewing, reading, driving or working at a VDU screen. It can usually be avoided by taking a break every now and then, or at least by looking up from the work you are doing every few minutes and focusing further into the distance.

If your eyes feel very tired try placing cold teabags or slices of cucumber over them – it can be very soothing. If they become sore or inflamed then a cool infusion of the herbs CHAMOMILE and EYEBRIGHT can be used to bathe them. You can also take EYEBRIGHT internally to strengthen the eyes. The homoeopathic remedy RUTA may be taken to relieve eye strain after reading or other, similar activities.

Fevers and Influenzas

You will only 'catch' an illness when your body's resistance is weakened and you are susceptible to certain bacteria and viruses. The body's defences against disease can be diminished by many physical and psychological factors. When we treat an infection or other acute illness, it is important to reassess any inadequacies in our diet, environment and lifestyles, as well as relieving the immediate symptoms of the disease.

If an infection lingers, or if you regularly contract illnesses, you will need to concentrate on improving your immune system (see the Immune System beginning on page 79). Any illness should be taken as a message from our body to slow down, or to look at what it is in our daily lives that creates the conditions for disease to occur. Suppressing the symptoms of an acute, infectious illness, for example with antibiotics or aspirin-type drugs, will tend to impair the immune system still further, and often means that we avoid investigating the underlying cause of the problem.

Fevers

A fever is part of the body's natural defence response to combat disease. A fever is marked by an increase in body temperature; as long as this does not rise too high, it is best to let the fever run its course and allow the body to heal itself. If you are caring for a child whose temperature rises above 40°C (104°F), then get emergency medical advice.

Mild fevers may be treated at home by drinking plenty of fluids, resting in bed, and using natural remedies to promote healing and ease any discomfort. Sponging down the body with tepid water will usually bring down the temperature effectively. If the fever is very high, or continues to rise despite attempts to bring it down, you should seek professional advice. It is especially important to keep a close watch on children because they can develop convulsions during a very high fever; emergency medical aid must be sought if there seems any likelihood of this occurring.

Herbal infusions can be an effective way of reducing a fever, promoting healing, and increasing fluid intake. Consider especially the following herbs: BALM, BONESET, CHAMOMILE, ECHINACEA, ELDERFLOWER and YARROW.

Essential oil of CHAMOMILE or LAVENDER may be added to tepid water to sponge down the body, or apply as a compress to the forehead. The essential oils of CLOVE, EUCALYPTUS and SAGE may be diluted in water and sprayed around the room in a plant spray to disinfect it.

The homoeopathic remedies most commonly indicated in the treatment of fever symptoms include: ACONITE, ARS ALB, BELLADONNA, CHAMOMILLA, FERRUM PHOS, GELSEMIUM, MERC SOL and PULSATILLA. Compare these in the Materia Medica section of this book to find the most suitable.

Glandular Fever

Glandular fever, also called infective mononucleosis, is caused by a virus, and is most common in teenagers. The symptoms are a very sore throat, fever, swollen lymph glands in the neck and often a general enlargement of the glands. There may be a red rash covering the body.

Glandular fever may drag on for weeks and the patient may feel 'run down' for months afterwards. The disease sometimes recurs after an apparently complete recovery. There is no orthodox cure for glandular fever, and antibiotics should not be given because they cannot kill the virus and they will impair the efforts of the immune system to fight the illness.

In severe cases of glandular fever there may be jaundice, in which case you should seek professional advice.

The herbal treatment for glandular fever in its initial stages will be the same as for Fevers (see page 75) and Sore Throats (see page 159). Once the acute symptoms are over, the most important herbs to use to promote healing and recovery will be the alteratives, including:

CLEAVERS, ECHINACEA, NETTLES and POKE ROOT. If depression and debility are part of the post-glandular fever picture, then also consider BALM, OATS and SCULLCAP.

Essential oils may be used in massage, or in the bath. They will act as anti-microbials and will encourage the immune system to fight off the disease. Consider especially EUCALYPTUS, LAVENDER, ROSEMARY, TEA TREE and THYME.

Homoeopathy can be really helpful in bringing a patient back to a full and rapid recovery following glandular fever. These remedies may be indicated in the initial stages or in a more mild attack; if the symptoms have dragged on for a long time you will get the best results by consulting a qualified practitioner. Look the following up in the Materia Medica section to see which is the most suitable: APIS, BELLADONNA, CALC PHOS, HEPAR SULPH, LAC CAN, LACHESIS, MERC SOL, PHYTOLACCA, PULSATILLA or SILICA.

Influenza

Influenza, commonly called flu, is an acute infection of the respiratory tract; it is often accompanied by symptoms of feverishness and aching. Different strains of influenza will produce different symptoms, such as sore throats, nausea and coughs, and these should be treated specifically.

Influenza normally lasts between two and five days, but more serious complications may develop, particularly in the elderly. People who do not respond well to home care should be referred to a practitioner. Increasingly, influenza tends to linger, leaving the person feeling debilitated and depressed afterwards. In order to strengthen the attempts of the body to fight off the disease, follow the general advice in the introduction to the Immune System on page 79.

A general mixture of herbs to combat flu can be made from: BONESET, ELDERFLOWER, PEPPERMINT and YARROW. Add ECHINACEA if your resistance to illness is generally low. Add BALM or SCULLCAP if you feel depressed alongside your other symptoms.

Essential oils may be diluted in vegetable oil and massaged into aching limbs and onto the chest, used in a compress or bath, or the vapours may be inhaled in the form of a steam inhalation. The effect of essential oils will be anti-microbial, decongestant and stimulating to the immune response. Consider especially: EUCALYPTUS, LAVENDER, ROSEMARY and TEA TREE. Essential oil of CLOVE may be combined with one or two of the others mentioned and diluted in water to spray around the room to disinfect and freshen it.

The main homoeopathic remedies to consider for flu symptoms include: ACONITE, ARS ALB, BRYONIA, EUPATORIUM PERF, GELSEMIUM and RHUS TOX.

The Immune System

The immune system is the mechanism by which the body protects itself from infection and disease. In fact, several different organs and mechanisms are involved in the immune process.

Micro-organisms such as bacteria, fungi and viruses enter the body continuously, and some live there permanently without doing any harm. But infection will develop when the conditions are right for certain invading organisms to reproduce and multiply within the body. Once a threatening micro-organism enters the body, a chain of events, involving a specialised group of cells known collectively as the white blood cells, is set in motion. This is known as the immune response. White blood cells are transported by the bloodstream but are found in large numbers in the lymph nodes, spleen, thymus and tissue fluids.

The lymphatic system plays an active role in the immune response by forming some of the white blood cells that manufacture antibodies to suppress the growth and activity of bacteria and viruses. The lymphatic system also filters out and drains the body of bacteria and other unwanted substances. During an infection the activity of the lymphatic system is greatly stimulated, and the accumulation of cells and bacteria may cause the lymph nodes to become enlarged. This is experienced as swelling and possibly tenderness in the neck, armpits and groin. See also pages 89–90 for specific recommendations on how to improve the function of the lymphatic system.

The adrenal glands also play an important role in the immune response by secreting hormones that trigger off some of the necessary processes. The vitality of the adrenals is depleted by exhaustion and stress, which is one reason why we have less resistance to illness when we are over-tired or under stress.

In western society, an increasing number of health problems are the result of either an under-active immune system, such as with ME or AIDS, or an immune system that has become deranged, as with allergies or rheumatoid arthritis. There are many reasons for this increasing prevalence of immune problems, including an unhealthy diet, exposure to pollution, over-medication and stressful lifestyles. By living in a society that allows pollution of the earth, air and water on a massive scale, we have undermined the health-sustaining capabilities of our environment, and as individuals we have become unable to defend ourselves against the levels of toxicity that we have created.

The best that most of us can hope for is an immune system which is sufficiently effective in eliminating enough of the daily chemicals and pollutants that we are exposed to, so that an intolerable level of toxicity does not build up in our bodies, and cause disease. If the level of toxicity in our system does become too great, we will not be able to maintain a balance of health, our immune system will be unable to cope, and illness will result.

In general, factors that tend to impede the body's attempts to eliminate what is not good for it, and increase the strain on the immune system, include: any foods containing additives, hormones, inorganic fertiliser or pesticide residues; refined sugar; polluted air and water; chemical drugs; vaccinations (for more information on vaccinations see page 48 in Children's Illnesses); constipation; smoking; anti-perspirants; and any creams, ointments or lotions that are put onto the skin and contain harsh chemicals or are suppressive. All these things should be avoided as far as is possible.

There are some positive steps that we can take to minimise the impact that living in a polluted environment has on our bodies. We can: eat fresh food, which is preferably organically produced; drink filtered or bottled spring water; use unleaded petrol; take regular exercise; use natural plant-based cosmetics and toiletries; and use natural remedies. Undertaking a cleansing diet for a period of time can be a good way of livening up the immune system: consult a dietary therapist or naturopath for advice, or follow the cleansing diet on page 395 of this book.

If your immune response is weak and your resistance to illness is low, there are some natural remedies which are known to generally strengthen and tone the immune system, and encourage it to eliminate waste products. In herbal medicine these will include: plants known as adaptogens, such as GINSENG; alteratives, such as BURDOCK, CLEAVERS and RED CLOVER; anti-microbials, such as ECHINACEA, GOLDEN SEAL, GARLIC and THYME; and general tonics, such as ELDERBERRIES, NETTLES and ROSEMARY. Certain essential oils are also known to strengthen the immune system: BERGAMOT, EUCALYPTUS, GINGER, LAVENDER, LEMON GRASS, ROSEMARY and TEA TREE.

AIDS

The letters that make up the abbreviation AIDS stand for Acquired Immune Deficiency Syndrome. This indicates the collapse of the body's immune system and hence the body's ability to resist disease. People with AIDS become highly susceptible to a wide variety of infections and various forms of cancer.

Theories about the spread of AIDS are constantly being reviewed, but it is generally believed that it probably develops in those people who have previously contracted HIV (Human Immuno-deficiency Virus). HIV can be transmitted via body fluids such as blood and semen, and it is most commonly contracted through sexual intercourse with an infected partner, from sharing a needle with an infected drug-user, or from receiving contaminated blood products.

The virus probably needs to enter the body via the bloodstream to be contracted. This means that sexual intercourse with an infected male partner will not always lead to the woman contracting HIV, but she may do so if there are any small breaks or tears in her skin or the mucous membrane of her vagina. During anal intercourse, penetration frequently does cause a tear in the delicate membrane of the anus or rectum, which is why HIV is more common amongst sexually-active homosexual men. Using a condom during intercourse greatly reduces the risk of contracting HIV during vaginal or anal intercourse.

To date about 30 per cent of people who are known to be HIV positive actually develop AIDS. In order to prevent HIV multiplying and developing into AIDS, the immune system must be in peak condition. AIDS will develop in those people whose resistance to HIV is low, and so the virus can multiply and become destructive to the system as a whole. In order for this to happen the virus needs to invade its host cells, which are the white blood cells known as T-Helper cells. T-Helper cells stimulate and co-ordinate the activity of the other white blood cells active during the immune response mechanism. If these T-Helper cells are invaded and destroyed in large numbers by the virus, the body is unable to resist infection and disease, and AIDS has developed.

Therapists working with people who are HIV positive try to help them to strengthen their immune system. As well as the measures and remedies discussed in the introduction to the Immune System on pages 79–81, many therapists of natural medicine have developed treatments which are particularly appropriate for people with HIV. Therapies that are popular, and have had notably good results, include aromatherapy, herbalism, homoeopathy and naturopathy. Some people have found that creative visualisation is greatly beneficial too, often in conjunction with other more physically-oriented therapies, like herbalism or homoeopathy. Most counsellors or therapists will be able to guide you through an appropriate creative visualisation programme.

The herbs and essential oils that are useful for treating people with HIV are those known as adaptogens, alteratives and tonics, for example: BALM, BURDOCK, CLEAVERS, ECHINACEA, GARLIC, GINGER, GINSENG, GOLDEN SEAL, LIQUORICE, POKE ROOT, ROSEMARY and THYME.

Once AIDS has developed, any treatment needs to be twofold: that is, it needs to attempt to rejuvenate the immune system while also treating symptoms of infection and disease as they arise. These symptoms are sometimes known as ARC (Aids Related Complex). Remedies to consider in addition to those mentioned above are those that combine the properties of strengthening the immune system with a marked anti-microbial effect: BERGAMOT OIL, EUCALYPTUS OIL, LAVENDER, MYRRH, TEA TREE and WILD INDIGO, for example.

Allergies

Our bodies react to the presence of foreign substances by bringing the immune response into action: this is the process designed to neutralise, kill and expel the invading substance. Part of the immune response involves the production of antibodies, which help to kill invading bacteria, and assist the white blood cells in their job of removing any dead and dying foreign substances. The body remembers the particular substance (antigen) that produced those antibodies, and introduction of the same substance in the future can provoke a much quicker response to even a tiny amount of the antigen.

This process can sometimes become over-active causing, in a susceptible person, an allergic reaction to a wide range of foreign protein substances. The reason for this is that a process similar to the antibody-antigen reaction is set off not only in the bloodstream, but also on the surface of the body cells. This antibody-allergen reaction damages the cell walls and liberates a substance known as histamine. Histamine produces two main effects: it allows the fluid part of the blood or serum to leak into tissues which results in swelling, blisters, and irritation of the skin and mucous membranes; and it can bring about a spasm of the bronchial muscle, resulting in asthma attacks.

There is often a hereditary component to allergic sensitivity, particularly with what are known as the 'atopic' diseases – asthma, eczema and hayfever. Stress is also known to play a significant role in predisposing people to allergic reactions. The number of people suffering from allergies has increased enormously in recent years, and is particularly noticeable amongst children. This is because our immune systems are being undermined by over-medication and over-vaccination, and the proliferation of chemical pollutants and additives in food, air and water.

The term allergy is now often used to describe reactions other than those caused directly by histamine production (such as itching, a runny nose, urticaria, wheezing and so on). These more recently recognised conditions have become known as 'sub-clinical' allergies, and include such symptoms as catarrh, cystitis, hyperactivity in children, migraine and a variety of skin disorders. It is increasingly acknowledged by people working in health care that certain foods and food additives are connected to these sub-clinical allergies. Special rotational diets, eliminating suspect foods for a week or more at a time, have been developed to try and establish which food substances are causing a particular problem. For more information, contact the relevant self-help group from the list of contacts on page 397.

While it can be useful to avoid specific allergens, such as milk or wheat, for a time, to give the body a chance to heal itself, the long-term aim of natural medicine must be to cure the individual, so that she or he no longer suffers from allergies. If you suffer from allergies, your immune system is no longer functioning smoothly and you will need to follow the general advice given in the introductory section to this section on pages 79–81. There are also a number of natural remedies that are particularly useful in the treatment of allergies.

Herbs to consider are: CHAMOMILE, ECHINACEA, ELDERFLOWER, BALM, LIQUORICE, RED CLOVER and YARROW. The most important essential oils are: CHAMOMILE, LAVENDER and MELISSA. The homoeopathic remedies for first-aid treatment of allergies, include: APIS, ARSENICUM, RHUS TOX and URTICA. For constitutional treatment to cure the tendency to allergic reaction, you should consult a qualified homoeopath.

See also Asthma on page 155, Eczema on page 164, Hayfever on page 158, and Urticaria page 167.

The Liver and Gall Bladder

The liver is the largest organ in the body and it carries out many important functions. The liver produces bile that is needed to emulsify fats; it stores glucose in the form of glycogen, which is one of the most important stores of energy in the body; it is needed for the metabolism of protein; it is active in the formation and storage of several vitamins; it deactivates a number of hormones when they are no longer needed; and it detoxifies the body of drugs and poisons.

The variety of these vital functions shows how important it is to have a healthy liver. Most people have experienced the effects of the liver working under pressure after a few drinks too many: the symptoms of a hangover (irritability, nausea, headache) all come on as it struggles to rid the system of the toxic effects of alcohol. These days, most livers are under even more strain as they detoxify and process the increasing quantity of chemicals and additives in modern foods.

A diet that is good for your liver includes plenty of fresh fruit and vegetables, preferably organically grown, whole cereals, such as brown rice, and proteins that are low in fat, such as white fish and chicken. Greasy and fatty foods should be avoided and so should foods which contain additives such as preservatives, flavour enhancers and colouring. Alcohol is particularly damaging to the liver and should not be taken by anyone with liver problems. Coffee is also bad.

Most cleansing diets are concerned with assisting the liver in the detoxification process; any dietary therapist or naturopath will be able to guide you through such a regime. Alternatively, follow the cleansing programme in the back of this book on page 395. Spring is a traditional time to undergo a liver cleansing diet, after the excesses of Christmas and the stodgy foods of winter.

There are several herbs that are considered liver tonics, these may be taken during a cleansing diet or when the liver is feeling sluggish. We recommend especially: BALMONY, BARBERRY, BLUE FLAG, BOLDO, DANDELION, FRINGETREE BARK, GOLDEN SEAL, VERBENA, VERVAIN, WILD YAM and YELLOW DOCK. The most important essential oil to strengthen and cleanse the liver is ROSEMARY. Other oils that may be helpful and should be looked up in the Materia Medica section are: CHAMOMILE, CYPRESS, GRAPEFRUIT, JUNIPER, LEMON and ORANGE.

The gall bladder is a pear-shaped sac attached to the liver. It acts as a reservoir for bile. Bile is used to break down large globules of fat into tiny globules so that they can be absorbed in the duodenum. Any diet prescribed for a condition of the gall bladder will involve cutting out fat.

Jaundice is the term given to the yellow discolouration of the skin and whites of the eyes caused by an excess of bile pigment in the bloodstream. This yellowness is a very common and marked sign of most diseases of the liver and gall bladder. Jaundice is a symptom rather than a disease – it is the underlying cause that needs to be treated and then the jaundice will clear.

In Chinese medicine the liver and gall bladder is known as the seat of anger. Anger causes certain tensions and also glandular secretions in the body that may in turn have an undesirable effect on the liver. Likewise, people often feel irritable and grumpy when they suffer from liver disorders. It may be that a two-way link develops between the emotions and the physical symptoms. It is worth considering whether people who develop liver disease are angry types, or if they have suffered a lot of frustration or suppressed anger in their lives. If this is the case, then as well as addressing the liver physically, a cure is going to be more permanent if these tendencies are also examined and dealt with as part of the treatment.

Gall Bladder Inflammation

Inflammation of the gall bladder (cholecystitis) causes severe pain in the upper part of the abdomen under the ribs. This pain can radiate through to the back and be felt under the right shoulder-blade and even in the tip of the right shoulder. Nausea and vomiting can accompany the bouts of pain. The attack may come on after a long period during which you have experienced much indigestion and wind.

This condition appears more often in women than in men, and

recurring attacks are usually treated by removing the gall bladder. This is a shame because the condition can often be successfully treated by natural medicine.

During an acute attack you should stay away from fats in your diet. The homoeopathic remedy MAG PHOS may be taken as often as you need to relieve the pain, or massage the diluted essential oils of LAVENDER and ROSEMARY over the painful area. Recurring attacks need to be cured with careful treatment by an experienced practitioner of natural medicine – a naturopath, herbalist, homoeopath or acupuncturist. A general herbal mixture that will relieve the pain and reduce the inflammation can be made from: DANDELION LEAVES, FRINGE TREE BARK, FUMITORY and MARSHMALLOW ROOT.

Gallstones

Gallstones form when deposits from the bile concentrate in the gall bladder. They may consist of cholesterol or bile pigment, and sometimes calcium as well.

Many gallstones are 'silent' and there are no symptoms, or there may be flatulence, a feeling of fullness after meals and a sense of discomfort after fatty food. If a stone enters the bile duct it causes biliary colic: a severe colicky pain in the right upper abdomen, which may make the sufferer roll about in agony.

Gallstones are more common in women than in men, and most common in women who are overweight. You should always reassess your diet if you have gallstones, and animal fats in particular should be excluded. Small stones may enter the duodenum and be passed with a bowel motion. A large stone may obstruct the bile duct and result in jaundice. This will require medical intervention.

It is well worth consulting a natural therapist to treat gallstones before resorting to the surgical removal of the gall bladder. For the acute pain of an attack, take the homoeopathic remedy MAG PHOS, although if you want to get rid of the stones and reduce inflammation permanently you must consult a homoeopath. The acute pain will also be relieved by massaging the diluted essential oils of LAVENDER and ROSEMARY over the area. Try the following herbal mixture to dissolve the stones, although this will need to be taken for some months to achieve a result: BALMONY, DANDELION LEAVES, FRINGETREE BARK and STONE ROOT. Check all these remedies in the Materia Medica section of this book to see if they are particularly suitable for you.

Hepatitis

Hepatitis is a term that is usually applied to an acute inflammation of the liver caused by a virus infection. Two strains of virus have been identified: Virus A and Virus B (serum hepatitis).

The symptoms of hepatitis are a marked loss of appetite, nausea at the sight of food, especially fats, and feeling off-colour generally. After a few days of these symptoms the urine becomes dark owing to the presence of bile, and the bowel motions become pale. The yellow skin and eyes of jaundice will also become evident.

General treatment includes bedrest and a light, low-fat diet. You should not drink alcohol for some months after your recovery. Most people suffering from hepatitis get a mild attack, but in a small number of cases the attacks are severe, with a high fever. If you suspect that you have hepatitis you should consult a medical practitioner for a diagnosis and to assess the impact of the disease on your liver.

The majority of hepatitis sufferers make a complete recovery with no permanent damage to their liver. However, it can take several months to feel totally fit again, and it is not uncommon to feel low and depressed for some time following an acute attack. If this is the case, consult an alternative practitioner such as a herbalist, homoeopath or acupuncturist. Some of the general liver tonics mentioned on pages 85-6 in the introductory section on the liver will also assist recovery.

The Lymphatic System

The lymphatic system moves lymphatic fluids around the body through the action of muscles and the lungs, via a one-way valve system, collecting waste products and toxins as it goes, and disposing of them through the bladder, bowels, lungs and skin. The lymphatic vessels are spread as a network throughout the body, but they are particularly concentrated in the groin, behind the knees, in the armpits, neck and upper chest.

Lymph fluid is involved in the absorption of fats from the intestines, as well as in the drainage and removal of toxic wastes from the body. Lymph fluid is also a reservoir for certain kinds of white blood cells that attack and ingest chemical and bacterial invaders, and clean out waste.

This system is one of the most important methods the body has of detoxifying itself, and it is also a vital part of the immune response. If the lymphatic system is not functioning properly, a very wide range of illnesses can develop. General symptoms of the lymph system not working effectively include a tendency to oedema (swelling), swollen glands, a susceptibility to infections and viruses, recurrent tonsilitis or sore throats, and a tendency to constipation. The function of the lymphatic system will often remain impaired following a bout of glandular fever.

Regular exercise is necessary to maintain a healthy lymphatic system because vigorous motion stimulates the dumping of wastes, and the flow of lymphatic fluid. Skin brushing is also considered to be an effective way of moving the lymph fluid and freeing any impacted lymph mucus from the nodes. Use a brush made from natural fibres, and brush towards the lymph nodes (up the arms and legs, and inwards on the chest) in long, sweeping strokes. For best results, brush on dry skin for at least five minutes each morning. Skin brushing is particularly good for getting rid of cellulite.

A cleansing diet can be very effective for toning and clearing the lymphatic system. Consult a dietary therapist or naturopath for advice, or follow the cleansing diet on page 395. Foods that should be avoided are: red meat, fatty food, dairy products, coffee, vinegar, alcohol, refined sugar and all artificial additives. All drugs, whether recreational or prescribed, should be avoided where possible, as the lymphatic system has to clear chemicals and toxic residues out of the system.

Foods that are beneficial include fresh fruit and green vegetables, preferably organically grown. Also, drink filtered or bottled mineral water, as the lymphatic system has to struggle to remove the chemicals and metals that are present in high levels in our tap water from the body.

There are known to be some effective lymphatic cleansers amongst herbal remedies, including: CLEAVERS, ECHINACEA, GOLDEN SEAL, MARI-GOLD, NETTLES, POKE ROOT and RED CLOVER. Consult the Materia Medica section to see which of these is most appropriate for you. Massage therapists have developed a specialised form of massage known as 'lymphatic drainage', and this can be particularly effective when essential oils are also used. The essential oils renowned for clearing the lymphatic system include: FENNEL, GERANIUM, JUNIPER, LAVENDER, LEMON and ROSEMARY. You could also consider the homoeopathic tissue salt KALI MUR for symptoms resulting from a poorly functioning lymphatic system.

The Muscular and Skeletal System

The muscular and skeletal system allows us to stand upright, keep our shape and move around. It is a truly wonderful achievement of natural engineering. The key to the muscular and skeletal system lies in the balance between structure (rigidity) and flexibility (fluidity). It will stay healthy if we look after ourselves, avoid strain and injury where possible, eat a good diet, take moderate but not excessive amounts of exercise, know how to relax and let go of stress, and have a reasonable posture.

Emotional stress will affect our posture and well-being as much as physical abuse, and joint problems are particularly affected by unexpressed anger and prolonged feelings of guilt. Learning to express feelings of anger and aggression, rather than suppressing them so that they turn inwards, is an important part of the healing process for anyone with joint problems (and this is indeed a challenging task for many women).

Most problems that involve the muscular and skeletal system develop for a period of years before they result in physical symptoms. Diseases of the bones and joints are the end result of a combination of physical, emotional, dietary, hereditary and environmental factors. Helping yourself to unravel these various factors, and reversing the degenerative process into a process of healing, will also take time, and a considerable commitment towards improving your health. Natural remedies will only be successful if they are part of an integrated approach aimed at healing the whole person.

Generally, people who suffer from muscular or bone and joint problems benefit from a diet based on wholefoods and plenty of fresh vegetables. You could try a detoxification diet for a limited period of time to help the body reverse the degenerative process: consult

The Muscular and Skeletal System

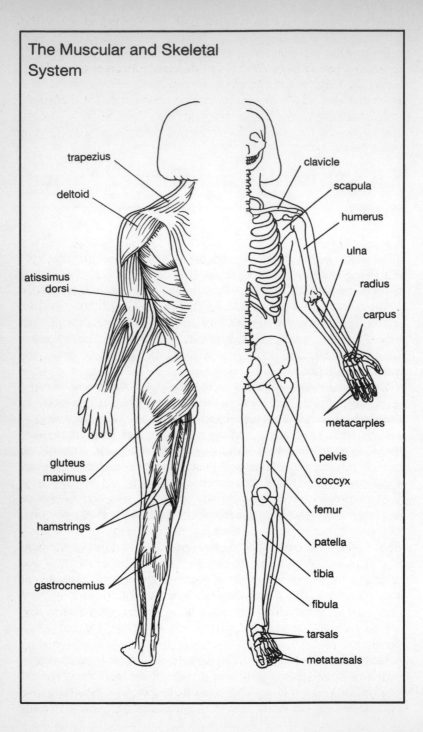

trapezius

deltoid

atissimus dorsi

gluteus maximus

hamstrings

gastrocnemius

clavicle

scapula

humerus

ulna

radius

carpus

metacarples

pelvis

coccyx

femur

patella

tibia

fibula

tarsals

metatarsals

a naturopath or dietary therapist for advice, or follow the suggested cleansing diet on page 395. Many different therapies have played a part in helping to cure chronic diseases of the muscular and skeletal system, including acupuncture, homoeopathy, herbalism and naturopathy. Visiting a therapist who can also help you to understand the physical and psychological patterns underlying your disease is the best way to get relief.

Arthritis and Rheumatism

Rheumatism is an inflammation of the connective tissues covering the muscles and tendons; it is sometimes called myalgia, fibrositis and lumbago. The muscles in the affected area tighten as a defensive reaction and when this happens the nearby joint may become deformed. Once a joint becomes inflamed or painful, the condition is called arthritis; and thus the various forms of rheumatism and arthritis tend to overlap and become confused.

Although defining the exact type of rheumatism or arthritis that you have can be interesting, it isn't usually vital in terms of being helped by natural remedies. It will be more useful if you try and unravel the various factors in your particular lifestyle that are contributing towards your disease. Factors that need to be investigated include: your diet, your genetic inheritance, physical stress or injury, environmental influences and your emotional patterns. While we can suggest some ideas and remedies here that will probably be of some help, to reverse a chronic degenerative process caused by arthritis or rheumatism, you will probably need to try to improve your health on every level over a long period of time, and you may need professional help to unravel the underlying causes.

On a psychological level, joint problems are often the result of friction in your relationships with other people that is being ignored or suppressed rather than actively dealt with. Ignoring problems in personal relationships does not tend to make those problems go away, instead it leads to a build-up of anger, resentment and guilt. If these tendencies are not expressed they are carried around in our emotions, and eventually they can poison the whole person, including the physical body. Holding on to negative emotions causes a lack of flexibility, stiffness and pain.

Many women feel very guilty about feeling such so-called negative emotions as anger, aggression and resentment. Guilt can lead to great restlessness and a tendency to overdo things to compensate; this over-exertion may place a further strain on the muscular and skeletal system. If you recognise this pattern in your own life at all, it is worth considering some form of counselling or psychotherapy, or at least try talking about it to your natural therapist, so that you can work on trying to reverse the trends.

Changes in your diet can also be an important part of healing rheumatic and arthritic problems. An unhealthy diet will tend to lead to a build up of toxins and waste products in the system. If the body cannot eliminate these waste products effectively, they may well be dumped in the joints, causing irritation, inflammation and pain. The foods that should be avoided are those that trigger an acidic reaction in the body, including: red meat, dairy products, vinegar, wine, most spices, oranges, refined carbohydrates and refined sugar. Coffee, strong tea and salt should be also be avoided, as they tend to add to the accumulation of toxins in the body.

Sticking to a cleansing diet for a limited period of time can be a great help, particularly if you use it to kick-off a concerted effort to improve your general diet. Consult a naturopath or dietary therapist for advice on cleansing diets, or follow the one on page 395. Fresh, organically-grown vegetables, both raw and cooked, fruit (other than tomatoes and oranges) and brown rice are particularly good if you suffer from rheumatism or arthritis. Fish and white meat may usually be safely eaten. Try drinking plenty of mineral water (particularly the low-sodium varieties) and a drink made from a teaspoon of cider vinegar and a teaspoon of honey in a cup of hot water, taken every morning, helps many sufferers.

Food supplements that have been found to help people who suffer with arthritis are COD LIVER OIL capsules and EVENING PRIMROSE OIL capsules. Herbs that may be taken to heal rheumatism and arthritis include: BOGBEAN, CELERY SEED, FEVERFEW, MEADOWSWEET and WHITE WILLOW. Look these up in the Materia Medica section of this book and make a mixture of the ones that look particularly appropriate in your case. A poultice to apply to the affected joints may be made from CAYENNE and SLIPPERY ELM.

To find a homoeopathic remedy to relieve symptoms of arthritis or rheumatism compare: APIS, ARNICA, BRYONIA, LEDUM, NAT PHOS and RHUS TOX. If the remedy only helps a little then it probably means that you require constitutional treatment by a qualified practitioner.

Essential oils help rheumatism and arthritis in a variety of ways. Detoxifying oils such as CYPRESS, JUNIPER and LEMON can be used in the bath and for massage to help the body to eliminate poisons from the joints and out of the body altogether. Anti-inflammatory and pain-relieving oils such as CHAMOMILE, LAVENDER and ROSEMARY may be used for local massage or compresses. Rubbing oils can be used to improve circulation in the area and relieve stiffness, try a combination of: BENZOIN, BLACK PEPPER, EUCALYPTUS and MARJORAM, diluted in a vegetable-oil base.

Backache

Back pain is one of the most common ailments referred to medical practitioners. Its causes are very varied, and the best method of treatment will vary accordingly. Pain caused by tensions arising out of bad posture can respond very well to the Alexander Technique. If the vertebrae or pelvis is out of alignment, then a manipulative therapy such as chiropractice or osteopathy can be of great help.

The most common cause of backache is overstraining or injury. In this situation, the remedies suggested here may well relieve the pain; if the problem does not clear up quickly then consult an osteopath, chiropracter or other therapist of natural medicine. If the problem keeps coming back, then you will need to redress the physical weakness and look at any underlying pattern of stress that is contributing to the back symptoms.

Pain in the back at waist-level may be due to spinal disorders or kidney and bladder problems (toxins that should be eliminated by the kidneys and bladder can be deposited in surrounding tissue, causing inflammation and discomfort). In many women's cases, low-back pain can be caused by disorders of the reproductive organs. If there is any doubt about the cause of your back pains it is vital to get a diagnosis to rule out any serious causative factor.

One of the most pleasant ways to relieve backache is a massage with essential oils. The most effective essential oils for relieving pain due to fatigue or tension, are: GINGER, JUNIPER, LAVENDER, MARJORAM and ROSEMARY. Any one of these may be diluted in a massage-base oil and rubbed into the back, or add a few drops to a warm bath. You can rub macerated herbal oils into the back to relieve pain; the most useful will be made from COMFREY or ST JOHN'S WORT. Herbs may also be taken internally to reduce inflammation and relieve pain, try a combination of: JAMAICAN DOGWOOD, ST JOHN'S WORT, VERVAIN and WHITE WILLOW. The homoeopathic remedies that should be compared to find the most suitable one for you, include: ARNICA, BRYONIA, HYPERICUM and RHUS TOX.

Osteoporosis

Osteoporosis literally means 'porous bones', and it occurs when the mass of the bones becomes reduced. Bone tissue is constantly being worn out, resorbed into the bloodstream and excreted, and replaced by newly-formed bone. Usually bone mass reaches its peak when we are in our early thirties; thereafter there is a tendency for more bone tissue to be lost than replaced. As the density of the bones decreases, they become fragile and brittle, and break more easily.

A decrease in bone mass is part of the general ageing process but it tends to occur earlier in women than in men, although by about the age of 80 men have caught up. Osteoporosis occurs earlier in women partly because our bones tend to be less dense to begin with, because we exercise less than men (and exercise seems to slow down bone loss), and because the body is less able to absorb calcium from the diet and assimilate it into bones, as a result of the decline in the hormone oestrogen after menopause.

Advanced osteoporosis can lead to hip, forearm and wrist fractures, backache and loss of height (due to the vertebrae in the spine collapsing). The orthodox management of osteoporosis in women includes Hormone Replacement Therapy (HRT) which boosts oestrogen levels and keeps the bones absorbing calcium. However HRT does not cure osteoporosis, it merely delays it for as long as the medication is taken, and there are other risks associated with taking it (see the entry on page 143).

The two most important things that we can do for ourselves to prevent osteoporosis is to take regular exercise and have a good diet. Exercising will actually slow down bone loss but this has to be built into our lifestyle before the problem has had a chance to develop. We need to have an adequate supply of calcium in what we eat. Foods rich in calcium include: dairy products, fish (especially sardines), watercress, soya bean flour, brewer's yeast, eggs, nuts, sunflower and sesame seeds, chickpeas and lentils.

There is not much point in taking calcium supplements unless you eat a very poor diet because it is the body's inability to use calcium properly that is the important factor. The homoeopathic tissue salt CALC PHOS may be taken from time to time to encourage the body to assimilate calcium well. Excessive amounts of phosphorous in the diet tend to disrupt the body's ability to use calcium, and foods which are particularly rich in phosphorous include: red meat, fizzy drinks and many processed foods.

If you have already developed osteoporosis it would help you to visit a practitioner of natural medicine who should be able to encourage your body to take in calcium more effectively. We particularly recommend that you visit either a herbalist or homoeopath so that she or he can deal with this problem properly.

The Nervous System

The nervous system is made up of the brain, the spinal cord, and the nerves and sensory receptors distributed throughout the body. It is one of the great communication and transport systems of the body (the others are the bloodstream and the lymphatic system); in diagrams it looks rather like a tree, with smaller and smaller branches departing from a larger central trunk.

The nervous system is the link between mind and body. This link operates in two ways: physical experiences are conveyed via the nervous system to the brain, where they are registered or translated into information and experience; the reverse flow occurs when either there is an automatic response or the will to act is transmitted from the brain to the body via the nervous system. For this system to remain healthy there needs to be a balance between the ingoing tendency and the outgoing tendency – between the receptive and active sides of our nature.

A disease, such as sciatica or shingles, may seem to rise directly out of the physical components of the nervous system, or it may appear to arise from the realm of the mind, as anxiety or depression seems to. The truth is that here, more than in any other of the body's systems, the distinction between the physical and the psychological is always complex, and usually it is only partially understood. Most ailments associated with the physical nervous system will have an effect on the mind of the sufferer. For example, shingles is often accompanied with depression, and many so-called psychological disorders will result in physical complaints, just as stress causes migraine attacks.

If you suffer from a problem of the nervous system, you must be prepared to examine and work towards healing on every level – physical, emotional and mental – in order to bring about a cure. You need to reassess the amount of stress you live with at home and

The Nervous System

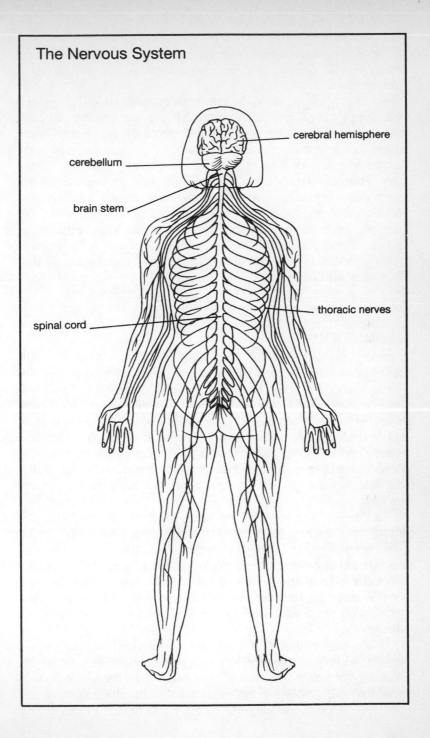

cerebral hemisphere

cerebellum

brain stem

thoracic nerves

spinal cord

at work. You also need to consider your ability to communicate thoughts and feelings, and also your capacity for putting ideas into action.

For many people, life in the twentieth century is stressful, and the barrage of stimuli and information that our nervous systems have to contend with is astounding (just think of the number of hours many people spend watching television). Driving a car, operating a computer or switchboard, even crossing a busy road, all require considerable powers of concentration and co-ordination. This creates extra stress for our nervous systems and increased stress may be one reason why people have suffered more from various diseases of the nervous system in recent years. A positive aspect of increased stress may be that all this stimulation is enlarging the capacity of this system (this is particularly noticeable in children), and this is one way that humanity may be continuing to evolve.

Addiction

Addiction occurs when we allow our inner or spiritual purpose to be satisfied on a desire level. The impulse to search for purpose, love, fulfilment and creative expression is an ongoing process in everyone's life; if we allow this search to become a craving for a substance, object or particular way of being, for example power, sex, money, alcohol, drugs, cigarettes or food, then we are in danger of becoming addicted. None of these things will be ultimately satisfying because they are all only substitutes for the thing we really crave or seek.

Breaking an addiction, like breaking any habit, is extremely difficult because we have to confront the empty space in our life that we were attempting to fill with whatever we were addicted to. Every time that we feel dissatisfied or unfulfilled, we will automatically crave the same thing. In addition, most addictive substances contain chemical compounds that alter the body's biochemistry, and removing the substance will create a reaction that is uncomfortable, and at times dangerous.

It is a great challenge in life to break an addiction, and success brings benefits in terms of both an improvement in your health and self-esteem. It will always be a lonely task because it is only you that can put in the effort and only you that can reap the rewards, although the support of family and friends should always be gratefully received, and they no doubt will also enjoy your increased well-being. Self-help groups, like those for alcoholism, can provide a supportive environment to communicate feelings and to share ways of dealing with the difficulties that arise. Counselling and psychotherapy can also help us to understand and deal with the patterns that are underlying the addiction.

Breaking an addiction successfully depends on your will to succeed. The need to be free from the offending substance has to be greater than your desire for it. Once you have made the decision to break the addiction, and if you have the necessary support available, there are natural remedies that can help. These strengthen the nervous system, and have an uplifting effect, supporting the body as it clears out the residual toxins. Acupuncture treatment has been shown to be particularly successful in treating certain forms of addiction, especially for alcohol, smoking and recreational drugs. The following suggestions may be used to support professional help, but they are not meant to replace it.

Amongst the herbal remedies used for treating addictions, the most useful is OATS, which is a nervine and is also said to help strengthen the will. LADY'S SLIPPER, SCULLCAP and VALERIAN all calm the nervous system and can help to overcome the initial reactions to coming off an addictive substance. ANGELICA ROOT is said to create a distaste for alcohol. If alcoholism is associated with suspected liver problems then read the section on the Liver and Gall Bladder on pages 85–8. A combination of COLTSFOOT and PLANTAIN may be taken to help strengthen and clear out the respiratory system after giving up smoking. ROSEMARY generally strengthens the nerves, physically, and can be combined with BALM and SCULLCAP to calm the mind and lift depression. CRAMPBARK helps nervous tension and anxiety.

It will probably be necessary to have constitutional treatment for homoeopathy to be successful. However, many people have found that taking NUX VOMICA in low potency helps them to give up smoking. KALI PHOS is also a useful homoeopathic remedy for strengthening the nervous system, and it is particularly useful to take each night if you are trying to come off tranquillizers for sleeping problems.

The Healing Herbs of Dr Bach can be very helpful for the underlying emotional causes of addiction. Consult the chart on pages 191–6 and make up a mixture of the most appropriate ones.

All the antidepressant essential oils help in breaking addiction, with BERGAMOT, CHAMOMILE, CLARY SAGE, JASMINE, ROSE and YLANG YLANG being among the most useful. Detoxifying oils such as FENNEL and JUNIPER can also be helpful with clearing the toxic residues out of the body.

Use essential oils for massage or in the bath. But you will get the most benefit by visiting an aromatherapist for massage treatment combined with counselling and support.

Anxiety

All of us have experienced feelings of anxiety at certain times during our life, often as a response to stressful events such as exams, an illness, or concern for a member of our family. If the anxiety becomes long term, remaining beyond a particular event, then some form of counselling may be necessary to help you break the habit that anxiety can become.

The symptoms of anxiety include feelings of uneasiness, apprehension and tension, and sometimes feelings of panic may also develop. You may experience tight breathing, palpitations, nausea, diarrhoea, perspiration and disturbed sleep. Continued anxiety may well result in physical disease, such as digestive disorders, headaches, backache or high blood pressure.

Tranquillizers and antidepressants are often prescribed for the orthodox treatment of anxiety. This is counterproductive because they rarely help in the long run. Drugs certainly don't cure the cause of the anxiety and, at best, they simply mask some of the symptoms; at worst, coming off the medication often aggravates all the initial symptoms, making it very difficult.

The following natural remedies will help to strengthen the nervous system and relieve the symptoms of anxiety, but if they are persistent you should seek constitutional treatment by a qualified practitioner. Curing anxiety should involve developing an understanding of the symptoms, redirecting the fears involved, strengthening the nervous system and dealing with any other contributory factors.

First, look at your diet to make certain that it contains sufficient sources of calcium, magnesium and Vitamins B and C (consult the tables on pages 392–4 for rich food sources of these vitamins and minerals). Herbs that can be used to treat anxiety include: BALM, CHAMOMILE, HOPS, LIMEFLOWERS, MOTHERWORT, OATS, ORANGE BLOSSOM, PASSIFLORA, SCULLCAP and VERVAIN. Consult the Materia Medica to see which herbs are the best indicated for you, and then make a mixture of the most suitable ones.

For chronic anxiety to be treated successfully by homoeopathy, constitutional treatment by a qualified practitioner is necessary. For more transient symptoms, the following homoeopathic remedies may be considered: ACONITE, ARG NIT, ARSENICUM, GELSEMIUM, IGNATIA, KALI PHOS and PHOSPHOROUS. The Healing Herbs of Dr Bach can be a very helpful way of treating anxiety – consult the table on pages 191–6 and make a mixture of the most suitable.

The essential oils that are most useful for treating anxiety include: BASIL, CLARY SAGE, GERANIUM, LAVENDER, MELISSA, NEROLI and ROSE. You will probably get most benefit from visiting an aromatherapist and having a regular consultation and massage. Any of the oils may be diluted in a vegetable-oil base and used in massage, or add a couple of drops of the oil of your choice to a warm bath.

Depression

The word depression means to be pushed down, and there are times when all of us have felt like this – when we feel 'low' and unhappy with ourselves and with life. Depression can develop after a stressful event like losing your job, a bereavement or housing difficulties, or it can be brought on by a physical condition such as an illness or from taking drugs. For some people, depression is chronic and it is a pattern that affects their whole life, and the immediate cause is not easily identified.

Symptoms of depression include an inability to feel pleasure, loss of appetite, sleep disturbances, fatigue, anxiety, poor libido, pessimism, thoughts of death, feelings of hopelessness and low self-esteem. The orthodox treatment of depression is to prescribe antidepressant drugs. This is counterproductive because the drugs don't cure the depression, or help you to come to an understanding of it. Furthermore, it can be extremely difficult to stop taking the drugs because all the symptoms they have masked will reassert themselves.

Although there are many natural remedies that can help to relieve depression, no single remedy, in isolation, will cure it because overcoming it is a learning process. Much depression springs from an attitude that is common in our society in which we tend to lose touch with our purpose for existence and our inner sense of creativity and self-esteem.

Difficult circumstances and various incidents may be the trigger for depression, but we only become its victim when we are unable to communicate our inner needs and feelings, and we are out of touch with our initial emotional impulses. Failure or inability to recognise and express these early, primary emotions leads to suppression; this develops into a confusion and complication of emotions and we lose touch with our sense of self-worth and purpose. We call this depression.

A consultation with a practitioner of natural medicine, psychotherapist or counsellor may well be one of the steps necessary to help an individual investigate and come to terms with the life patterns that are contributing to his or her depression. A professional practitioner should assess the severity of the depression, particularly if it is persistent or if the depressed person is suicidal. Severe depression may need more intensive intervention, possibly including twenty-four hour care under professional supervision.

Mild symptoms of depression may be relieved by questioning yourself about what is going on, and by treating yourself with natural remedies (such as those mentioned here) to strengthen the nervous system and relieve some of the more distressing symptoms.

The best antidepressant and nervine herbs include: BALM, BORAGE, CAYENNE, KOLA (these two for a boost), LIMEFLOWERS, OATS, ROSEMARY, SCULLCAP, ST JOHN'S WORT and VERVAIN. Make a mixture of the most suitable herbs after looking them up in the Materia Medica section of this book.

There are many homoeopathic remedies that can be used to treat depression, but because the particular symptoms tend to be so individual, a visit to a qualified practitioner may be necessary to find the remedy or remedies that will be of most value to you. You may find it interesting to look up the following remedies in the Materia Medica and then try one if it appears to be particularly appropriate: AURUM, IGNATIA, NATRUM MUR, SEPIA and STAPHYSAGRIA.

The Healing Herbs of Dr Bach can be very helpful in the treatment of depression. Consult the list on pages 191–6, and make up a mixture of those that look the most appropriate.

The essential oils that are used to treat depression tend to be divided into two categories: those that are mainly sedating, and those that are mainly uplifting. Overall, most of the oils have a balancing effect and should help to strenghten the nervous system, as well as relieving particular symptoms. The mainly sedating antidepressant essential oils are: CHAMOMILE, CLARY SAGE, LAVENDER, NEROLI and SANDALWOOD. The mainly uplifting antidepressant essential oils are: BASIL, BERGAMOT, GERANIUM, JASMINE, MELISSA and ROSE. Oils from the two groups can be combined if that seems appropriate. Consult the Materia Medica and choose two or three of the oils that look the most suitable, and that you enjoy using, and use those oils on a regular basis. The oils that you choose can be made up into a massage oil, or added to a warm bath.

Headaches

Nearly everyone gets a headache at one time or another. There are many possible causes. For example, a headache may be caused by stress, exposure to strong sun, having a cold or flu, pre-menstrual tension, overindulging in alcohol or drugs, or from poor posture. If a headache is very severe or persistent, or results from a head injury, then seek immediate medical advice.

If poor posture is causing your headaches then consider consulting an Alexander Technique practitioner or chiropractic therapist. If headaches are recurrent, then constitutional treatment by a qualified therapist will be necessary to help discover the underlying factors contributing to them. With tension headaches, it may be useful to reassess the balance between the head and the heart (or the rational thought versus the feeling element) in your life. Relaxation techniques including meditation and yoga can teach us to let go of tension and relax more effectively. For the occasional headache with an obvious, non-serious cause, the following remedies will be helpful.

Look up these herbs in the Materia Medica section, depending on the cause of your headache: BALM, CHAMOMILE, JAMAICAN DOGWOOD, LAVENDER, ROSEMARY, SCULLCAP, WHITE WILLOW and VERVAIN. Make an infusion to drink from the most appropriate ones.

The most effective essential oils for treating headaches include: EUCALYPTUS, LAVENDER, MELISSA, NEROLI and ROSEMARY. Add a few drops of one to a warm bath, or make up a massage oil to apply as a neck and shoulder massage.

A homoeopathic remedy may be chosen from the following list by comparing them in the Materia Medica section: ARNICA, BELLADONNA, BRYONIA, GELSEMIUM, KALI PHOS, NUX VOMICA, and PULSATILLA.

Insomnia

An inability to sleep may take various forms. You may not be able to 'drop off' to sleep or you may wake during the night or very early in the morning. Most people experience sleeplessness at some time in their lives, maybe before an exam, during emotional trauma or because of discomfort or pain. Usually this will pass after the obvious cause has gone, but if a pattern of sleeplessness becomes established it can be difficult to break.

The amount of sleep an individual needs varies. Some people are convinced that they can only operate effectively with ten hours a night; others appear to manage perfectly well on only a couple of hours. If you worry about not having enough sleep you have the double problem of making it more difficult to actually get to sleep and the anxiety.

Where there is a clear reason for your insomnia – if you are in pain or discomfort or you are anxious – it is obviously best to deal with the causes, if this is possible. It is more appropriate to treat the pain, indigestion, depression and so on, than deal directly with sleeplessness. The specific remedies for insomnia suggested here are appropriate if you need to function in the short term, during a period of known stress such as during exams, interviews or emotional traumas. Where sleep difficulties, particularly early-morning waking, are accompanied by dark moods, you should seek professional help to determine the possibility of underlying depression.

Most standard medications for insomnia are hypnotic sedatives that depress brain function. The principal 'sleeping pills' are benzodiazepines (tranquillizers), nonbarbiturates (bromides, chloral and so on) and antihistamines. All of them carry some risk of habituation and tolerance, so that the doses have to become ever larger to remain effective. Many people find also that they are drowsy or less able to concentrate during the day.

Insomnia is common during the later stages of pregnancy, when it can become difficult to find a comfortable sleeping position. Try a warm drink before going to bed and use extra pillows to find a more comfortable position. If all else fails, try and make the time to have a rest or nap during the day or after work.

It is worth bearing in mind that the body is basically a self-regulating organism and that given positive assistance, it will take the amount of sleep that is needed. Resting and relaxing generally will create the best conditions to encourage sleep and even if sleep is minimal, enable the body to cope better with that situation.

On a practical note, it is worth avoiding tea and coffee and other stimulants in the evening if you do suffer from sleeplessness. Similarly, try to avoid things that are intellectually stimulating or potentially stressful late at night. Physical exercise generally improves one's ability to sleep soundly, and for those of us who lead sedentary lives, a daily exercise routine can make a marked difference.

A great deal of sleeplessness is caused by an over-active brain, which will tend to dwell on worries and troubles and send them round in circles when you are tired. Meditation and visualisation exercises can be used to distract the brain from such worries and encourage it to let go into sleep more easily. Try concentrating on relaxing the entire body, muscle by muscle, from the feet upwards, or running through the day backwards without becoming unduly attached to any one event.

There are many traditional herbal remedies to assist sleep. BALM, BORAGE (for low spirits), CHAMOMILE, HOPS, LIME FLOWERS, ORANGE BLOSSOM, PASSIFLORA, SCULLCAP, VALERIAN and VERVAIN can be made into an infusion, either as a combination or separately, and drunk in the evening. Essential oils can be a particularly pleasant method of assisting sleep and a few drops of BASIL, CHAMOMILE, LAVENDER, MARJORAM or NEROLI either in an evening bath or dropped onto a tissue and placed on the pillow can be very effective. A useful homoeopathic remedy to try is KALI PHOS as a tissue salt, which is taken one each night on retiring, for up to a month. Homoeopathic COFFEA may also be indicated. The most frequently used remedy from the Healing Herbs of Dr Bach for insomnia is WHITE CHESTNUT which is indicated where there are persistent, unwanted thoughts or mental arguments preventing sleep.

Persistent insomnia may require psychological therapy if the cause is primarily emotional, or constitutional treatment, by an acupuncturist or homoeopath, if the body's energy is not readily able to establish a better sleep pattern to suit the individual.

Migraine

The pain experienced during a migraine is caused by a temporary spasm followed by considerable dilation of blood vessels in the brain. The symptoms are intense pain, usually only in one side of the head, nausea and visual disturbances. The length of the attack varies from between a couple of hours to several days. A migraine attack is normally accompanied by the desire for solitude, and to lie down in a quiet, dark room.

Factors known to contribute to migraines include stress, tension, hormonal changes during the menstrual cycle, congestive disorders, allergy, certain foods (commonly cheese, chocolate and red wine), and a hereditary predisposition. If your migraine attacks keep recurring, you should consider constitutional treatment or even psychotherapy to try and establish and change the more profound reasons for them. It is often necessary to help a migraine sufferer become more in touch with their physical body and particularly their sexuality, in order to bring about true healing.

For an infrequent or mild migraine attack, the following natural remedies may be of some benefit. Try an infusion made from the following herbs: BALM, FEVERFEW, JAMAICAN DOGWOOD, MEADOWSWEET, ROSEMARY and SCULLCAP. A warm or cold compress (whichever is preferred) may be applied to the back of the neck or forehead and temples, using one of the following essential oils: BASIL, LAVENDER, MARJORAM or MELISSA. Consult the Materia Medica section of this book to see if any of the homoeopathic remedies look particularly appropriate: BELLADONNA, BRYONIA, GELSEMIUM, KALI BICH, NUX VOMICA and PULSATILLA.

Neuralgia and Sciatica

Neuralgia is an acutely painful condition caused by the inflammation of a nerve. The trigeminal nerves in the face are the most common site of neuralgia. If the sciatic nerve in the spine is affected, then there is pain in the lower back and down the legs and the condition is called sciatica.

Neuralgia often seems to occur during a phase of life when there are a lot of worries and troubles around, and particularly when communicating or the sharing of problems is difficult. If it seems possible that these are underlying factors in your case then you should consider some form of counselling. Sciatica often occurs in someone who has taken on a lot and is burdened by family, life or work, and this should be assessed and dealt with if necessary.

There are some natural remedies that can be of great benefit while you are confronting any underlying factors. Firstly, however, make sure that you are getting the right nutrients in your diet, and particularly that you have a plentiful supply of B complex vitamins (check the food source charts on pages 392–4 if you are unsure).

Herbs that have a nervine and pain-relieving effect include: JAMAICAN DOGWOOD, OATS, PASSIFLORA, PEPPERMINT, ST JOHN'S WORT and SCULLCAP. Try a combination of these in an infusion three times a day. The essential oils of CHAMOMILE, EUCALYPTUS, LAVENDER, MARJORAM,

PEPPERMINT, ROSEMARY or SANDALWOOD may be applied in a compress, massage or bath. Look the following homoeopathic remedies up in the Materia Medica section to see if one of them looks particularly appropriate: CAUSTICUM, HYPERICUM, KALI CARB, KALI PHOS and RHUS TOX.

Shingles

Shingles, also called herpes zoster, is caused by a virus similar to the chickenpox virus. The distinguishing symptom of shingles is the very painful clusters of blisters on the skin at the site of the nerve endings, for example around the chest or on the thighs. The sufferer will feel generally unwell and he or she may have a fever during the acute attack. The pain may persist even when the blisters have gone.

An attack of shingles is often a sign of general debility, and patients should reassess their diet and take plenty of rest. Particular attention should be made to an adequate supply of B complex vitamins in the diet (check the chart on pages 392–4 for rich food sources of vitamins).

The following natural remedies will bring relief to shingles affecting the chest, back, thighs, buttocks and so on; shingles on the forehead or anywhere near the eyes should be treated only under the supervision of a qualified practitioner. Make a combination of the following nervine herbs and drink an infusion three times a day: LADY'S SLIPPER, OATS, SCULLCAP, ST JOHN'S WORT and VERVAIN. Diluted tinctures or cool infusions of the following herbs may also be used to bathe the affected area: MARIGOLD, PLANTAIN and ST JOHN'S WORT. Essential oils can combine analgesics with anti-viral properties, and may be applied as a compress, or by diluting them in a base-massage oil to gently massage in. Try combining a couple of the following oils after looking them up in the Materia Medica section: BERGAMOT, CHAMOMILE, EUCALYPTUS, GERANIUM, LAVENDER, MELISSA and TEA TREE.

The homoeopathic remedies to consider for the treatment of shingles include: ARSEN ALB, KALI PHOS and RHUS TOX.

Stress

Stress is not an illness in itself, but it is a response to any situation that puts us under pressure. Factors contributing to stress may be environmental, physical or mental. For example, environmental stress may be caused by pollution or poor housing; physical stress results from an accident or injury; and mental stress may arise from pressure of work, or difficulties within a relationship.

We seem to be able to adapt to a certain amount of stress in our lives without showing symptoms of disease, but at some point, if the stress continues, or a new one is added, the balance is tipped and we begin to experience symptoms of one kind or another as a result. The amount of stress involved in everyday life in our society is considered to be unacceptably high by many people; and certainly therapists see a great many diseases these days which have a clear correlation with particular stress factors in the sufferer's life. Diseases that often have an obvious relationship with stress include: allergies, asthma, eczema, headaches, migraine, digestive disorders, heart disease, insomnia and depression.

The only way that we are going to be able to reduce the amount of stress in our lives is to choose another way of doing things. For example, we must choose additive-free diets, reassess how hard we work, take steps where possible to improve our physical environment and develop our ability to communicate with others. Feeling helpless is in itself stressful, so it can be helpful to join an environmental pressure group or self-help group for the particular disease or problem that you have, in order to feel more empowered.

We need to be as healthy as possible so that our bodies can adapt efficiently to stresses. As well as dealing with any specific health problems, we must eat well, avoid excessive amounts of coffee and alcohol, avoid smoking or taking drugs, get enough sleep (which is the only time that the body can repair itself), and enjoy ourselves mentally and physically. There are a variety of different techniques that are known to help us deal with stress more effectively – such as yoga, meditation, music or art therapy, and certain exercises.

If we feel that we need some extra help during a particularly stressful phase of our lives, then there are some remedies that we can employ, but these should only be taken for a relatively short period of time, before we really reassess the habits and activities in our lives that are causing the stress in the first place. It is useless to relieve the symptoms while maintaining the stressful lifestyle.

Our bodies use up the B group of vitamins particularly rapidly when we are under stress, and so it is a good idea to check that our diet is rich in these vitamins (see the food source chart on pages 392–4), and consider taking a supplement such as brewer's yeast tablets. There are herbs that act as nervine tonics to feed and strengthen the nervous system, the best ones for treating stress in a general way are: BALM, BORAGE, CHAMOMILE, LAVENDER, LIMEFLOWERS, OATS, ORANGE BLOSSOM, PASSIFLORA, ROSE PETALS, SCULLCAP and VERBENA. Any of these may be drunk as an infusion on a regular basis.

GINSENG is known to be an adaptogen and it helps the body to deal with the effects of stress.

Essential oils that have an uplifting and relaxing effect can be helpful, for example: BASIL, BERGAMOT, CHAMOMILE, GERANIUM, JASMINE, LAVENDER, MARJORAM, NEROLI and ROSE. Essential oils that strengthen the adrenal system, which tends to be weakened by stress, may also be useful, for example: GINGER, LEMON GRASS and ROSEMARY. All of these oils should be checked in the Materia Medica section and then they can be used in massage, baths or by burning them in a room.

Pregnancy

The experience of pregnancy and childbirth is one of the most exciting and challenging times in any woman's life. The experience of your own body creating another human being is one that is on the leading edge of nature at her most miraculous. Every pregnant woman, and every mother, is brought into an awareness of her inherent creative power.

Most healthy women become radiant during pregnancy; it is a shame that in our society we have fallen into the habit of looking upon pregnancy as an illness, and the pregnant woman as a patient in need of treatment. With reassurance, and practical advice where there is not the experience already built in, most women can enjoy pregnancy and labour without the need for medication and intervention.

In many ways, this is an exciting time for all those concerned with pregnancy and childbirth, because as well as the privilege that goes with being involved in this field, there have been many positive steps towards reclaiming the experience as the immensely creative, feminine, personal and natural process that it should be. The days when women were subject to all the intervention, restrictions and personal idiosyncracies of the doctor or hospital concerned are hopefully numbered, as the numbers of women and midwives who demand the right to choose their treatment during pregnancy and the type of birth that they want, grow.

Prenatal classes in active birth and exercise are now increasingly easy to find. There is information available on how to arrange a home birth. More and more clinics and labour wards are responding to demands for facilities for an active labour, soft lighting in the delivery room, and the desire of the mother to remain in contact with the baby as soon as she is born. However, in some areas, expressing your

The Baby in the Womb at Term

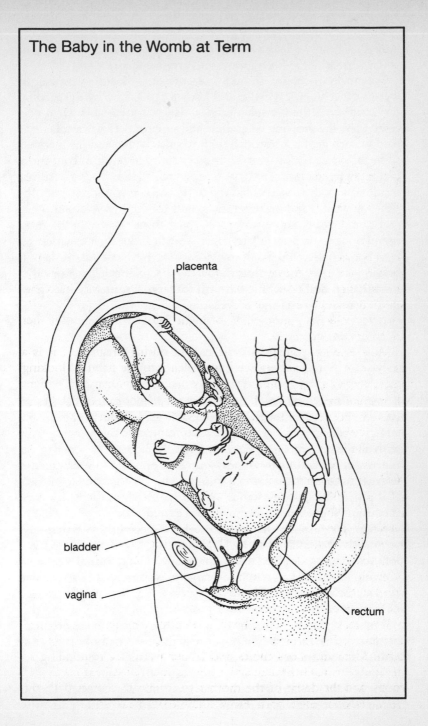

placenta

bladder

vagina

rectum

individual needs and wishes can still feel like a real struggle, at a time when what is needed is support and creative assistance.

Potentially then, we should have the best of both worlds: the wealth of technical expertise and knowledge gained by the medical profession over the last few decades, which is invaluable when necessary; and the growing awareness and support network available to help women get back in touch with what is natural and instinctually right for them. Unfortunately, choice can often result in confusion, and it can feel daunting to have to deal with all the changes occuring inside your body as well as having to try and run your pregnancy the way you want it and make arrangements for your own labour when you cannot really know how it is going to be. Probably the most useful thing to do is to talk to other women about their experiences, read books on natural childbirth, join an active birth class if there is one in your area, and contact the National Childbirth Trust or other organisation dealing with childbirth for more information (see page 398 for useful names and addresses).

Diet

The importance of a good diet during pregnancy cannot be stressed enough. It is vital for the mother to be able to maintain her health and energy while nourishing the fetus, and to provide the growing baby with all the nutrients necessary for a healthy body. It is better to get nutrients from their natural food sources as opposed to supplements, because these are naturally in a form suitable for the body to absorb. If it proves difficult to establish a well-balanced, nutrient-rich diet, then some supplementation may be required.

Vitamin E aids the development of the reproductive system and is needed for a healthy and well-toned uterus. The daily requirement for this vitamin is doubled during pregnancy. Good natural sources of Vitamin E are: wheatgerm oil, wheatgerm, sesame seeds, oats, brown rice, sunflower seeds, cabbage and lettuce. The Vitamin E content of foods is lost by most forms of processing, including freezing. Do not take a high dose Vitamin E supplement while you are pregnant because it can increase blood pressure in those women who are prone to high blood pressure anyway.

The growing baby will use up a lot of iron from the mother's supply, especially during the last two months of pregnancy. Unfortunately, most iron supplements are renowned for causing digestive upsets such as nausea, colic and diarrhoea or constipation, and they should be avoided. Foods rich in iron are: liver, lean meat, treacle and molasses, lentils, haricot beans, dried fruit, eggs and green leafy vegetables. If you suspect that you may be anaemic, or a blood test indicates that you are, then follow the recommendations under Anaemia in the section on the Circulatory System on page 55.

Zinc is an extremely important mineral for the growing child in the womb; it is important for the development of healthy skin, bones and teeth. Good sources of zinc are: shellfish, liver, cheese, lentils, haricot beans, sesame seeds, sunflower seeds, almonds, avocado and bananas. Herbal infusions that will provide a rich supply of zinc include: ALFALFA and RASPBERRY LEAF, both of which are suitable for drinking during pregnancy.

The need for calcium increases greatly during the last three months as the baby takes what it needs for forming healthy bones and teeth. A lack of it will cause leg and foot cramps in the mother and a susceptibility to tooth decay. Foods rich in calcium include: dairy products, fish, watercress, wheatflour, oats, millet, soya beans and green, leafy vegetables.

There are also things that should be avoided during pregnancy. Coffee reduces the availability and absorption of nutrients from your diet and should be avoided. Alcohol should be avoided or kept to a suitable minimum – such as half a glass of wine mixed with water. An excessive amount of alcohol during pregnancy has been shown to have a detrimental affect on the child. Smoking should be avoided for the sake of both the mother's and baby's health. Smoking greatly increases the risk of miscarriage, premature birth, still birth and neonatal death.

Medication and Remedies to Avoid During Pregnancy

Taking any medication in pregnancy is a matter of weighing up the benefits against possible damage to the fetus. For two-thirds of drugs commonly consumed by women, and for a third of those used in labour, there are no published reports showing that they do not carry any risk to the baby. Many other drugs that are taken regularly by women, for example some sleeping pills, tranquillizers, migraine pills and some antibiotics, are known to have a detrimental effect on the fetus.

Basically, it is better to avoid taking any medication during pregnancy that is not absolutely vital to maintaining the health of the mother, such as for the treatment of diabetes and epilepsy. The fetus is particularly vulnerable to damage from medication during the first three months of pregnancy, when major organs of the body and the skeleton are forming. This is another argument for getting as healthy as possible before becoming pregnant so that there is no need for medication.

There are also a number of herbs that should be avoided during pregnancy. Basically this list includes those herbs that act as abortifacients, emmenagogues and strong laxatives. Any herb taken in therapeutic dosage should be specifically checked for safety and use during pregnancy; the list of those that should definitely be avoided (unless specifically recommended by a medical herbalist), includes: ALOES, BARBERRY, BLACK COHOSH, BLOODROOT, BUCKTHORN, CASCARA SAGRADA, CINCHONA, COTTONROOT, GOLDEN SEAL, GREATER CELANDINE, JUNIPER, LIFEROOT, MALE FERN, MANDRAKE, PENNYROYAL, POKE ROOT, RHUBARB, RUE, SAFFRON, SAGE, SOUTHERNWOOD, TANSY, THUJA and WORMWOOD.

There are also some essential oils that should be avoided during pregnancy, these include: ANISEED, BASIL, CAMPHOR, CARAWAY, CEDAR, CINNAMON, CLARY SAGE, CYPRESS, FENNEL, HYSSOP, JUNIPER, MARJORAM, MYRRH, NUTMEG, OREGANUM, PEPPERMINT, PENNYROYAL, ROSE, ROSEMARY, SAGE, SAVOURY, THUJA, THYME and WINTERGREEN.

Miscarriage

The first symptom of a miscarriage (medically referred to as a spontaneous abortion) is bleeding, sometimes accompanied by cramping pains. Slight bleeding, although alarming, does not necessarily mean that you will definitely miscarry, and some women lose small amounts of blood regularly throughout their otherwise healthy pregnancies. You should seek urgent medical advice for persistent or heavy bleeding. Bleeding accompanied with cramping pains nearly always indicates that a miscarriage is in process and you should seek urgent medical advice.

There is no concrete evidence that bed rest will prevent a miscarriage once it has started, but rest will probably help you to adjust and deal with the stress better.

The emotional trauma experienced after a miscarriage can be considerable, and the support of an experienced and caring practitioner can be a very helpful addition to that of friends and family.

An estimated 15 to 20 per cent of known pregnancies end in miscarriage in Great Britain, and this figure is much higher in third world countries. The majority of miscarriages occur within the first three months of pregnancy. It is thought that many occur as the body's natural way of rejecting an unhealthy fetus. As a result, you should not take any form of treatment to prevent a miscarriage at any cost.

If you have a history of miscarriages, constitutional treatment by a qualified therapist of natural medicine should be sought from the beginning of the pregnancy, or preferably before. The following remedies may help, but should only be used in conjunction with treatment from a qualified therapist.

If a miscarriage is threatening, consider the herbs BLUE COHOSH, CRAMP BARK, FALSE UNICORN and WILD YAM. Compare these in the Materia Medica section of this book and take a mixture of the most appropriate ones as a decoction, three times a day. If you are suffering from a lot of stress and anxiety, add SCULLCAP to the mixture.

The homoeopathic remedies that you should consider for a threatened miscarriage include: ACONITE, ARNICA, BELLADONNA, CHAMOMILLA, IGNATIA, PULSATILLA and SEPIA. Compare these in the Materia Medica and select the most appropriate remedy for you. Remember that if the fetus is not viable, then the right remedy assists the mother through the miscarriage emotionally and physically, but will not save the baby.

The Healing Herbs of Dr Bach RESCUE REMEDY can have a very calming influence during this stressful time. Take a few drops as often as required.

For remedies to help to restore health following a miscarriage see the section on Abortion below.

Abortion

Some people have attempted to use herbs and oils specifically to induce an abortion; this is an extremely dangerous and irresponsible way of terminating a pregnancy. In some cases it can cause haemorrhage, epileptic fits, or an infection following a partial miscarriage; if

117

the abortion is not successful it can damage the growing fetus. If the decision is reached to terminate a pregnancy, it is far safer to have a mechanical abortion at a reputable clinic or hospital.

You should be aware that you will need ongoing emotional support and possibly counselling after an abortion. Be cautious about the possibility of an infection following an abortion, if there is an unusual smell to any discharge, pain or a general rise in temperature, seek immediate medical advice.

Herbs that may be used to re-balance the hormones and tone the uterus after an abortion (or miscarriage) include: AGNUS CASTUS, BLUE COHOSH, FALSE UNICORN, HOLY THISTLE, LIQUORICE and RASPBERRY LEAF. Check the herbs in the Materia Medica section and take the most appropriate ones as an infusion or as tinctures, for a month. If you are under a lot of emotional stress, consider adding BALM and SCULLCAP to the mixture.

The homoeopathic remedy ARNICA is useful to take following any physical trauma or operation. Other homoeopathic remedies to consider after an abortion are: BELLIS PERENNIS, IGNATIA and STAPHYSAGRIA.

The essential oils of LAVENDER, NEROLI and ROSE can help to ease stress and promote healing after a miscarriage or abortion. Dilute to use in a massage or add a few drops to a warm bath.

Tests and Scans

There are a wide range of tests than can be carried out during pregnancy these days; some of these, although valuable in special circumstances, are now routine.

Today, most pregnant women in the western world are subjected to one or more ultrasound scans. Ultrasound was invented during the Second World War and used to detect submarines at sea. It works on the principle that sound rays bounce off solid objects.

During an ultrasound scan, a probe that emits waves of sound too high for the ear to hear, is passed over the uterus. The sound is translated into dots, which are used to build up an image on a screen. The ultrasound scan can provide doctors with a great deal of information about the placenta and the growing fetus. It can be used to locate the position of the placenta, to establish whether the heart is still beating after a threatened miscarriage, to reveal certain congenital handicaps and to date a pregnancy more accurately. But ultrasound also has many disadvantages. It often diagnoses conditions, such as a low-lying placenta, which may have righted itself by the time labour starts. Results are not always accurately interpreted, and many women have suffered terrible stress and anxiety because they were told that something was wrong with the unborn child when there was not. Between sixteen and twenty-four weeks, ultrasound should be able to give an accurate dating of pregnancy, after that time it is very likely to be wrong.

At present there is no evidence that ultrasound is unsafe, but very little is known about its possible delayed and long-term risks. It has been suggested that ultrasound may produce changes in fetal cells which could lead to later health problems. It does also seem to affect the fetus in the womb, often by making it jump around wildly. It could be that while our ears cannot pick up the high-pitch sound waves, the sensitive ears of the developing fetus pick them up as intensely shrill and powerful noise. Because there is no evidence that the routine use of ultrasound benefits either mother or child, and because the possible long-term risks are not yet known, it seems wise to restrict its use to those cases where there are good reasons to suspect that all is not well.

Amniocentesis is a test carried out by inserting a needle through the mother's abdominal wall, into the uterus, and drawing off a sample of the amniotic fluid in which the baby floats. It cannot be done until you are sixteen to eighteen weeks pregnant because until then there is not enough fluid. Fetal cells from the fluid can be grown in a culture to reveal a range of abnormalities, including Down's syndrome, sickle cell anaemia, thalassaemia and spina bifida. Amniocentesis can also show the sex of the baby which is important if there are sex-linked diseases, such as haemophilia or muscular dystrophy, in the family.

If the amniocentesis test does reveal that the fetus suffers from a congenital abnormality, the mother must decide whether or not to have an abortion. It is an unfortunate problem with amniocentesis that if the pregnancy is to be terminated, it results in a late abortion, after twenty weeks, which can be very distressing. Another drawback is that many results take three to four weeks or longer for a result, which can be a very worrying time. If the mother has decided that she would not agree to an abortion there is no point in having the test.

Other risks involved with amniocentesis are a higher rate of miscarriage, and an increased incidence of newborn babies who have difficulties with breathing. However, the medical authorities will always recommend amniocentesis if you are over 35 because of the link between older mothers and Down's syndrome babies. The test is also recommended for women from ethnic groups that are more at risk of a genetic disorder such as sickle cell disease, and for those women who are likely to pass on an inherited abnormality.

Tests that should be carried out routinely when you are pregnant are: measuring your weight; blood tests to ascertain your blood group and the possibility of anaemia; blood pressure; urine tests to check for sugar and protein; and palpation of the abdomen to feel the size of the uterus and size and position of the baby. It is particularly important that weight and blood pressure are measured regularly throughout pregnancy.

Common Ailments of Pregnancy

We are going to discuss the issues and problems that may arise during pregnancy under three stages: the three trimesters (three-monthly periods) of a normal pregnancy. There may well be an overlap in many cases, for example, constipation may occur in any or all of the three trimesters, not just the second one as it is discussed here (although this is probably when it is most commonly experienced); in that case the information and suggestions given will still be relevant and can easily be applied to your stage of pregnancy.

THE FIRST TRIMESTER
The first three months of pregnancy can be the time when you experience some of its most distressing symptoms. After the initial excitement of discovering that you are pregnant, you can feel suddenly that you are out of control of your body and your life. Many women suffer with nausea in early pregnancy, and feeling exhausted is also common. If the pregnancy was unplanned these symptoms can be even harder to accept. It is as if your body is expressing the turmoil of preparing itself for the enormously creative task ahead.

Some women sail through their whole pregnancy without experiencing any uncomfortable symptoms; and indeed they may feel healthier than they ever have before. However, most women experience some tiredness in the first three months – fortunately these feelings of exhaustion do not usually get worse as the pregnancy progresses but improve considerably by the second trimester. If at all possible, the sensible thing to do if you do feel really tired, is to assist your body at this time of adjustment and get plenty of rest.

The need to urinate more frequently usually starts in early pregnancy, once the uterus begins to swell and press on the bladder. Try to avoid drinking anything just before you go to bed to reduce the number of visits to the toilet during the night. Also cut out tea, coffee and alcohol as these tend to stimulate urine production.

The one symptom that everyone associates with the early stages of pregnancy is morning sickness, and some morning sickness will be experienced by most women during the first few months of pregnancy. The symptoms include nausea, vomiting and a feeling of weakness. It seems to be caused by the massive upheaval of hormones occuring in the body, combined with low blood sugar. You generally feel it most in the morning, when the stomach is empty, although it may occur at any time of day. It is often helpful to get up slowly in the mornings, and try eating a dry biscuit before rising.

If you feel nauseous later in the day, try eating small snacks at frequent intervals. Your metabolism speeds up during early pregnancy, so you will probably find that your weight doesn't increase in the first two or three months even though you may be eating more. Foods that can aggravate feelings of nausea are fatty foods and milk, so try cutting these out.

The symptoms of morning sickness usually recede after the third month of pregnancy. In some rare cases they persist throughout pregnancy, and you should seek professional help. You should also seek professional guidance if vomiting is persistent, or if you develop a prolonged aversion to eating. Herbs that can be safely used to alleviate the nausea of morning sickness include: BALM, BLACK HOREHOUND, MEADOWSWEET, PEPPERMINT and RASPBERRY LEAF. Combine these, or use them separately, to make an infusion to drink three times a day. Ground GINGER may also be made into capsules to treat nausea, or take the tincture diluted in water.

The most commonly used homoeopathic remedies for relieving morning sickness are: IPECAC, NUX VOMICA, PULSATILLA and SEPIA. Look these up in the Materia Medica section of this book to see which one is the most suitable for you.

THE SECOND TRIMESTER

The second trimester is a time for becoming attuned to the baby growing within. Around the fourth or fifth month you will feel the first movements of the baby. Actually, the fetus has been moving around for months, but the movements can only be felt from this

121

stage. Most women feel very well during this time and the nausea and exhaustion of the early stages often recedes.

Your pregnancy is also beginning to show at this stage. The fetus has begun to grow bulkier and your waist starts to thicken. The line from your naval to your pubic region becomes dark, as does the area around your nipples. Sometimes the facial pigment also becomes darker, but this will fade after the birth.

As your abdomen grows larger, the skin over it will stretch. If you do not have very supple skin, pink or reddish streaks may appear, called stretch marks. To reduce the likelihood of stretch marks developing, massage the abdomen regularly with the essential oils of FRANKINCENSE (OLIBANUM), LAVENDER or ROSEWOOD, diluted in a base of combined almond and wheatgerm oils.

A homoeopathic tissue salt that is very useful to take during pregnancy is CALC FLUOR. This remedy will increase the suppleness of the skin to prevent stretch marks, give elasticity to vein walls thus reducing the likelihood of varicose veins or haemorrhoids developing, and it will also be good for the developing baby's teeth and bones. It is easily available in health food shops and many chemists and should be purchased in the 6X potency. Take one dose three times a day for ten days, then have a break for a few days and repeat the course once or twice more if required.

A herbal tea that has been taken by many of thousands of women during pregnancy to tone the uterus is RASPBERRY LEAF. This is a pleasant tasting herbal tea that can be taken by drinking a cupful at least once a day throughout the second half of pregnancy. SQUAW VINE is an American Indian herb that is taken in the same way as RASPBERRY LEAF: to tonify the uterus in preparation for labour. This may be taken as an alternative or take them together. Check the Materia Medica section for dosage and more information on its actions.

One unpleasant symptom that can develop once pregnancy is established is indigestion and heartburn. This may be due to progesterone and other hormones softening the valve at the top of the stomach, and thus allowing digestive acids to rise into the oesophagus; or from the uterus pressing on the digestive organs later in pregnancy. To relieve this eat small meals at more regular intervals, or eat slowly and chew everything well and avoid fatty and fried foods. It is also advisable not to eat late in the evening; and if the problem comes on at night try sleeping well propped up on a number of pillows.

Remedies that will relieve symptoms of heartburn and indigestion include the homoeopathic remedies: KALI MUR, NUX VOMICA and

PULSATILLA. Check these in the Materia Medica section to see which is most suitable and take as required. An infusion of the herbs BALM, MEADOWSWEET or PEPPERMINT can also bring relief: try sipping a cupful after each meal. Or take SLIPPERY ELM half an hour before a meal.

Constipation is another symptom that can prove troublesome during pregnancy. This is sometimes due to hormone changes slowing down intestinal action, and sometimes occurs when the uterus presses against the large intestine. Your diet is very important here and the problem can be solved by eating more fibre-rich foods such as oats, pulses, raw fruit and vegetables, and also more dried fruit, especially figs and prunes. Avoid all refined foods, particularly white flour and sugar. Do not take iron tablets. Constipation can be caused by the bowel absorbing more fluid during pregnancy, so try drinking more water (you should be drinking 6–8 glasses of fluid a day).

If constipation becomes persistent consult the Materia Medica to see if one of the following homoeopathic remedies looks appropriate: BRYONIA, NATRUM MUR, NUX VOMICA and SEPIA. The herbs FENNEL, LIQUO-RICE and MARSHMALLOW ROOT all have a mild laxative action and may be taken as an infusion before bedtime. Do not take stronger laxative herbs during pregnancy, and do *not* take LIQUORICE if you suffer with high blood pressure.

Partly as a result of pelvic pressure, and partly due to the tissue-relaxing effect of progesterone and other hormones present in pregnancy, many pregnant women suffer from haemorrhoids and varicose veins. It is really important not to get constipated if you are trying to avoid haemorrhoids; if you do get them follow the advice under Haemorrhoids in the Digestive System (see page 68). Continuing to take exercise during pregnancy, combined with regular rest with the legs raised, should prevent varicose veins developing but if you do get them see Varicose Veins in the Circulatory System on page 61 for advice.

THE THIRD TRIMESTER
The third trimester takes you from the twenty-ninth week of pregnancy to the birth. During this time your abdomen will be becoming very large as the baby puts on weight in preparation for the birth. Movements by the unborn child can be seen and felt from the outside by this stage. Many women begin to feel impatient to see and hold the child towards the end of pregnancy, and the last few weeks can seem like a very long time. The sheer extra weight that is being carried around by late pregnancy – as much as 11½–13½kg

(25–30lbs) – can make a woman feel very tired and in need of plenty of rest and sleep.

Small, irregular contractions will be felt across the uterus from the second half of pregnancy. These are called Braxton-Hicks contractions and are thought to prepare the uterus for labour.

Cramps in the legs are commonly experienced by pregnant women, particularly in the third trimester. It is thought the cramps are caused by metabolic changes that cause an imbalance of calcium and phosphorus. If you have had plenty of calcium in your diet throughout your pregnancy you are less likely to suffer with cramps. If you get a cramp, flex your foot upwards toward your knee, and rub the calf. If cramps do become a problem, try drinking a decoction of the herb CRAMP BARK once a day, or take the homoeopathic tissue salt MAG PHOS 6X one dose three times a day for ten days and repeat the course after a few days break, if necessary.

It is not uncommon to experience shortness of breath in the last trimester, as the uterus can put pressure on your lungs, and your diaphragm may be pushed up. If the problem is worse when you lie down, try propping yourself up with several pillows. The pressure of the uterus upwards can also cramp the stomach and cause indigestion; in this case, try eating small meals at more regular intervals.

Usually sometime between six and two weeks before the birth, the baby's head drops or 'engages' into your pelvis. This usually eases any pressure on the lungs or stomach and some women say that they feel lighter, although it can then feel as if there is large lump protruding between your legs. In mothers who have already had two or three children, engagement may not occur until labour starts, because the baby is not such a tight fit in a uterus that has already been stretched by childbirth. If a baby engages bottom down (breech), or any position other than head down, then ask an experienced midwife to suggest exercises to turn the baby, or to consider turning the baby by easing it round from the outside (external version).

Some water retention (oedema) is common in pregnant women, and often this will cause swollen ankles. Water retention can be reduced by cutting out salt from the diet. If oedema is associated with high blood pressure and protein in the urine, then a condition called pre-eclamptic toxaemia is developing. Mild pre-eclampsia in the last few weeks of pregnancy is common – around 25 per cent of all women get it; but pre-eclampsia that starts before thirty-six weeks, or that is severe, is very serious.

If the mother actually develops eclampsia and has fits, there is grave danger to both the mother and the baby. Some doctors advise all mothers with pre-eclampsia to agree to the baby's induction, but this should only be necessary for those women whose blood pressure is dangerously high. There is no evidence to suggest that diuretic drugs do relieve pre-eclampsia, although they are often prescribed; however, there is no harm in consulting a medical herbalist, acupuncturist, homoeopath, aromatherapist or other natural therapist of your choice who may be able to prevent a serious situation developing.

Generally there is no reason why you can't continue to enjoy a regular sexual relationship throughout pregnancy, and sensitive lovemaking can be a good way of continuing to develop a loving relationship between your partner and yourself and the child. Most women find that being pregnant does affect their libido, but this varies in different women from having no desire at all for sex to an increased sex drive and heightened sexual response.

Many women find intercourse difficult during the last weeks because they feel bulky and tired, and find it difficult to get into a comfortable position anyway. With a gentle and patient partner it is often possible to find a position that enables intercourse to be enjoyable, probably by the women being on top, or by both partners lying on their sides with the man entering from behind. If you don't feel like having intercourse it is better to express this; and try encouraging your partner to give you a massage and to stroke your abdomen if you both enjoy this.

Intercourse should not be attempted once the waters have broken, or for a few weeks after any bleeding, because it may increase the risk of an infection entering the uterus. If you are near term, or past the date when your baby is due, intercourse may help labour start, especially if it is combined with nipple stimulation.

The Reproductive System

It is the female reproductive system, more than any other sphere of bodily activity, that needs to be claimed back by the individual woman, away from the domain of male attitudes and invasive treatments. Attitudes and expectations about the processes of the woman's reproductive system have an enormous effect on the functioning of this system, and how these functions are experienced. The dominance of male attitudes over female processes has even led to certain natural functions being treated as illnesses or indispositions, as in the case of pregnancy and menstruation. It has become very difficult to have a positive attitude to certain natural and life-enriching experiences because of negative expectations around them. For example menstruation is treated as a 'curse' and 'proof' of a woman's changeability and unreliability.

The woman's sexual system connects her to the ever-changing rhythms of life. Just as everything in our universe is cyclic – the change from day to night, the yearly seasons, the cycle of life and death itself – so every aspect of a woman's reproductive system is cyclic: from the menstrual cycle itself to the cycle of pre-pubescent non-fertility through the fertile phase and on to post-menopausal non-fertility. The importance of staying in touch with these cycles, and hence in touch with the processes of life itself, cannot be overstressed. Forms of control that take a woman out of her natural cycles, such as the birth control pill, HRT and other forms of hormonal intervention, are removing her from her individual contact with the rhythms of life.

The woman's reproductive system is particularly susceptible to disease. The probable causes of this are partly psychological and partly physical. A woman's relationship with her creativity and her sexuality is tied up within this one system. In our male-dominated

The Reproductive System

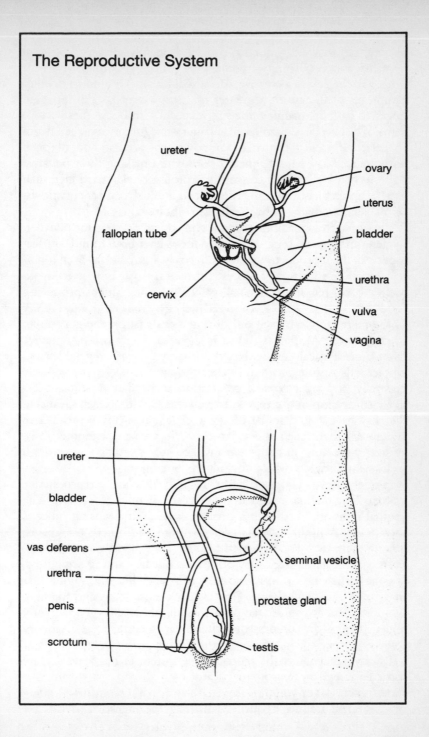

society, negative attitudes towards a woman's creative role and sexuality abound. Things are changing, but any woman who is at odds with herself as a creative and sexual being is bound to develop symptoms of disease to a greater or lesser extent, as tensions and negative patterns manifest themselves in her body. As these symptoms of disease develop and cause pain or irregularity, you can begin to feel less and less in control of your own processes, and out of touch with yourself as a naturally healthy woman. Breaking these negative patterns may well include consulting a professional practitioner, such as an acupuncturist who can redirect and unblock poor energy flows, or a skilled aromatherapist, herbalist or homoeopath.

Physical factors that influence the reproductive system include diet, hygiene and general lifestyle. Certain foods have been found to affect aspects of the reproductive system adversely. Caffeine has been found to contribute to fibroid and cyst formation, so it is wise to avoid coffee, coke, tea and other sources of caffeine. Mucus-producing foods such as dairy products and red meat generally reduce the ability of the uterus to clean itself out during menstruation and contribute to congestion. Alcohol is found to aggravate certain inflammatory complaints. Basically, a diet based primarily on fresh vegetables and wholefoods is going to reduce the amount of toxicity in the body generally, and symptoms of congestion and inflammation are less likely to develop in the reproductive system. A thorough cleansing diet has been found to be of great benefit in many reproductive system disorders, such as ovarian cysts, fibroids and endometriosis. A dietary therapist or naturopath will be able to guide you through a cleansing programme, or consult the one on page 395.

Hygiene is an important factor in the health of the reproductive system. The vagina is a delicately balanced mini-ecosystem. The vaginal walls are lined with a protective and self-cleansing mucous membrane. A healthy vagina contains numerous micro-organisms, among them lacto-bacilli, which help to create slightly acidic conditions that prevent infection by numerous disease-causing organisms. It is important not to introduce any substance into the vagina that may upset this pH balance. This includes most soaps and foaming bath products. If you use tampons they should be changed regularly and if there is any dryness or irritation it is better to use sanitary towels.

Lifestyle may affect the reproductive system in many ways. Any form of stress or tension may cause you discomfort during the menstrual cycle, or you may feel more aware of discomfort. Anxiety or emotional trauma frequently disrupts the menstrual cycle. An

128

irregular sleeping pattern or other life-cycle disturbance can also upset it. If the symptoms of discomfort or irregularity are prolonged it is advisable to consult a professional practitioner to find out the causes of the problem.

Birth Control

A method of birth control that truly enhances a woman's overall health and well-being is not always easy to find. It often requires conscious commitment and sustained effort to employ the methods that are known not to harm your health. The positive side to this is that those unharmful methods tend to encourage us to be more aware of our bodies and to discuss and share responsibilities in our relationships.

The most simple-to-use and unharmful methods of contraception that are effective are the barrier methods: the condom (sheath) and the diaphragm (cap). Both these methods are very effective if they are used carefully and properly. The condom must be rolled onto the man's penis before there is any contact between it and the woman's genital area, as some sperm may come out with the drops of liquid that are emitted by the penis well before ejaculation (orgasm) occurs. Either partner may put the condom onto the penis as part of foreplay. Care should be taken not to tear the condom when rolling it onto the penis. When the man withdraws, one partner should hold the condom in place so that it does not fall off until withdrawal is complete.

In recent years condoms have escalated in popularity because they offer significant protection against the transmission of venereal infections, including AIDS, in addition to their use as a contraception. Used properly, a good quality condom is 97 per cent effective as a method of contraception; in combination with a spermicidal jelly or cream, it offers close to 100 per cent protection. It may be advisable to use a condom in conjunction with a spermicide or diaphragm during the woman's fertile mid-cycle phase. Condoms are easily available in chemists and in many public lavatories, and they are free from Family Planning Clinics.

The diaphragm is made of soft rubber and is shaped like a shallow dome that fits snugly over the cervix. It needs to be the right size and shape for each woman, so it should be fitted by someone with experience, such as a doctor or nurse at your local Family Planning Clinic. It must always be used with a spermicidal cream or jelly to be effective, and must be inserted before there is any contact between the penis and the woman's genital area. If the diaphragm is used properly it is about 97 per cent effective, but if you are not very careful, its effectiveness drops to about 85–90 per cent. For extra protection, the man can wear a condom during his partner's fertile mid-cycle phase.

The disadvantages of the diaphragm and the condom are that you need to plan ahead or interrupt your lovemaking – which some people find off-putting. The added disadvantage of the diaphragm is that the spermicide is rather messy, and it can cause irritation in a small number of women. The disadvantage of the condom is that some men say that it reduces the penis's sensitivity during intercourse.

Both the condom and the diaphragm may be used in conjunction with another, totally unharmful method of contraception called 'natural birth control'. In fact, there are several ways of working out this method, but the aim of them all is to establish when the woman is ovulating, and to avoid intercourse at that time.

The most traditional form of natural birth control is that advocated by the Roman Catholic Church and known as the rhythm or calendar method. This is based on the fact that ovulation usually occurs about fourteen days before the start of the next period, so if a woman has a fairly regular cycle she can use the length of past menstrual cycles to calculate the probable time of ovulation. This method has quite a high failure rate because it cannot take individual cycle fluctuations into account. In recent years, far more accurate methods of working out the time of ovulation have been developed, including the basal temperature chart and the cervical mucus chart. There are several good books on the market explaining how these methods work and how to draw up a chart for yourself; one of the clearest books is *Natural Birth Control*, by Katia and Jonathan Drake (Thorsons).

In practice natural birth control methods mean that for just over half of the monthly cycle no extra contraceptive protection is needed; and for the rest of the time lovemaking which does not involve intercourse can be explored, or one of the barrier methods of contraception should be used. The success rate of natural birth control depends greatly on how carefully the cycle is worked out and followed, and the statistical success rate varies accordingly. It was found to be 98 per cent effective when the basal temperature chart method was carefully used, and around 90 per cent effective for women who stated that they intended to use this method to space the births of their children rather than to avoid pregnancy totally.

In contrast to the effective methods of birth control that are unharmful, there are those methods that are effective but carry a risk to the health of the woman using them. The intra-uterine device (IUD or coil) is a thin piece of bent plastic, metal or some other material, that is inserted into the uterus for months or years, to prevent pregnancy. It is not known exactly how the device works but it seems that it causes an inflammation of the endometrium (uterine lining), which probably prevents the fertilised egg from implanting itself in the lining.

An IUD must be fitted by a qualified nurse or doctor; it is effective against pregnancy immediately, although spontaneous expulsion from the uterus is not uncommon during the first few months after insertion. If the IUD remains in position, it is about 96 per cent effective in preventing pregnancy. For those women who do become pregnant with an IUD in place, the consequences are often serious: There is a 50 per cent chance of miscarriage. If a woman with an IUD does get pregnant it should be removed immediately to prevent infection.

There is also considerable risk of an ectopic pregnancy if you use an IUD (this is when the fertilised ovum implants itself in the fallopian tube instead of the uterus). Ectopic pregnancies are far more common amongst IUD users; they usually mean the loss of the affected fallopian tube and they can be life-threatening. Any woman who has an IUD and suspects that she may be pregnant should seek urgent medical advice.

Apart from pregnancy, the main complication of the IUD is a much higher incidence of pelvic infection. Such infections can be mild but if they are severe they can also become life-threatening. Any woman with signs of pelvic infection such as abdominal pain or tenderness, fever or an unusual discharge, should seek urgent medical attention.

An IUD should never be used by women who have previously had an ectopic pregnancy, pelvic inflammatory disease, gonorrhoea, fibroids, endometriosis, endometrial hyperplasia, heavy periods, heart disease or diabetes. In addition, young women who have had no children should not be fitted with an IUD because of the greatly increased risk of pelvic infection which often leads to sterility. Despite their disadvantages, about 50 million women throughout the world currently use an IUD, and for those who experience no complications it represents a reliable, convenient and reversible form of contraception.

The birth control pill (oral contraceptive) is a hormone preparation taken to prevent pregnancy that has been available since 1961. It was the first convenient method of contraception that offered nearly 100 per cent protection against pregnancy and it has been hailed as being responsible for the revolution in sexuality that has been occuring since its introduction. While the loosening up of old-fashioned and rigid attitudes to sex is arguably a good thing in many ways, unfortunately this has been at a cost to the health of a great many women.

The most common birth control pills combine the hormones oestrogen and progesterone, and are taken daily on a monthly cycle. The synthetic oestrogen released by the pill raises the woman's oestrogen levels enough to simulate pregnancy and checks the natural cyclic process that would normally result in an egg being released by the ovary. This means that during the time a woman is on the pill, her ovaries are relatively inactive and no egg is released to be fertilised by a sperm. The synthetic progesterone component of the pill provides two extra contraceptive criteria: it increases the viscosity of cervical mucus and alters the development of the uterine lining.

In theory the pill offers 99.5 per cent protection against pregnancy, but in practice it is more like 95 per cent. This is usually because women forget to take the pill for a day or the hormone content is lost before it can be absorbed because of vomiting or diarrhoea. The effects of the pill are supposed to be totally reversible: if a woman wants to become pregnant she simply stops taking the pills at the end of a packet. However, it is not uncommon to miss several periods when you stop taking the pill, and it can take several cycles before the ovaries function regularly again. The long-term incidence of infertility is higher for those women who have been on the pill, particularly for those women who have not had any children before taking it.

Much of the evidence about the risks and side-effects involved in taking the birth control pill appears to be contradictory, and sometimes it varies greatly according to the source of the information. Unfortunately, the medical profession does not receive ongoing training specifically in contraception, and most of the information that they do receive is given out by the drug companies that produce the pills, which can hardly be expected to be impartial. Some women feel that the Family Planning Association itself often plays down the risks involved in taking the pill, and this may be because they consider that their most important role is to advise women on how to avoid pregnancy, over and above any other factors.

The pill enters the bloodstream and travels around the body affecting many tissues, glands and organs as it goes – just as natural hormones do. It is not surprising then that the side-effects and complications of taking the pill are very varied. Some women experience side-effects, such as nausea, headaches and weight gain, immediately; others may not have any at all until a great deal of damage has already been done. The more serious side-effects are: an increased risk of blood clots, high blood pressure and other circulatory diseases, cervical cancer, thrush, depression, increased susceptibility to venereal infections, gall bladder disease, epilepsy and liver tumours. It seems that women on the pill suffer from viral infections more than others, so there is evidence that the pill generally undermines the immune system.

In addition to the physical side-effects, all hormones, whether they are natural or taken in artificial form, have an effect on emotional balance (just as they do during pregnancy or with premenstrual tension), so we are also manipulating our emotional well-being by taking the pill.

When you come off the pill it can be good to take some herbs to help the body re-adjust its hormonal balance. Some useful herbs to consider are: AGNUS CASTUS, BLACK COHOSH, BLUE COHOSH, FALSE UNICORN, SARSAPARILLA and WILD YAM. You can take a mixture of these herbs but look them up in the Materia Medica section to check dosage, and that they are particularly suitable for you.

Genital Herpes

Genital herpes is usually caused by the herpes simplex virus type II, although the herpes simplex virus type I that normally causes 'cold sores' around the mouth can also cause genital herpes. The symptoms of both types of virus are similar – the appearance of a group of small, painful, itchy blisters in the vaginal or anal area. The blisters are moist with red edges and when they burst they form a soft, acutely painful open sore. In addition to the local sores, there may also be the symptoms of feverishness, general malaise and swollen glands.

Genital herpes is one of the most common venereal diseases in Britain, particularly among women who contract it far more often than men. Most women feel extremely angry and depressed when they first discover that they have contracted the disease, but although

133

it is often a recurrent condition, the first attack is usually by far the worst, probably because no antibodies have built up in the body.

Untreated, the outbreak will usually clear up in two to three weeks. Individual outbreaks tend to be more likely during menstruation, pregnancy, emotional stress or when you are generally run down. Genital herpes can only be transmitted to someone else during an outbreak, so it is crucial to avoid sexual contact if there is any sign of a sore.

There appears to be a link between genital herpes and an increased risk of cervical cancer, so regular cervical smears are advised for herpes sufferers. Pregnancy is another complication for genital herpes sufferers. The baby is not normally affected before birth, but if the mother has a sore during labour the baby may become infected as he passes through the birth canal. The herpes virus can be dangerous for a baby, so if the mother has an attack at the time of the birth doctors normally advise her to have a caesarean section.

All the medical prescriptions used to treat herpes are toxic to some degree so natural remedies can be very helpful. Probably, the best approach is to use remedies locally during an outbreak to relieve the symptoms, and boost the immune system with appropriate internal remedies and a cleansing diet to lessen the likelihood and/or severity of recurrent attacks.

To boost the immune system and help fight infection drink a decoction of CLEAVERS, ECHINACEA and POKE ROOT (or take them as tinctures) three times a day for six weeks. Externally, dab on a strong dilution of the tinctures of GOLDEN SEAL, MARIGOLD and MYRRH. Essential oils may also be applied locally, try dabbing on either BERGAMOT, LAVENDER or TEA TREE. The main homoeopathic remedies to consider are NAT MUR and RHUS TOX; although best results will come from consulting a qualified homoeopath.

Infertility

When a woman finds out that she is not going to conceive easily it is often a devastating discovery. Most women assume that after a few months of unprotected intercourse the natural result is a pregnancy. When this does not happen, a woman often needs time for a profound and often prolonged reappraisal of her life's purpose and role as a woman.

A great deal of good can come out of such a reappraisal, whether or not the woman then goes on to have a baby. After all, to achieve a sense of fulfilment and satisfaction from one's own existence, without relying on one's children or the role of motherhood to provide it, is a very great achievement. This kind of self-reliance, however, is likely to be the very end result of learning to cope with a lot of disappointment, feelings of alienation and emotional realignment.

Some doctors state that infertility should be suspected after a couple have been having regular, unprotected intercourse for twelve months, although many others say that two years is a more realistic time-span. The age of the woman is a significant factor in terms of her fertility; in general, the older a woman is, the less fertile it is considered she will be. It seems that fertility usually declines throughout a woman's twenties, often to have an upsurge in her early thirties, and then declines more rapidly after the age of 35. With many women postponing starting a family until their late twenties or early thirties these days, infertility is becoming a common situation, affecting an estimated 15 per cent of couples.

Women over 30 who are anxious about not conceiving immediately, can feel a lot of extra pressure because of the sense that they are running out of time. In fact, although many doctors and clinics start running tests and offering treatment to women in this age-group after only a year of unprotected intercourse, in one large study of women over 30 who became pregnant, three-quarters of them had not been using contraceptives for two to three years.

The orthodox treatment of infertility has rapidly become a highly technological and specialised branch of medicine based on a great deal of research and experimentation. The success rates of the most technologically-advanced techniques for establishing pregnancy – those involving in vitro fertilisation (IVF) – are very poor (around 10–15 per cent). Unfortunately, the combination of many women's desperation to become pregnant and the prestige of genetic research within the field of science, has led to a burgeoning of commercial clinics and drug-company interest to find highly-technological solutions to infertility. In very many cases, it is not primarily the overall well-being of the individual woman concerned that is considered before these methods are employed. This is especially surprising when you consider that it will be her body and hormonal system that will be controlled and manipulated by the processes involved, with only a slim chance of the result that she desires.

There are many natural methods of improving the chances of conception. Timing intercourse to coincide with ovulation is very important. Ovulation usually occurs about fourteen days before the next menstrual period, so if your periods are fairly regular you can work out roughly which day of the cycle ovulation is likely. There are many books on the market on infertility or natural birth control that show how to draw up a fertility basal temperature chart, which can be used to determine on which day ovulation occurs, if you want to be more exact. If possible, it is ideal to make love on alternate days for the few days preceding and around ovulation. The temperature chart can also be used to establish whether or not you are ovulating and if not, then steps to stimulate ovulation should be considered.

The position you choose during lovemaking is also important to maximise the chances of conception. Generally, the best position is for the woman to be on her back, with her knees raised in the air, and for her partner to be on top, penetrating as deeply as is possible and comfortable for both of them. She should remain on her back, with her legs raised for half an hour afterwards. A pillow placed under the woman's hips either during or just after intercourse encourages the sperm to come into contact with the cervix. If the woman has an orgasm after the man, the uterus acts like a vacuum during the contractions of her orgasm, and actually sucks up the sperm into the fallopian tubes hundreds of times faster than they could swim there under their own steam.

Putting these suggestions into practice can make sex seem rather mechanical, but the important things are to be patient with your body and to remember that sex is a fun and sharing experience, just as it probably was before you started trying to get pregnant. If, after a year or more of trying these methods, you are still not conceiving it is time to consider visiting an infertility clinic to try and establish if there is anything preventing conception. If you are an established couple, it is important for both of you to attend the clinic from the outset, because the chances of a man having reduced fertility are about the same as for a woman. In about 40 per cent of cases infertility is attributed to the woman, and in about 40 per cent of cases it is attributed to the man; in the remaining 20 per cent of cases problems are found in both partners, or no cause is discovered at all.

The most common cause of infertility in men is a low sperm count. There may be several factors involved here. One of the main causes is an excess of alcohol: even two or three pints of beer a day is enough to affect a man's sperm. Obviously if a couple is trying to conceive it is advisable for both partners to drink small amounts of alcohol only occasionally. Another frequent cause of reduced fertility in men is that they wear underpants or trousers that are too tight: the testicles need to be a degree or two cooler than the rest of the body to be able to manufacture sperm efficiently, and if they are close up against the body they can become overheated.

Herbs that will increase the sperm count are: HE SHOU WU (FLEECEFLOWER ROOT) and SAW PALMETTO BERRIES. These may be combined with known aphrodisiacs, if appropriate, such as: DAMIANA, GINSENG and SAVOURY. Consult the Materia Medica for individual suitability and dosage. To treat the more serious causes of male infertility such as obstruction of the sperm ducts or endocrine problems, professional advice by a qualified therapist of natural medicine should be sought.

Treating infertility in a woman by natural means should involve both the treatment of any specific problem inhibiting conception, and maximising her general health. Improving her overall well-being will often increase her chances of conception because a generally toxic system reduces fertility.

A diet to improve fertility should include plenty of fresh fruit and vegetables, wholegrains and seeds to strengthen the conception vessel. If symptoms of toxicity are present (such as a dark, clotted menstrual flow, a tendency to colds and infections, constipation and so on) then a cleansing diet can be of great benefit: consult a dietary therapist or naturopath for guidance or turn to the one in this book on page 395. Foods containing chemicals and additives, excess salt, excess red meat and coffee should generally be avoided. Alcohol should be kept to a minimum, and smoking and the taking of any kind of drugs should be avoided. Sufficient Vitamin E is particularly important for the reproductive organs, so eat lots of wholegrain cereals such as brown rice, oats and wheatgerm. It can also be helpful to take wheatgerm oil capsules which are a naturally rich source of Vitamin E.

If there is a specific problem which is known to be inhibiting conception, such as endometriosis, blocked fallopian tubes, fibroids, an absence of ovulation, or polycystic ovaries, then careful treatment by a qualified practitioner of natural medicine should be sought so that it can be overcome. Most practitioners of alternative medicine have had patients who came to them because they were infertile, often after many tests and treatments, and then went on to conceive after a course of treatment by homoeopathy, acupuncture, aromatherapy, naturopathy or herbalism, to name a few. Obviously, this depends on the severity of the factors inhibiting fertility, but most practitioners have had some seemingly miraculous results.

If there is no known specific cause of infertility then consult the following remedies in the Materia Medica section of this book and try them out if they seem appropriate. The herb AGNUS CASTUS will promote fertility in cases where a hormonal imbalance is suspected. FALSE UNICORN ROOT helps to regulate the ovaries and strengthen the endometrium. HE SHOU WU, MOTHERWORT and WU WEI ZI are all good general tonics for the reproductive system. If a woman is suffering from stress either generally or because she is not conceiving, BALM, PASSIFLORA and SCULLCAP should also be considered.

The main essential oils that are traditionally used to treat infertility, are: GERANIUM, MELISSA and ROSE. These may be combined and diluted in a vegetable-oil base and massaged over the abdomen on a daily basis, or add a couple of drops of the most appropriate oil or combined oils to a warm bath on a regular basis. It should be said, however, that the best results will probably come from a regular massage by a trained aromatherapist, who can choose specific oils on an individual basis, and combine the aromatherapy treatment with dietary advice and stress counselling.

Menopause

The menopause is potentially one of the most exciting and challenging transitions in every woman's life. It can herald the shift from a focus on caring and nurturing others, to an emphasis on self-development and personal satisfaction. Normally, the child-bearing and rearing years are over; after the menopausal phase itself, the biological reminders of our reproductive capacity are also in the past. For many women it is truly a liberating experience not to have to cope with pre-menstrual changes, and menstruation itself, each month.

However, like all periods of transition, this time of change can throw up problems and symptoms that need to be dealt with before we can move on to the new phase in our lives. Just as puberty can be a time of stormy emotional upheavals as we make the transition from child to young woman, so menopause can throw up both emotional and physical symptoms as we adjust physically and emotionally from being someone who is probably younger looking and fertile, to being a more mature woman who is unable to bear children.

A woman's ability to adjust emotionally to life following the menopause will be greatly influenced by how much she values her life and role within society beyond being a mother. If she has identified herself only as a mother – in the valuable role of caring for and nurturing her children – and hasn't developed other abilities and interests sufficiently, then the menopause, which probably coincides with her children becoming independent, may seem to be a time when everything fulfilling in life disappears. Women who have managed to combine an interest in the world and society with their family life, can look forward to life beyond the menopause as a time of greater freedom when they pursue their personal wants and needs.

How you cope with the menopause physically is determined by the body's ability to ride the huge hormonal changes that are sweeping through the system at this time. As hormones strongly affect our moods this can have a marked knock-on effect on our emotional well-being as well. Some women go through the menopause with few or no inconvenient symptoms. Many experience symptoms to the extent that they recognise the need for some assistance in helping their bodies to make the adjustments, or they put up with the bothersome symptoms and discomforts until they subside. But for a number of other women, the symptoms are severe enough to considerably disrupt their lives and pose a serious threat to their health. These women need careful and professional treatment to help them through this time.

The menopause usually occurs between the ages of 45 and 53, but it can happen quite normally several years earlier or later than that. Menopause beginning before the age of 40 is considered to be premature and requires investigation to rule out any underlying disease. A sudden menopause will occur if both of a woman's ovaries are removed (oophorectomy).

The symptoms that herald the onset of the menopause are often changes in the menstrual cycle. A variety of menstrual changes may be experienced: periods may become lighter and/or less frequent, or periods may become heavier and/or more frequent. These irregularities are caused by the hormonal changes that are occuring. During menopause the pituitary gland signals to the ovaries to produce less oestrogen, ovulation also becomes less frequent and eventually menstruation tapers off. The menopause is usually complete when there has been no sign of menstruation for one year.

Although ovulation happens less frequently during the menopause, it is still possible to become pregnant. Birth control methods are necessary until you have not had a period for at least twelve months, to prevent an unwanted conception. There is a health risk involved in taking the birth control pill or using an IUD during the menopause, so it is advisable to use one of the safer, barrier methods, such as a diaphragm or condom.

Some irregularity of the menstrual cycle is common during menopause. But if you experience extremely heavy bleeding, periods that are more frequent than every twenty-one days, prolonged staining between the periods or bleeding after there have been no periods for twelve months, you should get a medical diagnosis to rule out serious disease.

Obviously, the fitter a woman is generally, the better equipped she is to deal with menopausal changes. However, if you are experiencing specific symptoms that are distressing, or severe, or persist despite following the suggestions that we outline here, then professional treatment with a qualified therapist is necessary. One basic but crucial factor that can ease the passage through this time is sufficient rest. Giving yourself permission to rest more while your body is accommodating these massive hormonal changes can make the world of difference to your well-being. Regular although preferably not excessive exercise, such as walking, cycling or swimming, will help your body to remain fit and supple.

Diet is another part of your lifestyle that can help considerably during this time. Some foods actually contain hormone-like substances that can help to cushion the adjustment of the menopause. These foods include: wholegrains, seeds, carrots, ripe bananas, apples, royal jelly and bee pollen. Foods to be avoided are: any containing chemicals, coffee and salt, and excessive alcohol.

We do not advise you to take synthetically-produced vitamins or minerals because an individual's response to and requirement of these potent supplements is very variable. However, there are some food supplements from natural sources that can be very beneficial during the menopause. WHEATGERM OIL CAPSULES provide a natural source of Vitamin E which helps to keep the reproductive organs healthy, and also helps to keep the skin supple. KELP TABLETS are a useful source of iodine and a range of other minerals that can help improve your general vitality and help to prevent weight gain and depression. ROYAL JELLY contains beneficial hormone-like substances and the Vitamin B complex, and can be taken as a tonic either in capsule form or preserved naturally in honey. The amount of Vitamin B complex in your diet may need to be increased to help combat stress and depression. Foods naturally rich in the Vitamin B complex are: fish, liver, free-range eggs, brown rice, wheatgerm, sesame seeds and brewer's yeast.

Herbal remedies can prove to be very useful in assisting the body through the menopause. A useful mixture of herbs to help balance the hormones and tone the reproductive system, contains: AGNUS CASTUS, BLACK COHOSH, FALSE UNICORN, OATS, ST JOHN'S WORT and WILD YAM. Make a decoction of the herbs and drink it twice a day for six weeks, or take as tinctures. Check all these suggestions in the Materia Medica section of this book to see that they are particularly suitable for yourself. If anxiety or depression is present with other menopausal symptoms then consider adding SCULLCAP and VERVAIN to the above mixture. Both acupuncture and homoeopathy have had excellent results in helping women to overcome problems associated with the menopause, but you really need constitutional treatment by a qualified practitioner to get the best results.

Essential oils can be a very pleasant way to ease menopausal symptoms. GERANIUM essential oil is said to be a hormonal balancer and should be used regularly, diluted in a vegetable-oil base as a massage oil or added to a warm bath. ROSE essential oil has useful tonifying and detoxifying effects on the reproductive system and will work well combined with GERANIUM. If you are particularly anxious or depressed then consider using CHAMOMILE or NEROLI by comparing them in the Materia Medica. If you are in doubt about which oils are the best to use, then consult an experienced aromatherapist who will give you a wonderfully soothing massage, as well as helpful advice about diet and lifestyle.

HOT FLUSHES

One very common symptom of the menopause is hot flushes. These can be bothersome but easily tolerated, or they can become frequent, severe and very distressing. Hot flushes are caused by the body's struggle to adjust to the hormonal changes occuring at this time. The flushes usually cease once the body has adjusted to its lower oestrogen levels, but they may persist for several years.

The process of a hot flush usually begins when the body gets overheated. It seems that the brain over-reacts to the fact that the body is warm and initiates a series of changes in the nervous system which cause the body to try to cool itself down. To do this the blood vessels near the surface of the skin dilate and blood pours through the vessels, bringing heat and redness to the skin. In this way, the heat radiates outwards, there is perspiration, and evaporation of the sweat cools the body down again. The experience feels like a sudden flush of heat, usually to the face, neck and chest, often followed immediately afterwards by perspiration, shivering and a chilled feeling.

The flushing process can occur even if a woman doesn't feel herself to be hot initially, but being overly warm, wearing tight clothing and emotional stress all tend to increase the likelihood of a hot flush coming on. Women who are prone to hot flushes often find it helpful to wear fairly loose-fitting clothes, preferably made from cotton, and to wear layers of clothes that may be discarded and then replaced after the flush. Alcohol, very hot drinks and spicy food can also trigger off the flushing process, and these are best avoided by anyone who finds hot flushes very uncomfortable or distressing. They can also occur at night. A woman usually wakes because she is feeling very hot or because the sheets are soaked from the subsequent sweating.

There are many natural remedies that are excellent for relieving any tendency to hot flushes. If the flushes are not very severe then the following suggestions may be of help; if the flushing is severe or has continued for many years, you should consult a qualified alternative medicine practitioner for proper treatment. A helpful herbal mixture to relieve hot flushes can be made from BLACKCURRANT LEAVES, HAWTHORN TOPS and SAGE; combine the herbs and make an infusion to drink three times a day for six weeks. This mixture may be even more beneficial if AGNUS CASTUS is added to balance the hormones. The essential oils of CLARY SAGE or CYPRESS may also be used to alleviate hot flushes; add three or four drops of either to a warm bath and repeat every other day for several weeks. Compare all these remedies in the Materia Medica section of this book to check that they are suitable for your individual case.

GENITAL CHANGES

The decline in oestrogen and other hormonal changes during the menopause begins to affect the rate of cell growth in all our tissues and body organs. This means that there is a gradual thinning in the tissue of the vulva and the vagina. As the labia gradually lose some of their fatty layers, the clitoris begins to become more prominent.

Lower oestrogen levels also mean that there is less protective natural lubrication on the vaginal tissue and this can mean that some women are more vulnerable to vaginal infection and irritation. For specific remedy suggestions refer to the entry on Vaginitis on page 150.

A woman's sex drive is not necessarily affected by the menopause and a healthy sex life can be enjoyed for many years afterwards. Indeed, many women enjoy sex even more after the menopause because they are free from the risk of getting pregnant. Genital

THE REPRODUCTIVE SYSTEM

changes may mean that physical sensitivity in that area slowly decreases, and lovemaking may need to become less vigorous to remain comfortable as the vaginal tissues become less elastic and less moist. But many women adjust to these changes while maintaining a pleasurable physical relationship with their partner. The use of a lubricating agent such as K-Y Jelly (available over the counter at any chemist shop), can help to make penetration easier and more comfortable if vaginal dryness does become a problem.

The orthodox treatment for irritation or recurrent infection resulting from vaginal atrophy (the name for the natural ageing process that affects the female genital area), is oestrogen creams. However, these are readily absorbed by the body and carry the possibility of serious side-effects, including an increased risk of cancer, and so we would not recommend this treatment.

HORMONE REPLACEMENT THERAPY (HRT)

A controversial orthodox treatment for menopausal symptoms is HRT (hormone replacement therapy). This treatment introduces synthetic hormones into the bloodstream to replace the oestrogen supplies that are waning naturally as part of the menopausal process. Sometimes the oestrogen comes from the urine of pregnant mares.

HRT comes in the form of creams, tablets or implants; all of which are absorbed into the bloodstream. While it does relieve certain menopausal symptoms, including hot flushes and vaginal atrophy, and it slows down osteoporosis (see page 96), it does not prevent cardiovascular disease, arthritis or depression. Moreover, it only postpones menopausal symptoms and they will reassert themselves whenever HRT is stopped. Indeed, it can be argued that the adjustments that are occurring during the menopause are taking place at the natural time for the woman concerned, and postponing them with HRT could upset the delicate hormonal balance and rhythm completely by overriding the body's natural processes.

Another argument against the use of HRT is that there are serious side-effects associated with it. There is evidence that the use of oestrogen increases the risk of serious cardiovascular disease, especially potentially fatal blood clots. HRT is also linked to an increased risk of cancer, particularly cancer of the breast and uterus. Gallstones are also much more common among women who take HRT.

Menstruation

AMENORRHOEA

Amenorrhoea, or the absence or cessation of menstrual periods at an age when regular menstruation is the norm, may have several causes. Many women will miss one or two periods during the fertile phase of their lives, perhaps during a time of emotional stress, and if periods then return to normality there is nothing to worry about. Obviously amenorrhoea is normal during pregnancy.

Primary amenorrhoea refers to the failure to begin menstruating by the age of 18. A physical examination should be carried out if a young woman has not begun to menstruate by this age to rule out the presence of a physical blockage or other obvious physiological reasons, preventing menstruation. If there is no physical blockage then constitutional treatment by a qualified practitioner of natural medicine should be considered to stimulate the sexual development and onset of menarche (the start of menstruation) of the young woman concerned.

Secondary amenorrhoea refers to when the menstrual periods disappear for more than three months after normal periods have been established, but before the onset of menopause. Missing periods during the several months following menarche is very common – it takes many young women months or even a couple of years to establish a regular cycle. This should be taken into account when secondary amenorrhoea is being considered, as should the possibility of pregnancy and the early onset of menopause. Other causes of secondary amenorrhoea include: damage to the pituitary following postpartum haemorrhage or shock; ovarian cysts; drugs; extreme weight loss; very vigorous physical activity and severe stress. Obviously, to successfully treat the amenorrhoea the cause or causes need to be established: any professionally-qualified practitioner should be able to diagnose the likely cause and suggest the appropriate treatment.

Occasionally you may miss a period because of a cold or a chill, in which case it may be brought on if you drink an infusion of PULSATILLA, ROSEMARY and YARROW. If periods are missed due to anorexia, weight loss or general debility, then nutritious herbs will help; try a mixture of ALFALFA, FENUGREEK and NETTLES. Compare all these remedies in the Materia Medica section of this book before you use them. If the symptoms persist for more than two months consult a qualified practitioner.

One other common cause of amenorrhea is as an after-effect of coming off the birth control pill. As well as contributing to heart disease, thrombosis, vaginal infections and weight gain, the pill suppresses the natural glandular activities of the normal menstrual cycle and this can be difficult to re-establish. The following mixture of herbs may be taken three times a day for six weeks to help recover the hormonal balance after coming off the pill, but be certain that you are not pregnant first: AGNUS CASTUS, BLACK COHOSH, BLUE COHOSH, FALSE UNICORN and SARSAPARILLA. A regular massage with the diluted essential oil of ROSE may also help to re-establish the hormonal balance. If regular periods do not come back despite these remedies, consult a qualified practitioner.

HEAVY MENSTRUATION

Heavy menstrual flow, also called menorrhagia, is normally defined by the use of more than eight sanitary towels or tampons a day. Some women tend to have heavier periods than other women normally, so it is a marked change in a woman's own pattern that is considered more significant than a general tendency in this direction.

There are a number of causes behind heavy menstrual periods, including: fibroids, polyps, pelvic inflammatory disease, cysts and thyroid disturbances. It is usually necessary to find out what the cause is before treatment is possible, so the best course of action is to get a medical diagnosis and then consult a qualified practitioner for constitutional treatment.

It is not uncommon for heavy periods to result from the hormonal upheavals of menopause. In this case, you could try taking herbal astringents for a month or two, and if that does not work consult a qualified practitioner. Herbal astringents that may be taken for the odd heavy period include: LADY'S MANTLE, PERIWINKLE and SHEPHERD'S PURSE. They work best if they are taken as an infusion, three times a day, for six to eight weeks. If your heavy periods persist, consult a qualified therapist. Essential oils that can help to normalise heavy periods include: CYPRESS, GERANIUM and ROSE. Add a few drops to a warm bath or dilute in vegetable oil and massage over the abdomen. All these remedies should be checked in the Materia Medica.

IRREGULAR MENSTRUATION

The average length of the menstrual cycle is twenty-eight days, but for many women it is several days shorter or longer than this. The length of cycle does not matter, within reason (that is between twenty-three days and forty-five days), but if the cycle is widely varying, with some very short and some very long breaks between periods, this can indicate a hormone imbalance. Other possible causes of irregular periods are stress, crash dieting, anaemia and uterine growths (both benign and malignant). Obviously, the cause should be established before treatment can begin.

It is not uncommon for periods to be irregular at the beginning and the end of a woman's fertile life, during the first couple of years of menstruating and during menopause – times of great hormonal upheaval. A useful herb that you can take during these times, and that acts as a hormonal balancer, is AGNUS CASTUS. This may be taken three times a day for several weeks and may be combined with FALSE UNICORN ROOT, another hormonally toning and equalising herb. An essential oil that has the ability to regulate hormones is ROSE. This may be used regularly in a warm bath or diluted in vegetable oil for a massage. All of these remedies should be looked up in the Materia Medica section of this book before use.

PAINFUL MENSTRUATION
A lot of women experience some discomfort during their periods at one time in their lives. If discomfort becomes real pain, and especially if that pain is experienced month after month, it is an indication that there is some definite imbalance that should be dealt with. It really is not necessary to have painful periods on a regular basis because there is so much that natural remedies can do to help – both at the time of the period and to treat the causes of the pain.

If the cause of the painful periods (also called dysmenorrhoea) is due to some specific condition or disorder, such as endometriosis, fibroids or pelvic inflammatory disease, then constitutional treatment of the condition is necessary to clear that cause. Acupuncture, naturopathy, herbal medicine and homoeopathy can be excellent for treating these conditions, so consult a qualified practitioner. If painful periods are the result of having an IUD (intra-uterine device or coil) fitted then the only cure may be to have it removed.

Repeatedly painful periods will occur if there is a lot of toxicity and congestion in the system as a whole. Many women find that their periods are less painful after a good cleansing diet; consult a naturopath or dietary therapist to assist you through a cleansing regime or use the one on page 395. A diet that is full of fresh fruit, vegetables and whole cereals, and low in all meat, dairy products, sugar and processed foods, will generally help to reduce the toxic burden on the uterus during its cleansing process. Caffeine tends to aggravate any muscle tension and increase sensitivity to pain, so it is best to avoid coffee, chocolate and cola drinks if you suffer from menstrual pain.

Women who are not very physically active do seem to suffer more than those who take regular exercise – so assist the flow of circulation and muscle tone with regular swimming, cycling or walking. Gentle exercise can also help to get the circulation moving and relax the muscles during your period: one of the best exercises is to lie flat on your back, bring your knees towards your chin and hold them there for a few minutes before lowering them again; repeat this several times.

There are lots of natural remedies to help with menstrual pain, and we suggest several here, but if the pains return each month do consider consulting a practitioner to work at really improving your experience of your menstrual cycle and the quality of your life.

Herbs to take during the month to tone the uterus are: BLACK COHOSH, CRAMP BARK, FALSE UNICORN ROOT, RASPBERRY LEAF and WHITE DEADNETTLE. Make an infusion of these to drink three times a day for two cycles, or take them as tinctures. Herbs to relieve the cramps during the period include: BLACK HAW, CHAMOMILE, CRAMP BARK and VALERIAN. Make an infusion to drink three times a day when needed. All these remedies should be looked up in the Materia Medica section to check if they are suitable for you. The homoeopathic remedy MAG PHOS will help to relieve the cramping pains: dissolve a couple of the 6X potency in a little warm water and sip it at regular intervals. Other homoeopathic remedies that may be considered to relieve painful periods are: APIS, BELLADONNA, CHAMOMILLA and NUX VOMICA.

Using essential oils can be a particularly pleasant way of relieving menstrual pains. You can add a few drops to a warm bath, or dilute one or two of the essential oils in a vegetable-oil base and gently massage the abdomen. Choose from the following essential oils by comparing them in the Materia Medica: CHAMOMILE, LAVENDER, MARJORAM, MELISSA and ROSEMARY.

Pre-Menstrual Tension (PMT)

Pre-menstrual tension, also called congestive dysmenorrhoea, occurs as a result of the hormonal changes that take place between ovulation and the next menstrual period. The pre-menstrual symptoms most women commonly experience include: bloatedness, nausea, headaches, swollen breasts, spots, fatigue and irritability. Many of these symptoms are a result of the increase in water retention in the body's tissues that occurs at this time, because of the higher levels of oestrogen and aldosterone hormones.

An individual woman's response to these hormonal changes will vary according to her physical and emotional health; and so the impact of pre-menstrual tension will also vary. Women who suffer distressing emotional symptoms before their periods should take this as an opportunity not to suppress these feelings and to reassess their well-being as a woman in our stress-filled society, perhaps with the help of a professional counsellor or therapist.

There are many natural remedies that can alleviate the symptoms of pre-menstrual tension but if the condition persists after a couple of months of trying them, we suggest that you consult a professional practitioner of natural medicine. All the remedies that we suggest should be cross-checked in the Materia Medica section of this book to assess how suitable they are for you.

EVENING PRIMROSE OIL has helped many women with their pre-menstrual symptoms, particularly those who suffer with swollen and tender breasts. We suggest that you take 500mg a day for two months and then just for the ten days preceding each period. Vitamin B6 is also helpful for some women, this may be taken in conjunction with EVENING PRIMROSE OIL.

The herbs AGNUS CASTUS and FALSE UNICORN have a balancing effect on the hormones; these may be combined and infused (or taken as tinctures) three times a day for two or three months. Other herbs to use if there are symptoms of stress and anxiety present, are: MOTHERWORT, OATS, PASSIFLORA and VERVAIN. If your water retention is marked and you feel bloated then make an infusion of COUCHGRASS and DANDELION to drink three times a day during the pre-menstrual phase.

The essential oils of GERANIUM and ROSEMARY can greatly relieve the physical symptoms of pre-menstrual tension including the bloating and water retention. If you feel particularly irritable and depressed then consider CLARY SAGE, NEROLI and ROSE. These essential oils may be diluted in a suitable vegetable-oil base and massaged in, or add a couple of drops of the oil of your choice to a warm bath when required. A course of lymphatic drainage massages by an experienced aromatherapist may be particularly good for pre-menstrual tension (see page 90).

In general, a poor diet can contribute to these symptoms by adding to congestion in the body and lowering your overall vitality. Women suffering from pre-menstrual tension should avoid food additives, caffeine (coffee, coke and so on), refined foods, salt, smoked foods and alcohol.

Thrush

Thrush is caused by a yeast-like fungus called *Candida albicans*. This organism normally resides in the vagina of most women and does not produce symptoms unless it multiplies more than normal. Factors likely to result in the Candida organisms multiplying are taking the birth control pill, pregnancy and following a course of antibiotics. Many women find also that making love after a period of abstinence can trigger off an attack of thrush if they are prone to it. The symptoms of the infection are vaginal itching and a thick, white discharge.

A one-off attack of thrush is usually quite easily dealt with by using natural remedies. However, the problem can keep recurring and this will require constitutional treatment by a professional therapist. Women who suffer persistently with thrush symptoms may need to follow an anti-Candida diet which means avoiding all sugars and yeast: things which the organism tends to thrive on. For advice on such a diet consult a naturopath or dietary therapist.

If you are sexually active with a male partner it is advisable for him to wear a condom during intercourse when you have thrush symptoms. The organism can live under the foreskin of the penis and be passed backwards and forwards between partners during intercourse.

An easy home remedy that has been found by many to relieve a bout of thrush is natural yoghurt. Eat plenty, and also apply it to the vaginal area either by dabbing it on and then using a sanitary towel to prevent too much mess, or with a vaginal applicator which can be bought in any major chemist.

To treat thrush with herbs it is advisable to take them internally to boost the immune system, and use them externally to relieve discomfort and clear the infection. Drink an infusion or take the tinctures three times a day for up to six weeks, of: ECHINACEA, LADIES' MANTLE, MARIGOLD and WHITE DEADNETTLE. For external use make an infusion, to use as a douche or for bathing the area with cotton wool, consisting of: GOLDEN SEAL, LAVENDER and MARIGOLD.

Essential oils may also be used as a douche, but make sure they are well-diluted or they may irritate the delicate mucous membranes. Add four drops of LAVENDER or MYRRH essential oil and two drops of TEA TREE essential oil to one litre of boiled warm water for a douche. For a mild attack of thrush, just adding ten drops of LAVENDER essential oil to a warm bath once a day can bring great relief. It is also worth comparing the homoeopathic tissue salts of KALI MUR and NATRUM MUR to see if either of these seems appropriate, in which case take a course of one three times a day for ten days. The homoeopathic remedy PULSATILLA can also be well indicated.

Vaginitis

Vaginitis is the term applied to vaginal irritation and inflammation; these symptoms may be found in association with a vaginal infection. The symptoms of a vaginal infection are an unusual discharge, an unpleasant smell from the genital area, a sensation of dryness, and itching and/or burning of the vulva. All women secrete mucus and moisture from the vagina, it is only if this changes, becomes smelly, blood-streaked or irritating that it should be considered abnormal or unhealthy. Similarly, many useful bacteria live in the vagina of all women, and it is only if these multiply too rapidly, or other harmful bacteria are introduced, that the symptoms of an infection will develop.

There are many possible causes of vaginal irritation: using a diaphragm, an IUD string, spermicidal creams, tampons, deodorant sprays, bubble baths, douching or vigorous sexual intercourse can all cause inflammation and lead to an infection developing. Your resistance to infection can be undermined by stress, certain drugs or general ill health. Women who have passed the menopause or who have had their ovaries removed experience vaginitis more frequently because of the reduced supply of hormones needed to maintain healthy vaginal tissues.

There are certain venereal diseases, such as gonorrhoea or chlamydia, that can cause vaginitis symptoms, and if they are left untreated they may cause long-term problems. If you suspect that your symptoms may have been sexually transmitted, it is advisable to visit your local VD clinic to have a test (see pages 151–2 for more information).

There are several preventative measures that are helpful if you are prone to vaginitis: wash regularly and gently pat yourself dry; wear only cotton underwear and avoid clothes that fit closely against the crotch; avoid strongly-scented soaps and bubble baths; avoid all vaginal sprays and 'deodorant' tampons; and always wipe from front to back after bowel movements.

We recommend several natural remedies here to treat vaginitis, however, if the symptoms are very uncomfortable or persist for more than a few weeks, you should seek professional advice. Externally, herbs may be used as washes or douches. Try a mixture of COMFREY, GOLDEN SEAL, LAVENDER, MARIGOLD and WHITE DEADNETTLE infused, and apply when cool. Internally, herbs can also be helpful to reduce inflammation and fight infection, try a decoction of: BLUE FLAG, ECHINACEA, PERIWINKLE, ST JOHN'S WORT and WHITE DEADNETTLE. Drink this three times a day for up to six weeks. Many women have found that a whole clove of GARLIC, peeled without knicking the surface with your fingernail or knife, dipped in olive oil and then inserted into the vagina overnight, can help to clear the early signs of an infection.

Homoeopathically, there are three main remedies to choose from, if none of these seems appropriate, or if you have tried one and it hasn't worked, seek professional guidance. KREOSOTUM is the main remedy for vaginitis that has an irritating or corrosive discharge and a feeling of rawness in the vaginal area. PULSATILLA can be helpful where there is a thick, white or creamy-yellow discharge that is either bland or causes itching. SEPIA will be indicated when the discharge is yellow or greenish and has an offensive smell, and particularly when there is also an uncomfortable, heavy feeling in the lower abdomen. Try taking either the 6th homoeopathic potency once three times a day for ten days, or just two doses of the 30th potency eight hours apart. All these remedies should be looked up in the Materia Medica section of this book to check that they are generally well indicated.

A few drops of the essential oils of CHAMOMILE or LAVENDER in a warm bath can be very soothing for the symptoms of itching and irritation. If there are symptoms of infection present then SANDALWOOD, TEA TREE and THYME should also be considered (look them up in the Materia Medica to see which is most appropriate). These may be used as a douche but make sure they are well diluted (two or three drops of essential oil dissolved in a teaspoon of vodka and diluted in one litre of water).

Venereal Infections

It is a legal requirement in Britain to have the main venereal infections (syphilis and gonorrhoea) treated by the orthodox medical profession. VD clinics tend to be better equipped to deal with these infections than your doctor, but both should be able to do tests and prescribe the appropriate treatment. Ask at your local health centre or look under Venereal Diseases in the telephone directory to find your nearest VD clinic.

Suspicious signs of a venereal infection include an unusual discharge, soreness, redness, sores, itchiness or a foul smell in the genital area. There are many different infections that can be sexually transmitted, and a test will be necessary to establish which are present. Many women feel acutely embarrassed and humiliated when they suspect they may have contracted a venereal infection, but it is very important to have any infection treated as quickly as possible to prevent complications developing. Do get any suspicious symptoms checked as soon as they arise. Both syphilis and gonorrhoea can cause permanent damage, including sterility and heart disease, so it is particularly crucial to have these treated if there is any possibility that you may have one of them. The standard treatment for these diseases is high doses of antibiotics.

There are ways of reducing the risk of contracting a venereal disease. The most direct way is to sleep only with people that you already know and who you can ask in advance whether they have any infection. Failing that, condoms for both vaginal and anal intercourse greatly reduce the risk of contracting a venereal infection (and also of contracting AIDS, of course). The use of spermicidal cream, film, foam or jelly also reduces the risk, preferably with a diaphragm for added protection. No method is 100 per cent effective – if you do suspect that you have an infection, avoid sex until you have a test, and until the disease is cleared.

It is not uncommon for some symptoms to remain, for example dryness and a slight discharge, even when tests show that the disease had been cleared by antibiotics; this is particularly true of non-specific urethritis (NSU). In this case, constitutional treatment by a qualified practitioner of natural medicine can often clear the symptoms and get you back to feeling healthy again.

The Respiratory System

The function of the respiratory system is to take air into the lungs; it allows the absorption of oxygen into the blood, and the excretion of carbon dioxide from the blood into the alveoli and out through the nose and mouth. The respiratory tract can be divided into the upper and lower parts. The upper respiratory tract includes the nose, nasal cavity and pharynx and larynx; the lower respiratory tract includes the trachea, two bronchi, two lungs and pleura.

Our breath connects us to the earth's atmosphere, and symbolically as well as practically to the trees and forests, which have been called 'the lungs of the earth' because of their oxygen creating capacity. As well as concentrating on healing a specific respiratory complaint, it is worthwhile considering our relationship to the air we breathe, and by its extension as the 'breath of life', to our enthusiasm for and positive attitude to life itself. There is nothing more likely to prolong a respiratory complaint than a negative and pessimistic attitude to life.

Air pollution is a problem that needs to be dealt with directly and urgently. There are two sides to the problem: what we are putting into the atmosphere, and the decimation of rain forests that purify it. While those of us who are in good health are able to cope with a certain level of air pollution, at least in the short term, those of us who are very young or elderly or already suffer from a respiratory complaint such as asthma, are at great risk from the increasing levels of air pollution. Smoking cigarettes does not only pollute your own lungs, it also pollutes the air of those around you to dangerous levels.

The Respiratory System

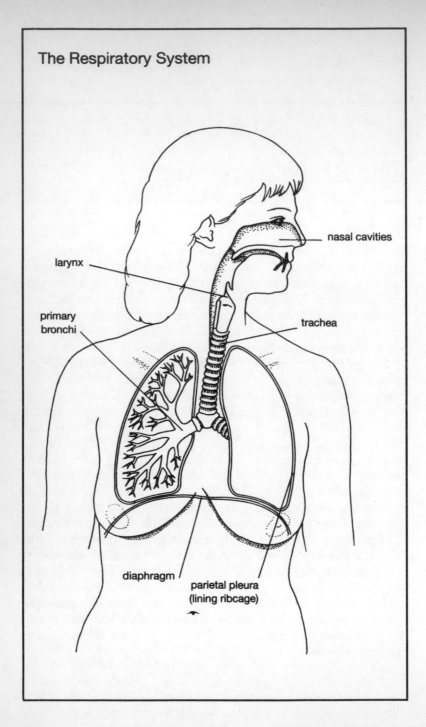

nasal cavities

larynx

primary bronchi

trachea

diaphragm

parietal pleura (lining ribcage)

Asthma

Asthma is a disease of the respiratory system which makes it difficult to breathe out, and is caused by the spasm of the smaller air passages in the lung. The spasm makes it difficult to cough away mucus which collects in the small bronchi, which impedes the breathing further.

There is often a hereditary factor to asthma and attacks can be triggered by allergies, chest infections, stress and anxiety in different people. Like other allergic diseases, asthma seems to be very much on the increase in recent years, particularly amongst children. A diet eliminating all mucus-stimulating foods (particularly dairy products) may be of help.

Conventional treatment for asthma includes the use of drugs which dilate the air passages of the lungs (bronchodilators), usually given in the form of inhalers, such as salbutamol (Ventolin). Steroid inhalations may be given to relieve the congestion of the bronchial lining; these are also usually given in the form of inhalers such as beclamethasone (Becatide). The medicines are usually given to children as a syrup. For very severe asthma attacks corticosteroids, for example Prednisolone, may be given for a limited period of time. Increasingly, it is recommended that asthma sufferers should use their medication continually, instead of just during an acute attack, as a means of preventing them from coming on.

The main drawback with the conventional treatment of asthma is that it aims to 'control' the disease, or to relieve an acute attack, but not to cure the illness. It is for this reason that many sufferers and parents of children with asthma turn to alternative medicine for help.

The treatment of chronic or recurrent asthma is a difficult, complicated problem and should be handled by an experienced practitioner. Constitutional treatment by an alternative therapy can be very rewarding and a cure is possible, depending on the severity of the case and the amount of medication that has been used in the past. The switchover from orthodox inhalers and medication should not be attempted unless it is under the supervision of a suitably qualified practitioner.

Herbs that may help during a mild attack include COLTSFOOT, ELECAMPANE, GRINDELIA, HYSSOP, MULLEIN and WILD CHERRY BARK. If there is stress and anxiety then MOTHERWORT and SCULLCAP should also be considered. TURMERIC has a bronchodilatory effect, and a teaspoonful stirred into a glass of warm water may be sipped at frequent intervals to help relieve an attack. The most commonly indicated homoeopathic remedies for an asthma attack are ARSENICUM, IPECAC and NATRUM SULPH. MAG PHOS may be given as a tissue salt to relieve the spasm of an acute episode. Steam inhalations with essential oils can also be of benefit, try: CHAMOMILE, EUCALYPTUS and LAVENDER. The Healing Herbs of Dr Bach RESCUE REMEDY can be taken at frequent intervals to relieve anxiety and panic during an attack.

The general management of an asthma attack should involve rest, preferably propped up in bed, and plenty of liquids to prevent dehydration from increased perspiration.

Colds

The essential feature of a cold is an inflammation of the nasal passages, known as rhinitis, which produces a running nose and sneezing. Watering eyes are also common, and the inflammation often spreads to the pharynx to cause a sore throat. The occasional cold is best looked at as an opportunity for the body to have a good clear out and, most importantly, a good rest. But frequently recurring colds are a sign that your resistance is very low, and that your diet and lifestyle are probably out of balance in some way.

When you have a cold it's sensible to make sure that you are getting enough Vitamin C. Eat more fresh fruit and vegetables and avoid mucus-stimulating foods such as dairy produce and concentrated orange juice. GARLIC capsules, or eating plenty of fresh garlic, will assist the body to fight the infection; it can also help to relieve problems with catarrh.

Take regular baths with a few drops of GINGER essential oil in the water at the beginning of winter – it is said to increase the body's resistance to cold viruses. The essential oils of EUCALYPTUS, PEPPERMINT, ROSEMARY, TEA TREE and THYME will all help to fight the infection and reduce congestion. They will also help to relieve the catarrh that can often follow on from a cold. It is particularly useful to use essential oils as a steam inhalation for congestion, but they may also be diluted in vegetable oil and massaged onto the chest.

For an acute cold the most frequently used homoeopathic remedies are: ACONITE, ALLIUM CEPA, EUPHRASIA, FERRUM PHOS, NATRUM MUR and

PULSATILLA. If catarrh is persistent then KALI MUR or KALI SULPH can also be helpful.

Our favourite herbal mixture for colds is ELDERFLOWER, PEPPERMINT and YARROW. A course of ECHINACEA will help make those of us prone to recurrent colds more resistant to them.

Coughs

The air passages of the lungs are lined with cells secreting mucus, which normally traps particles of dust. When the membranes are infected and inflamed, the secretion of mucus increases and the lining of the air passages is irritated; coughing is the reflex action by which excess mucus is driven out.

A cough may be due to a temporary external cause (for example, fumes), an allergy (such as asthma), an infection (bronchitis) or a chronic complaint (emphysema). These remedies will help to treat a mild cough, such as that following on from a cold or mild bronchitis; a more serious infection or a chronic complaint should be treated by a suitably qualified practitioner.

General care for a cough includes avoiding mucus-stimulating foods such as dairy produce, and increasing the intake of foods and drinks which are rich in Vitamin C. A soothing drink like hot lemon and honey can be very helpful.

For an unproductive, irritating cough the herbs to try are: ANISEED, COLTSFOOT, MARSHMALLOW, MULLEIN and WILD CHERRY BARK. For a more productive cough useful herbal expectorants include: BALM OF GILEAD, ELECAMPANE, LIQUORICE and WHITE HOREHOUND. If there are signs of an infection, as with bronchitis, then you should also use anti-microbials such as: GOLDEN SEAL, PLANTAIN and THYME. In this case take GARLIC capsules as well.

The best way to treat a cough with essential oils is by steam inhalation. EUCALYPTUS is particularly useful because it combines expectorant and anti-microbial properties. Other useful expectorant oils include: BENZOIN, FENNEL, HYSSOP and SANDALWOOD. THYME is good where there are signs of infection.

The most commonly indicated homeopathic remedies include: ACONITE, ANT TART, BELLADONNA, BRYONIA, CAUSTICUM, IPECAC, PHOSPHORUS, PULSATILLA and SULPHUR. The tissue salt CALC PHOS is useful during the convalescent period after a cough.

Hayfever

Hayfever seems to be becoming more common along with other allergic disorders, particularly amongst children. It is characterised by the irritation of the mucous membranes of the eyes, nose and air passages. This is caused by the pollen of various grasses and plants, so it is a seasonal allergy. Most cases of hayfever occur in spring and summer, when the antigen is grass pollen, but some occur in autumn when the pollen of ragweeds is usually the cause.

Conventional treatment consists of desensitisation injections which usually only last for one season, or antihistamine tablets or nasal sprays, which may temporarily relieve the symptoms. But these often cause side-effects, such as drowsiness, and also tend to deepen the imbalance in the natural defence system.

It is wise to eliminate all mucus-stimulating foods from the diet during the hayfever season, particularly dairy produce. You should also avoid sugar as this seems to impair the effectiveness of the immune system. Foods and drinks that are rich in Vitamin C are helpful.

Constitutional treatment from a qualified practitioner is probably necessary to cure hayfever, but the following suggestions will relieve the symptoms. EYEBRIGHT is a particularly useful herb to use as a soothing eyewash or to drink internally. Other herbs to take internally for hayfever include: GOLDEN SEAL, ELDERFLOWER, HYSSOP and MULLEIN. The essential oils that will be of help are: CHAMOMILE, EUCALYPTUS and LAVENDER; the vapours may be inhaled from a few drops placed on a handkerchief. The main homoeopathic remedies to choose from include: ALLIUM CEPA, ARSENICUM, EUPHRASIA, NUX VOMICA and SABADILLA.

Sinusitis

The sinuses are air spaces in the bones above the eyes and around the nose. Inflammation of the mucous membrane lining these cavities is called sinusitis. The symptoms of inflammation and infection in the sinuses are throbbing pains and tenderness over the area, and if the lower sinuses are involved, the teeth may also hurt. There is often an increase in mucus secretion which makes you feel stuffy and 'full'.

Home care will usually help a mild attack of sinusitis. But if the pain is severe or if you have a generalised fever you should go to a qualified practitioner. Home care should include rest, drinking plenty of liquids and avoiding mucus-stimulating foods like dairy products. GARLIC capsules or fresh garlic help fight any infection and relieve the build up of catarrh.

The main homoeopathic remedies to consider are BELLADONNA, BRYONIA, HEPAR SULPH, KALI BICH, and SILICA. Herbally, it is best to have a mixture that includes some herbs to fight the infection, such as ECHINACEA and GOLDEN SEAL, anti-catarrhals, such as ELDERFLOWER, EYEBRIGHT, GOLDEN ROD and PEPPERMINT, and an anti-inflammatory such as MARSHMALLOW.

Steam inhalations with essential oils can be very helpful in the treatment of sinusitis. The most useful oils are EUCALYPTUS, PINE and THYME.

Sore Throats

This section includes pharyngitis, laryngitis and tonsillitis. Pharyngitis and laryngitis generally appear with the common cold virus, and infections affecting the throat can frequently recur in some people. As well as a slight feverishness, you may feel a general malaise and other cold symptoms with a sore throat, and have a hoarse, husky voice. If the fever is very high, or if the sore throat is very severe, then you should get professional medical advice. Laryngitis symptoms which last for a long time should also be professionally assessed.

Tonsillitis is another common type of sore throat, and often the bacteria Streptococcus is present. In this case, you are usually struck by a sudden fever, sore throat and difficulty in swallowing; the throat often feels very dry. A mild case of tonsillitis will clear up with home treatment. However, with young children, or if any of the symptoms mentioned are very severe, urgent professional advice should be sought.

Steam inhalations with essential oils are a useful anti-inflammatory and antiseptic method of treating sore throats. Amongst the most effective oils, you should try BENZOIN, LAVENDER, SANDALWOOD or THYME. The homoeopathic remedies of FERRUM PHOS or ACONITE are good for the first stages of a sore throat. Other homoeopathic

159

remedies that may be useful are: BELLADONNA, HEPAR SULPH, MERC SOL and PHYTOLACCA. One of the best herbs to use is RED SAGE; this may be taken as a gargle or as an infusion to drink several times a day while the symptoms last.

The Skin

Our skin helps to define us as individuals. As well as providing us with a primary physical boundary, it allows for tremendous individual variation in terms of texture, colour, smell, temperature and sensitivity.

The skin is both protective and semi-permeable. It acts as an interface between the interior and the exterior world, and it has the dual ability of absorbing some things and excreting others. We should be very careful about what we put onto the skin because it readily absorbs substances which then pass into the bloodstream to be transported around the whole body. Similarly, we should help our skin in its excretory function by keeping it clean, allowing it to 'breathe' by wearing natural fibres, and by not using substances such as anti-perspirants which hamper its efforts.

An enormous amount of money and effort goes into creating and advertising beauty products for the skin and hair each year. This is not really surprising because the skin is the part of us that we present to the outside world, and our society places great importance on external appearances. Even healthy skin is judged as beautiful or not according to the dictates of culture, fashion and taste. If we have a skin problem it can be very difficult not to feel self-conscious about it, and not to let it affect our general confidence. Coping with a skin disease without suppressing it with strong medication is a real challenge for many people switching to natural medicine.

The actual causes of skin disease can be very difficult to unravel. They are often a complex combination of diet, environment, general health, hereditary factors, stress and individual susceptibility. The length of time it takes to cure a skin disease will largely depend on how long medicated ointments or drugs have been used to suppress the condition in the past, and the state of health of your other bodily organs. The remedies that we suggest here will improve most skin conditions, but for deep-seated skin diseases finding a real cure can take time, and it may only be possible by working at it for several years with the help of a professional therapist.

Generally, maintaining healthy skin and hair starts with a good diet. This means a varied diet with plenty of fresh fruit and vegetables, and based on whole grains. Avoid too much fatty, greasy or refined foods, and additives. Drink plenty of pure spring water to help to keep the skin clear. Too much alcohol and smoking has an extremely detrimental effect on the skin.

Clean, fresh air is a must for healthy skin, and this can be a real problem for anyone living in a city or by a busy road. Regular cleansing is very important to clear the pores of city grime. Apply a good plant-based moisturiser regularly to help to protect and nourish the skin.

Acne

Acne is a skin complaint that is characterised by blackheads and pustules that are usually found on the face and back. This problem is most commonly associated with adolescence, and is linked with a hormonally-induced hyperactivity of the oil-producing glands.

There is a dietary factor in acne that is related to how well the body can metabolise fats and carbohydrates. The condition can often be helped considerably if you cut out fats, sweets and refined carbohydrates from what you eat, and eat more fresh fruits and vegetables.

A combination of alterative and anti-microbial herbs can be helpful to clear acne. Try drinking a decoction of the following herbs three times a day for several weeks: BLUE FLAG, BURDOCK ROOT, CLEAVERS, ECHINACEA and YELLOW DOCK. Or look up the following remedies in the Materia Medica section to see if one of them looks appropriate: CALC SULPH, SILICA and SULPHUR.

Skin cleansing is an important aspect of the treatment of acne, and regular facial steams are a good way of healing the skin and cleansing the pores without adding more grease to the skin. Make a facial steam with the herbs CHICKWEED, ELDERFLOWER and MARIGOLD. Alternatively, add a few drops of one of the following essential oils to hot water for a facial steam: BERGAMOT, CHAMOMILE, LAVENDER or LEMON GRASS. These essential oils may also be well-diluted in a vegetable-oil base to massage into the skin.

Once the acne has cleared up, massage COMFREY OINTMENT into the old sites of the spots to help to reduce any scarring.

Boils

A boil is an infection of a sweat gland or hair follicle of the skin. They are most often found where clothes rub the skin – on the back of the neck, in the armpits or on the buttocks. Crops of boils may appear simultaneously or a succession of single boils may follow one another. They are more common among those people who suffer with diabetes.

A boil normally starts as a painful red lump, this grows bigger and then breaks down in the middle for pus to collect. It is important not to squeeze a boil, or interfere with it other than to apply a compress or dressing, and keep the surrounding skin clean.

Boils usually indicate that you have a toxic condition. If you keep getting them you should consider a cleansing diet (try the one on page 395), and particularly eating more fresh fruit and vegetables. Add plenty of GARLIC to your diet or take GARLIC CAPSULES to help you to fight the infection.

A poultice of either powdered SLIPPERY ELM or chopped CABBAGE LEAVES will draw out the poison. Or apply a compress made by adding a few drops of one or two of the following essential oils to warm water: BERGAMOT, CHAMOMILE, LAVENDER, LEMON or THYME. Dip a clean cloth into the solution and apply over the boil.

You can take herbs internally to purify the blood and fight the infection. Make a decoction from ECHINACEA and POKE ROOT, and drink a cupful three times a day for two weeks. The homoeopathic remedies that help to clear up a boil, include: ARNICA, BELLADONNA, HEPAR SULPH, SILICA and TARANTULA. Compare these in the Materia Medica section to see which one is the most appropriate.

Cold Sores

Cold sores are caused by a virus that is retained in the body and produces a sore when the body's resistance is lowered. The cold sore will form around the mouth, or occasionally nose and eyes. It develops from a reddish lump into water-filled blisters which then form a scab. It is the watery discharge that is infectious, so you should prevent anyone else touching the cold sore at this stage.

If cold sores are recurrent you will need constitutional treatment to clear them up, but the odd cold sore may be treated yourself by using natural remedies. Try dabbing on one of the following tinctures: CALENDULA, GOLDEN SEAL, HYPERICUM and MYRRH (or make up a combination). Alternatively, the essential oil of LAVENDER may be dabbed undiluted onto the sore. Homoeopathic remedies can be used to help a cold sore outbreak clear up more quickly, consult the Materia Medica section of this book to see which of the following is best indicated: ARSEN ALB, HEPAR SULPH, NATRUM MUR and RHUS TOX.

Dandruff

Dandruff is caused by dead skin cells flaking off the scalp. Strong detergents, including medicated dandruff shampoos, tend to irritate and dry out the scalp if they are used frequently, and may make the problem worse in the long run. Any hair, scalp or skin problem is generally an indication of poor health, so if you suspect an underlying cause you need to deal with that to find a cure.

Dandruff can be improved by applying an infusion of MARIGOLD and NETTLES to the scalp and hair as the final rinse. It is also possible to buy mild shampoos that contain extracts of these herbs. The essential oils of CEDARWOOD, LAVENDER and ROSEMARY can be diluted in a suitable vegetable-oil base, such as ALMOND or COCONUT OIL, and massaged into the scalp to eliminate dandruff.

You can take a combination of the herbs BURDOCK, HEARTSEASE, KELP and NETTLE internally to improve the condition of the scalp. Alternatively, see if the homoeopathic remedies KALI MUR or KALI SULPH look appropriate.

Eczema

The symptoms of eczema include redness, flakiness and weeping skin. It may start as tiny blisters that burst and leave a red, raw surface. Eczema can cause intense itchiness during its dry and wet stages, and sufferers often scratch the affected areas until they bleed. Things can be made even worse if an infection starts up in skin damaged by eczema and scratching.

Unfortunately, the incidence of eczema has increased dramatically in recent years, especially amongst children. This is probably because the vitality and natural immunity of our children's health has been impaired by pollution, food additives, over-medicated parents and over-vaccination. Eczema often forms part of the inherited 'atopic' diseases, like hayfever and asthma. Different members of the same family will often display one or more of the illnesses in this group. It is particularly tragic that suppressing eczema with medicated ointments greatly increases the chances of asthma, hayfever or other respiratory problems developing later in life.

The standard treatment for eczema is steroidal ointments such as Betnovate or Hydrocortizone. These ointments will usually relieve the symptoms temporarily but continued use will actually damage the skin by 'thinning' it; at the same time they are absorbed into the bloodstream, potentially causing a wide range of side-effects which are common to all steroids (such as impaired adrenal function and a predisposition to infection). Steroidal ointments in no way cure eczema, and the condition will often return in an even worse form when they are discontinued.

Curing eczema using natural remedies is definitely possible. But it will take time, and in some cases even years, although some improvement should be obvious after several months of treatment. Basically, the length of time that it takes to cure eczema depends on how long you have had it, how many years you have been suppressing it by using medicated ointments, and on your general state of health. If a cure requires general detoxification, then the eczema may even get worse before it begins to clear up, as the body struggles to eliminate more through the skin, and becomes generally healthier.

Many people find that certain foods aggravate their eczema. The most common foods that have this tendency are dairy and wheat products. The best way to find out if this is a factor for you or your child is to avoid all dairy products for three months and see if it makes a difference, then try the same with wheat products.

While we can recommend some natural remedies here that will help to relieve the symptoms, and may even cure a mild case, you will probably need constitutional treatment by a qualified natural therapist for long-standing cases of eczema.

A combination of herbs that combine alterative and anti-inflammatory properties will be most helpful. Try drinking an infusion of the herbs: BURDOCK, CHAMOMILE, FIGWORT, FUMITORY, HEARTS-EASE, MARIGOLD and RED CLOVER. You need to take these herbs three times a day for six weeks, then take a break for a couple of weeks before repeating again. Check the herbs in the Materia Medica section of this book to see that they are all suitable.

A soothing wash can be made by infusing the herbs CHICKWEED and MARIGOLD in boiling water, and bathing the affected parts when the solution has cooled down. Alternatively, you can buy an ointment made from the same herbs. Essential oils can be added to the bath, diluted in a vegetable-oil base to apply to the skin, or used as a compress. The essential oils that are most suitable for treating eczema include: CHAMOMILE, LAVENDER and MELISSA.

Psoriasis

Psoriasis is a common skin disease, in which red, scaly spots and patches appear on the skin of the bony areas of the body, such as the shins, elbows, eyebrows or scalp. The patches of psoriasis occur because the body is over-producing skin cells in those areas. The skin tends to flake off from the affected areas, and it can become itchy.

There is definitely a hereditary tendency with this disease, although the symptoms may not appear until adult life. Psoriasis can be triggered off by a shock or trauma, and flare-ups often occur during stressful times of life. The symptoms are often alleviated by sunshine and sea bathing.

The condition is notoriously difficult to treat by any method of medicine. However, more severe cases will often be considerably improved by natural remedies, and children tend to be easier to cure. We do mention some remedies here that may be a help, but if they don't seem to help after several weeks, we recommend that you consult a qualified practitioner who can take into account any other health problems that may be underlying the psoriasis, and also offer assistance if stress is a contributing factor.

Alterative herbs can help to clear psoriasis out of the system, try taking a decoction of BURDOCK ROOT, RED CLOVER, SARSAPARILLA and YELLOW DOCK ROOT three times a day for up to three months. An ointment made from COMFREY ROOT can be massaged into the patches to help reduce flaking. Essential oils can be diluted in a vegetable-oil base and massaged into the patches of psoriasis to improve the skin and reduce scaling. Try either a mixture of the essential oils of BERGAMOT, LAVENDER and SANDALWOOD, or a 1 per cent dilution of BIRCH TAR in a vegetable-oil base.

When psoriasis occurs on the scalp it tends to be more itchy than elsewhere. An infusion of CHICKWEED, MARIGOLD and NETTLES, combined and used as a final hair and scalp rinse after washing, often helps to reduce flakiness and itching.

Ringworm

Ringworm is a fungal infection of the skin that can occur on various parts of the body. The infection tends to spread outwards in a circle, the centre heals while the edges are still active, and a reddish ring-like eruption forms.

Scrupulous hygiene is required alongside local healing applications to eliminate ringworm. If the problem persists after following these suggestions, you should seek constitutional treatment from a qualified practitioner.

Combine the tinctures of ECHINACEA, MARIGOLD and MYRRH and dab the patches of ringworm twice a day. Add a few drops of the essential oils of LAVENDER, MYRRH or TEA TREE to your bath, and also dab on one of them undiluted to the patches of ringworm twice a day. Consult the Materia Medica section to see if the homoeopathic remedies of GRAPHITES, SEPIA or SULPHUR look appropriate.

Urticaria

Urticaria (also called nettle-rash or hives) is an allergic reaction set off by being sensitive to various substances such as shellfish, sunlight or penicillin. The red, raised lumps or weals that result are caused by the body releasing histamine into the skin, and are often intensely itchy. Flare-ups can be associated with stress and this should be taken into account during treatment.

Herbs may be taken internally for a soothing and anti-inflammatory effect. Try drinking an infusion of BALM, CHAMOMILE and HEARTSEASE three times a day. An infusion of CHICKWEED and CHAMOMILE may be used to bathe the affected area. If the urticaria covers a large area of the body, a warm bath with a couple of drops of essential oil of CHAMOMILE or MELISSA will be very soothing to the skin, and will help relieve any associated stress. Alternatively, add a couple of drops of one of the oils to a bowl of warm water and bathe the affected part.

Homoeopathic remedies can be very helpful in relieving the symptoms of urticaria. Consult the following remedies in the

167

Materia Medica section of this book to see which one is most suitable for your symptoms: APIS, RHUS TOX and URTICA URENS.

Warts

Warts are fleshy growths on the skin that are found in association with a virus. Only a person who is susceptible to the virus will produce a wart after coming into contact with one.

The most common sites for warts are the fingers, knees, face and genitals. Plantar warts, also called verrucae, are found on the soles of the feet. These usually have a visible dark core, and they may become painful.

External remedies will be successful where the warts are superficial in nature. If the warts do not disappear after several weeks of treatment you should seek constitutional treatment by a qualified practitioner. It is not a good idea to 'burn' off warts using acid and so on because this tends to thwart the body's attempt to express symptoms in a simple, direct way by using the skin as an outlet (anyway, they usually just return!).

A traditional way of eliminating a wart is to squeeze the milky sap from the stalk of fresh DANDELION onto it every day. Rubbing it every day with a slice cut from a clove of GARLIC can also be effective. The essential oils of LEMON, TAGETTES and TEA TREE all have marked antiviral properties. Try dabbing one of these on neat to the wart every day. For verrucae, make a footbath by adding a few drops of one of the essential oils to warm water and soak the foot every day (this will also help to soften corns or hardened skin on the feet).

The Urinary System

The urinary system consists of two kidneys which filter the blood to form urine, their ureters which propel the urine to the bladder, and the urinary bladder where urine is temporarily stored until it is discharged via the urethra.

The essential function of the kidney is to remove the waste products of metabolism from the body in the urine. In addition to this function, by excreting certain minerals and retaining others, the kidneys maintain the acid–alkali ratio of the blood at a constant level. The kidneys also regulate fluid balance. If a large amount of fluid goes into the body, the kidneys excrete more. In very hot weather, when a lot of fluid is lost in perspiration, the kidneys excrete less urine.

The urinary system as a whole is the physical expression of our relationship with fluids. This relationship is determined by our ability to deal with the 'water' aspect of our lives: water is traditionally a symbol of the emotions, which may be expressed clearly and be a source of joy, or become negative and murky and a reflection of inner discontent. Symbolically, water represents our ability to 'go with the flow of life': when we achieve this we feel purposeful and content, but when we feel at odds with the direction of our lives resistance and tension can set in, which may become expressed in the body as symptoms of disease.

The role of the kidneys in detoxifying the body is like that of the running waters of a river that in normal conditions are self-purifying and support great life. But once the toxic overload of pollution becomes too great the waters become poisonous and nothing can thrive. The kidneys and urinary system cleanse and purify the body and keep it healthy, but once they become diseased and prone to infection the body as a whole becomes weakened and less healthy.

The Urinary System

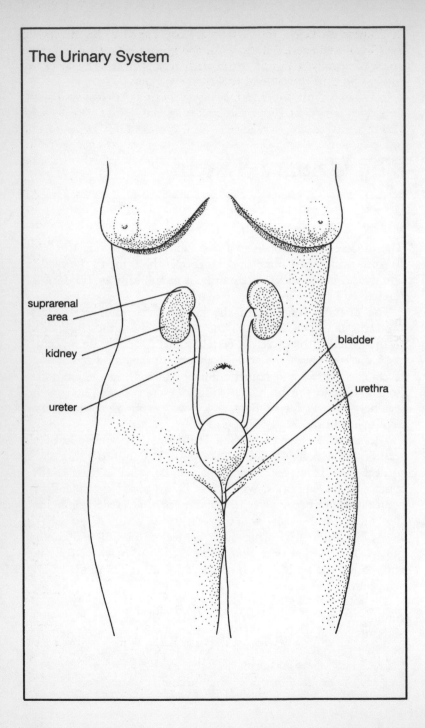

suprarenal area

kidney

ureter

bladder

urethra

In Chinese medicine, the kidneys are considered to be the seat of the *Chi* or vital energy of the body, and prolonged exhaustion or an excess of negative emotion, particularly fear, will weaken the kidney energy and thus the general vitality of the body.

In order to cultivate and maintain a healthy urinary system we should be confident about the quality of the liquids that we take into the body. Many people only drink stimulants, such as tea and coffee or sweet, fizzy drinks, and never pure water. The quality of the water that we drink is also important; it may be better to drink bottled spring water or filtered water because these days tap water is so often contaminated with chlorine, nitrates and unacceptably high levels of heavy metals. Food that is produced without an excess of chemicals and processing will be better for the body as a whole, and less likely to create high levels of toxins for the body's various systems to deal with. The use of salt in the diet tends to inhibit the action of the kidneys and so a low-salt diet will help to maintain a healthy urinary system.

If disease has already developed in the kidneys or urinary system, then professional advice should be sought as quickly as possible, before any further damage is done to this delicate and vital system.

Cystitis

Cystitis is an inflammation and/or infection of the bladder. It is one of the most common ailments in women; nearly every woman suffers from it at some time in her life. A woman's bladder is only about one inch from her urethra; in a man the distance is six or more inches and thus cystitis is much less common in men.

The symptoms of cystitis include: feeling an urgent need to urinate, urinating frequently, pain (often burning) during urination and possibly the presence of blood or pus in the urine. Cystitis is not normally a serious condition and it will clear up quickly with the suggested remedies. However, if you have a fever or lower back pain, you should seek urgent medical advice as the kidneys may be involved. Also, get professional advice if the cystitis keeps coming back, so that the underlying causes are dealt with.

Sometimes cystitis or urethritis (inflammation of the urethra) is triggered off by having sex, particularly if it is with a new partner or after a period of abstinence. This is often referred to as 'honeymoon cystitis'. Urinating before and after intercourse and washing afterwards with cool water can help to prevent this. It can also be more frequent during pregnancy when the foetus is pressing down on the bladder, preventing it from emptying.

The general treatment of cystitis includes drinking an increased amount of water and avoiding stimulants and irritants such as tea, coffee, alcohol and spicy food. Food additives, particularly food colourings, have been found to trigger cystitis symptoms in young girls.

Drinking home-made barley water can be very helpful in treating cystitis: boil pot barley in plenty of water for about forty minutes, then strain off the liquid and drink several cupfuls a day, with lemon juice (and honey if desired) added. Another natural cure is to soak a tampon in natural yoghurt for an hour, then insert the tampon into the vagina and leave it in overnight.

The herbs used to treat cystitis include urinary antiseptics and diuretics; decide on a combination from the following herbs, after you have looked them up in the Materia Medica section, and make an infusion to drink every few hours: BUCHU, CORNSILK, COUCHGRASS, MARSHMALLOW LEAVES, UVA URSI, YARROW. Essential oils can also bring great relief to cystitis symptoms, choose from BERGAMOT, LAVENDER and SANDALWOOD, or combine them and add a few drops to a warm bath for a soothing and antiseptic effect. The homoeopathic remedies to compare in the treatment of cystitis include: APIS, BELLADONNA, CANTHARIS, MERC SOL and NUX VOM.

Kidney Stones

Kidney stones, also called renal calculi, are fairly common. They may remain silent in the kidney, without symptoms; however, if they move they may give rise to renal colic. Renal colic causes severe pain over the kidney area, with restlessness, sweating and maybe vomiting. If you have these symptoms consult a medical practitioner immediately for a diagnosis.

Kidney stones can respond well to natural remedies, and they can be dissolved and passed out of the system during urination. For the best results, visit a professional practitioner, although the following remedies may be tried in a mild case or during a painful attack of renal colic.

It is important for anyone with kidney stones to drink plenty of water (about three litres a day) in order to flush the kidneys through regularly. The herbs that may be taken to dissolve the stones include: CELERY SEED, GRAVEL ROOT, PARSLEY PIERT, PELLITORY-OF-THE-WALL and STONE

ROOT. A decoction of these should be drunk twice a day for several months in order to obtain a result. During an acute attack of renal colic, try an infusion containing CORNSILK, COUCHGRASS, MARSHMALLOW LEAVES and YARROW. The essential oils that have been used to treat kidney stones include: FENNEL, GERANIUM, JUNIPER and LEMON. Compare them in the Materia Medica section, then blend a chosen combination and dilute in vegetable oil to massage over the kidney area or use in the bath. You should consult a qualified homoeopath to rid the system of kidney stones by homoeopathy; if you want to treat the acute pain of renal colic BERBERIS, CANTHARIS or MAG PHOS may be tried.

Water Retention

There are many causes of water retention ranging from heart failure to pre-menstrual tension. It is noticeable when the tissue under the skin becomes swollen and puffy, usually around the feet and ankles, although it may occur in the abdomen or the hands. Obviously the treatment depends on what is causing the fluid retention and this must be established so that treatment can follow accordingly.

The intake of salt will tend to make water retention worse, whatever the cause, so a salt-free diet is advisable. If the cause of the water retention is of a serious nature, such as heart or kidney failure, then you must seek professional treatment. If the cause is not serious and the water retention is temporary, as it is with pre-menstrual tension, then there are several natural diuretics to try. Herbal diuretics include: DANDELION, UVA URSI and YARROW. Make up an infusion of these to drink three times a day when required. The essential oils of CYPRESS and JUNIPER are effective diuretics that you can dilute and massage in where required, or add to your bath. Diuretics should not be taken during pregnancy without professional recommendation.

Materia Medica

Introduction to Materia Medica

This section contains the remedies that are described to help relieve the illnesses and problems mentioned within the systems. Remedies that have been suggested are outlined here so that you can become familiar with the remedy before a choice is made.

We are all individuals, with our own set of symptoms and with our own tendencies and personalities, so choose the remedy that is appropriate for you and your problems. We have selected the most common natural medicines, but there are a lot more: this selection is primarily a useful introduction. Also, the descriptions are not comprehensive – we have merely tried to present a picture that is wide enough for you to be able to use. They are intended to be a guide to some of the options available as opposed to a complete treatise on Homoeopathy, Herbalism or Aromatherapy.

The therapies need to be understood and the remedies experienced. The best way of gaining knowledge is through the process of decision. The importance of making choices is discussed in the Lifestyle section. It is true here. Look up and read the remedy that you are interested in using and if it seems appropriate, try it. What are the results? By trying the remedies you will learn which ones work.

The choice may be quite easy: you scald yourself making a cup of tea but you don't have a handy tube of ointment or Lavender Oil. However, there is the aloe vera plant sitting in the window. Use it. Likewise, your child is hot, dry, flushed with a high temperature, you think she needs Belladonna but you only have Ferrum Phos in the cupboard. Give this while you phone round for the right remedy. We also suggest that you combine remedies. Neuralgia, for example, may well be helped by mixing a couple of drops of Lavender and Chamomile essential oils into a macerated oil of Hypericum, and gently rubbing the mixture onto the areas where the nerves are inflamed; it may also be a good idea to take repeated doses of Kali Phos or Mag Phos, which are known to help nerve tissue. Knowing these natural remedies will take a lifetime, but becoming familar with them is part of a processs of involving yourself in your own well-being. Each remedy has its own secret – we can discover it by using it.

Please note: Throughout this section of the book, 1ml is equal to 25 drops. This is an approximation, as are the quantities given throughout the Materia Medica.

Herbs

Herbalism: this is part of the ancient art of healing. Traditionally, we used plants because they grew around us and we knew of their healing properties. They were part of our lives. We used plants for nourishment, for healing, for ritual. Nowadays, we are able to decipher a train timetable, road map or instructions to assemble a chest of drawers, but then we were familiar with our natural environment. We lived according to the changing seasons, we were skilled in healing, in collecting, drying and storing plants. Knowing plants was one of our skills and we knew which plants to use. In western industrialised society, our knowledge of herbs has been generally lost. But it is not just this knowledge that has disappeared, we no longer keep in contact with our natural environment and, in the same way, with our own bodies.

Over the centuries, the medical profession has became dominated by men, and the use of herbs has given way to developments in science. Herbalism in many parts of Europe and the industrialised world has lost credibility. But now, as the awareness about our planet grows, so herbalism is returning. How many plant species are we destroying with the forests of South America, Indonesia and elsewhere? What healing potential is disappearing? How long is it before the indigenous people of these regions lose their skills? For example, as desertification increases and families are forced to move in search of food, so traditions in natural medicine are replaced by quick, easy solutions, western drugs and inoculations.

Herbalism is a way to communicate with each other, all over this planet. Although there are different herbs and different names

INTRODUCTION TO MATERIA MEDICA

for herbs, each plant has adapted to its environment and the local diseases and needs: Arnica grows on high rocky mountains and is good for sprains, broken limbs etc. The herbal systems of China have been established for centuries, similarly, in areas of the Soviet Union, Africa, Australia, North and South America and elsewhere, they are part of the indigenous way of living. Throughout the world plants were or are used as medicines. What we all had in common was the knowledge that plants are effective healers and we shared the skills to use them.

But today, herbalism is returning. In the West, herbs are the basis of many modern drugs. The active components are isolated and synthesized to respond to particular symptoms. This is a very different process to using the whole herb as a remedy (for example, see Meadowsweet).

Herbs support the healing processes of the body rather than directly attacking disease. They have specific areas of action and these are traditionally classified. Some of the terms are used here to describe the herbs:

ALTERATIVES
These herbs are commonly known as blood cleansers. They are herbs that help with the elimination and detoxifying processes of the body, e.g. Burdock, Echinacea, Cleavers, Red Clover, Blue Flag, Nettles, Yellow Dock.

ANALGESIC
Pain reducing herbs, e.g. Jamaican Dogwood, Scullcap, Valerian. Chamomile, Willow.

ANTI-INFLAMMATORY
Herbs that help reduce inflammation, e.g. Chamomile, Meadowsweet, Comfrey, Marigold, Witchazel.

ANTISEPTIC
Herbs that help combat infections, e.g. Marigold, Lavender, Thyme, Tea-tree oil, Chamomile.

ANTI-SPASMODIC
These herbs relax or ease spasms or cramps, e.g. Chamomile, Balm, Lavender, Lime, Passiflora, Valerian, Scullcap, Crampbark, Wild Yam.

APERIENT	These herbs have a mild laxative effect, e.g. Rhubarb Root, Cascara Sagrada.
ASTRINGENT	These herbs contain a constituent called tannins and these have the effect of contracting the cells. This can have a drying effect on the mucous membranes and other tissues, e.g. Agrimony, Avens, Eyebright, Periwinkle, Golden Seal, Plantain, Witchazel, Raspberry.
BITTER	These herbs should taste bitter to be effective. They stimulate the digestive system, e.g. Wormwood, Barberry, Chamomile.
DEMULCENT	These contain mucilagenous matter, they can protect and soothe internal tissue, e.g. Slippery Elm, Marshmallow, Linseed.
DIAPHORETIC	These herbs promote sweating and elimination of toxins, e.g. Boneset, Ginger, Yarrow.
DIURETIC	These herbs promote the elimination of urine, e.g. Buchu, Couchgrass, Dandelion, Pellitory-of-the-Wall, Parsley Piert, Juniper.
EMMENAGOGUE	These herbs stimulate the period to start, e.g. Black Cohosh, Blue Cohosh, Sage, Yarrow.
EXPECTORANT	These herbs help the process of elimination of phlegm and mucus from the respiratory tract, e.g. Elecampane, Heartsease, Violets, Coltsfoot, Liquorice, Thyme.
LAXATIVE	These herbs help the process of elimination from the bowels, e.g. Cascara Sagrada, Rhubarb Root, Senna, Buckthorn.

NERVINE	These herbs have a strengthening and relaxing effect on the nervous system, e.g. Balm, Chamomile, Lavender, Oats, Limeflowers, Rosemary, Vervain.
SEDATIVE	These herbs have a calming and relaxing effect on the nervous system, e.g. Jamaican Dogwood, Lady's Slipper, Passiflora, Scullcap, Crampbark.
STIMULANT	These herbs speed up processes in the body, e.g. Cayenne, Garlic, Peppermint.
TONIC	These herbs have a restorative and strengthening effect on the body, e.g. Nettles, Thyme, Rosemary, Hawthorn, Cleavers, Aniseed, Balm.

All the herbs mentioned in the Materia Medica are available from herbalist shops. A dried herb should look and smell fresh. Try to buy organically grown herbs that are approved by the Soil Association. These herbs will also be free of any fumigation processes that imported herbs may be subjected to. It is of course preferable to gather fresh herbs and to use them before they have dried. It is best to gather them first thing in the morning. Herbs can be cultivated and collected and used when needed. Place your herb garden as far away from car and diesel fumes as possible. Drying herbs need dry air circulating around them so hanging bunches of herbs in ventilated attic rooms works quite well. Dried herbs should be stored away from light and in airtight jars.

USING HERBS:
Herbal preparations can be taken hot or cold. A hot infusion or decoction will encourage sweating so use for treating flu, fevers, etc. You may well prefer the taste if you add honey to sweeten it. Cold preparations tend to be more diuretic.
INFUSIONS
Make an infusion as you would tea. Pour 570ml (1 pint) of boiling water onto a heaped tbsp of herb or herbal mixture, cover it and let it stand for 7–10 mins. If you want to make an individual cup

the general rule is a tspful per cup of boiling water. Use twice the quantity if you are using fresh herbs.

DECOCTIONS

When the herb being used is woody, such as barks, roots and berries, it is necessary to place the herb or mixture of herbs in a saucepan. Don't use an aluminium pan or a chipped enamel one. Add 570ml (1 pint) of water to each 30g(1oz) of herb and bring to the boil, allow to simmer for 10 mins. The mixture can be stored in the fridge, as only a small wine glassfull will be needed 2–3 times a day.

TINCTURES

A tincture is an extraction of the herb using water and alcohol. If you want to avoid the bother of boiling up herbs or making infusions, this is a much easier way to take a herbal treatment. The usual amount is between 1ml and a teaspoonful (4ml) in a glass of water taken three times a day.

COMPRESSES and POULTICES

When you are making a compress, use a clean cloth and soak it in the hot infusion or decoction of herbs that you require. Apply the cloth (as hot as you can bear it) to the area where it is needed. When it cools down it can be changed. If it is appropriate, a sheet of plastic and a hot water bottle may keep it warm for longer and enhance the action of the herb. A poultice is similar but you apply the fresh or dried herb directly onto the skin. Make a paste with hot water and apply as hot as possible. It may be a good idea to apply a little oil to the skin beforehand so that the poultice is easier to wash off afterwards.

HERBAL SALVE

An ointment or salve can be useful where you need a healing yet protective covering, and you can make it according to your needs. Use for cuts, blemishes, dry skin, rashes and other complaints. It can be a good barrier for a baby's nappy rash. One that we make is very easy and effective:

40g (1½oz) Beeswax
104g (3½oz) Soya Oil
16g (½oz) Apricot Kernel Oil   } Melt together in a double boiler
8g (¼oz) Wheatgerm Oil
(these oils can be changed – use almond, avocado, jojoba, etc., according to your needs)
Plus: 8g (¼oz) Macerated Oil (St John's Wort, Comfrey, etc.)
3.5ml Tincture (Marshmallow, Golden Seal, etc.)
Add to the melted wax mixture and simmer until the liquid

from the tincture or infusions has evaporated. Remove from heat and add up to 2g of an essential oil. Mix well and pour into sterilised jars.

DOUCHE

When there are local infections in the vagina, a douche may be used, in conjunction with a course of remedies taken internally. Make an infusion of 15g (½oz) of herb, 570ml (1 pint) of water, or decoction, and sieve very carefully. Check that no bits are left before putting it into the container of the douche or drawing it up into the receptacle. Do check that it is the right temperature (36–37°C); if it is too hot or too cold it will be very uncomfortable. Insert the applicator into the vagina and let the liquid rinse the area. It is probably best to do this in the bath or on the toilet as all the liquid will run out. Do not persist with douching if there is no improvement after a few days, and consult a qualified practitioner. Do not use a douche when you are pregnant.

USING HERBS IN THE BATH OR FOOTBATH

Herbal infusions can be absorbed through the skin. A pleasant way to use herbs is to put them into the bath. A muslin or cotton bag can be made quite easily to hold either a herb or herbal mixture, tie it tightly at the top and place under the running hot water. It can also be left in the bath while you lie there soaking up the benefits. 30g (1oz) will be needed to have a reasonable effect. This method is especially good for nervine tonics or anti-inflammatory herbs for the skin. A particularly good mixture for the skin is Rose petals, Lavender, Chamomile, Borage and Cleavers, though of course put in the herbs that you feel are particularly appropriate for you. A relaxing herb bath can be made from Orange Blossom, Chamomile, Lavender, Limeflowers and Lemon Balm.

A warming foot bath can be made by adding Ginger and Yarrow when you feel a cold coming on. Add Peppermint, Marigold and Marshmallow when the feet are tired and aching.

Do not use herbs for a prolonged period of time unless otherwise indicated by a practioner. Because a herbal remedy is a natural remedy it doesn't necessarily mean that it is safe to use on a continuous basis or in large quantities. Use care and common sense and always consult a herbal practitioner if you feel unsure about what you are doing.

Chinese Herbs

A number of Chinese Herbs are mentioned in the book which we know to be beneficial in the ways mentioned. They should be seen within the context of the whole of the Chinese Herbal system. We can recommend a very good booklet on Chinese tonic herbs written and produced by Michael McIntyre. This can be obtained by writing to 'Midsummer Cottage', Nether Westcote, Near Kingham, Gloucestershire, UK.

Essential Oils

Treatment using essential oils is generally known as Aromatherapy. This term was first used by a French chemist, Gattefosse, in the 1920s, although the use of the oils is recorded as far back as records go. It was the fragrance that was significant as well as the healing properties of the plant. Generally, smell is the least valued of all the senses largely because it has escaped description. Perhaps because of our inability to categorise it, smell often has the power to evoke memories and associations more directly than other senses, and to affect us on a sub-conscious level. Different smells trigger different feelings and reactions. Essential oils can be very useful tools in healing, often because of this effect on our emotions. Research is now being done on various oils and they are coming to be recognised as valuable anti-bacterial and anti-viral agents.

Oils are produced by distillation from plant material that contains volatile oils. This can come from roots such as Orris (from the rhizome of the Iris), barks such as Cinnamon, seeds, berries and fruits such as Cardamon, Juniper and Bergamot, leaves such as Melissa, wood such as Cedar, flowers such as Ylang Ylang or gums and resins such as Myrrh. It is only the oily part which is separated out. An essential oil is therefore a highly concentrated plant substance. An oil varies enormously according to the type of distillation process, the variety of plant used, the growing conditions, etc. Distillation is done by either water, steam or steam *and* water; different methods produce different results, and although generally it is known which type of distillation method is best for the particular plant, it can vary from country to country.

Other methods of extraction include the use of solvents in the flower oils, and cold pressing the rinds of the citrus fruit.

The variety of the plant can make a great difference to the oil. Eucalyptus Oil is an obvious example with over 700 known species. Be aware too of the difference in oils made from different parts of a plant. Clove Oil can either be extracted from the bud, the stem or the leaf.

These are all ways in which the oils can vary. Until recently the market for which the oils were produced was almost exclusively for the perfumer and flavourist. Their particular sciences require their oils to be exact, predictable and often highly refined. Therefore the oils that are produced for them are not always appropriate for the aromatherapist who needs a pure essential oil which is properly distilled from fresh and, if possible, organically-grown plant material.

These oils are often very expensive because of the small quantity of oil present in a leaf or flower. The collection of flowers such as Neroli (Orange Blossom) is very labour intensive and it needs to be distilled quickly to prevent deterioration. Often a distillation of the Neroli is followed by a distillation of the leaves to produce Petitgrain. It is not surprising that a less expensive Neroli Oil can contain some Petitgrain. Unfortunately, adulteration is common with many of the oils. The main problem is the lack of accurate information available which someone using essential oils for therapeutic purposes needs to know. Our advice, when purchasing an oil, is to ask for exact information. You need to know what you are getting: the variety of the plant, type of distillation, country of origin and part of plant used.

MASSAGE

One of the best ways of using essential oils is by diluting them in a base oil. There are a range of vegetable oils that are suitable to use: **Sweet Almond Oil** is easily obtainable, good for sensitive skin, light and with little or no smell. **Apricot Kernel Oil** is similar. **Grapeseed Oil** is especially light and not quite so oily as Almond Oil. It is also very easily absorbed into the skin. **Soya Oil** is inexpensive and makes a good base. It is good to use when you want to include a heavier oil such as Avocado, Wheatgerm or Olive Oil. These three oils are thicker, with their own fragrance, and are probably best included to make a richer base. **Avocado** is a thick, rich, green oil that is very nourishing to the skin. It is good to include when the skin is very dry and papery.

Wheatgerm Oil is good to add where there is scarring and acne, etc. Being an anti-oxidant it can also help act as a preservative. It can be used on its own (rubbing it on the abdomen during pregnancy can help prevent stretch marks) but it is sticky and difficult to use, so it is generally mixed in with a lighter oil. **Olive Oil** is another vitamin-rich oil and is excellent to keep the skin supple. Use to prevent dehydrating skin in the summer or during a cold winter. It is good to mix with Coconut Oil as a base oil when the skin is exposed to the sun. It does have a strong smell and is less versatile when only a few drops of essential oils are required. **Hazelnut Oil** has a beautiful rich, nutty fragrance and again is very nourishing. **Evening Primrose Oil** is excellent to add to mixtures for skin treatments because it is very healing. Care must be taken though, as it is one of the quickest oils to oxidize and will make the whole mixture go rancid if it is kept for some time. **Jojoba Oil** is good to use when the skin is oily. It gives the skin a smooth, waxy feel.

Here are some suggested blends:

Soya	60%	
Almond	30%	An all round base oil
Wheatgerm	10%	
Grapeseed	80%	
Macerated oil of Calendula	10%	A very light oil where
Evening Primrose	10%	the skin needs healing
Olive	40%	
Coconut	50%	For dehydrated skin
Macerated oil of Calendula	10%	exposed to sun
Olive	50%	
Calendula	25%	For sunburnt skin
St John's Wort	25%	
Macerated oil of Comfrey	50%	A base oil for muscular
Calendula	25%	aches and stiffness
Grapeseed	25%	with bruising
Hazelnut	35%	
Avocado or Wheatgerm	15%	For ageing, dehydrated
Almond	50%	skin

MACERATED OILS
The main ones available are: St John's Wort Oil
                               Calendula Oil
                               Carrot Oil
                               Comfrey Oil
It is quite possible to make your own macerated oil by covering

the plant material with oil, leaving it in a warm place, such as a sunny window ledge, and shaking it from time to time. It will be ready to use when the oil has taken on the colour and smell of the herb. At this stage, take out the herb by passing the oil through a fine sieve. Borage and Chamomile oils may be produced for skin problems.

Adding essential oils to your base will vary according to the base, the oil and the person, but generally the proportion of essential oil to base should be 1–3 per cent. This roughly means that 20–60 drops of essential oil (or combined oils) should be added to 100ml of base oil. For one massage, pour a little base oil into a saucer and add 2–3 drops of the essential oil.

There are many good books and courses available on massage. Massage can be a relaxing, tension and stress-relieving process, it can also be stimulating, toning and re-energising, or it can be a mixture of both. It is a skill that we feel all of us can have and it is a method of communication. Giving someone permission to touch your body requires trust and a willingness to be receptive and vulnerable. When you are working on a person's body you are giving to them of yourself and are communicating that you care. Learn to express yourself through massage for therapeutic reasons as well as for enjoyment.

There are several other ways essential oils can be used, for example:

BASE CREAM
Use in a similar way as a base oil, although a lower percentage of essential oil should be added – not more than 1 per cent. It may be easier to use when a very oily base is not required.

OIL BURNER
Oils can be a very effective way to help clear the atmosphere. They mask unpleasant smells, can be used to fumigate a room from contagious diseases or create a change in the atmosphere. Put 2–3 drops of essential oil into a water-filled receptacle above a candle and the room will be slowly fragranced. Olibanum (Frankincense) is particularly good, and Sandalwood, Cedarwood and Rosewood are all excellent to help atmosphere change. Use antiseptic oils for fumigation: Eucalyptus citriodora is particularly good when combined with Lavender or Lemon. Try out different combinations: mixing a citrus oil with a sweeter or woody oil will give a more rounded, fuller scent, for example Mandarin with Ylang Ylang or Sandalwood.

INHALATIONS
Add 3–4 drops of oil to a bowl of steaming water and cover the head and bowl with a towel to inhale the oils. This is particularly useful for

respiratory complaints and congestion. It can also be good for skin problems. One suggestion for spotty, clogged pores is to pour boiling water onto 30g (1oz) of Chamomile and Elderflower herb mix before adding the oil of your choice, such as Lavender or Rose.

BATHS

One of the easiest ways to use oils is to add a few drops (5–10) to a hot bath. If you want to nourish the skin dilute the oils in a base oil or a dispersing base oil beforehand. But adding the oil of your choice just before you get in will give you the benefit of the aroma. Allow yourself at least 15 mins in the bath to derive full benefit. It is especially good to help relieve tension. If you are feeling too detached or overwhelmed or find yourself ignoring outside needs or not coping with affection – all signs of stress – a bath with oils such as Rosewood and Lavender can be of great benefit. It can also be good when a really cleansing bath is required. Combine with a bagful of herbs and a few drops of Walnut or Crabapple remedies made according to Dr Bach when you wish to rid yourself of outside influences and regain contact with yourself. Adding a blend of oils to a bath can help eliminate toxins and help sluggish conditions – Rosemary is especially good for this.

Oils can be used in compresses in similar ways to that described in the general information on herbs on pages 178–84 but extra care must be taken as they are so concentrated.

Caution: Always remember that essential oils are highly concentrated, never apply directly to the skin. Some should only be used after some experience and knowledge of the oils and the person you are treating. In general, treat all oils with caution, but in particular the spice oils: Black Pepper, Cinnamon and Clove can irritate the skin. Citrus oils must be used with care, and the following oils should be avoided during pregnancy: Basil, Camphor, Caraway, Cedar, Chamomile, Cinnamon, Clary Sage, Fennel, Hyssop, Juniper, Marjoram, Myrrh, Nutmeg, Oreganum, Peppermint, Penny Royal, Rosemary, Sage, Thyme and Wintergreen.

Do not use essential oils on babies, and be very careful with children – never use more than 1 per cent dilution. Do not continue using an oil over a prolonged period of time: once a day for 3 weeks is the maximum unless directed otherwise by a qualified practitioner.

Never take the oils internally, unless a qualified aromatherapist has directed you to do so.

Homoeopathic Remedies

Unlike herbalism and healing with essential oils, homoeopathy has not been known as a system of healing for longer than 200 years. The 'law of similars' though, on which the principles of homoeopathy are based, was a concept understood amongst ancient civilisations. What creates imbalance is also that which can create balance. It has been well known amongst herbalists that a herb given in small amounts will cure symptoms that it will create in larger doses. For example, Valerian in small doses relieves tension; larger amounts can cause headaches. Datura is an excellent remedy for lung complaints but in larger quantities it is a poison. Belladonna, a major homoeopathic remedy, will cure violent, sudden complaints, headaches, sweating, fever, convulsions, etc., whereas in its plant form it will cause these symptoms. Apis Mel is another remedy, made from the sting of a bee, which is a homoeopathic cure for painful red swellings.

In recent medical history, we have come to separate the person from their symptoms; treatments have been directed towards specific ailments, and these are often detrimental to the whole body. Medical practitioners have failed to understand what a cure is. Dr S Hahnemann (1755–1843), who devised the system of homoeopathy as we know it, defined cure as 'a recovery undisturbed by after-suffering'. With homoeopathy, the aim is to restore balance to the person.

There are a great many homoeopathic remedies. The skill of the homoeopath is to match the most appropriate remedy 'picture' to that of the person. This is done by accurate observation of the individual. All the tiny details are noted and are seen as clues to choosing the right remedy. It is important to include the whole person, and their habits on every level.

CHOOSING A REMEDY

In this Materia Medica section, the homoeopathic monographs give a rough outline of the main problems that are covered by the remedy. Before selecting one that has been mentioned in the section on systems, make a note of all the changes that have taken place while you or the person you are treating has been ill. Carefully observe the symptoms. Your friend has a bad cold; is there an accompanying headache? Aching limbs? A flushed face? Do they feel very cold or hot? Are they feeling congested? Check whether they feel better or worse lying down, sitting up, etc. Also, learn to observe changes in mood and thought patterns – everything you notice will lead to making the right decision. When you read through a monograph, remember that it does not matter if you do not have all the symptoms covered by a particular remedy. What does matter is that all the symptoms felt by you, or the person you are treating, are included in the homoeopathic remedy picture. Unlike herbs, it is best not to combine homoeopathic remedies.

CHOOSING A POTENCY
Homoeopathy is a very subtle form of healing. A remedy is made from a substance from one of the three kingdoms – animal, vegetable or mineral. It is reduced to such an extent that it does not contain sufficient matter to act directly on the tissues. An amount of the original substance is taken, mixed with alcohol and made into a tincture (mother tincture). One tenth of this is taken out and added to nine-tenths of alcohol, it is shaken (succussed) and this results in a 1X remedy. A 6X potency has therefore been diluted and succussed six times. A 30th or 30C is based on a different method of division. One part in a hundred is taken out each time and added to another ninety-nine parts. This is done 200 times to produce a 200th (200C) potency. The more times the remedy is diluted the higher the potency. It is paradoxical to our materialistic way of thinking that the more reduced the original substance becomes, the more profound the action of the remedy. Do not let these processes put you off using homoeopathic remedies: it is safe to use the lower potencies and these can be given on a repeated basis.

DOSAGE
When the symptoms are very acute a 6X potency can be given hourly or even more frequently. But for longer term, chronic conditions give one dosage in the morning and one at night. A 30C potency can be given for more dramatic, acute symptoms, where the whole body is involved and a more profound reaction is needed. Give one or two doses.

For example, Arnica 6 can be given repeatedly for bruising, aches and pains. When the injury involves some shock to the body use Arnica 30. This can be repeated once or twice, preferably eight hours apart, but it is advisable not to use any 30 potency over a prolonged period of time. Arnica 200 would be much more effective if the person is in a severe state of shock after an accident, and one dose should be sufficient. It is important to remember to *stop* taking the remedy when the symptoms start improving. If the symptoms return, repeat the remedy, or it could indicate that a higher potency is needed if you gave a 6X potency. Keep an eye on the symptom picture, if it changes, change the remedy. If there is no change in the condition after about six doses, look for a better alternative or get advice. Do not give a high potency of one remedy and then follow it up with a lower potency of the same remedy.

Homoeopathic remedies do work, they are used very effectively by vets on animals, and recently a few controlled tests have been done to prove their effectiveness. We cannot really explain *how* they work other than by suggesting that they encourage the natural forces of the body to restore a healthy balance by stimulating the person's vitality and directing energy where it is needed. It is a truly holistic form of healing. The fact that the more refined (i.e. diluted) the remedy the more profound the effect suggests it may be possible, in the future, to stimulate the body's healing processes without any remedy at all. This takes us into the area of spiritual healing which is in fact the basis from which shamans and witch doctors operate in non-materialistic societies. It is an ability that has been largely lost, but perhaps it will be acknowledged more in the future.

Until then it is worth remembering that homoeopathic remedies have no side-effects, they are cheap to produce and do not deplete natural resources. This makes them ideal for countries such as India, where homoeopathy is widely practised and recognised.

A final comment on homoeopathic medicines: they are sensitive and need to be treated with care – store in a cool, dark place away from strong smells. It is advisable to avoid taking coffee, peppermint, menthol, camphor or eucalyptus while using a homoeopathic treatment. They may antidote it, and it would be a shame to risk this happening.

The Healing Herbs of Dr Edward Bach

Dr Edward Bach (1886–1936) discovered flower remedies that would help such feelings as fear, anxiety and irritation. His medical researches led him to the understanding that much of our ill health has its origin in our emotional and mental state rather than in the physical body. He found plants that bring hope to the desolate, strength to the exhausted and comfort to the distressed.

Each of the remedy states that Dr Bach described has a positive and negative aspect – he saw the negative conditions as the true cause of illness and disease. The flowers embody the positive state – their natural vibrations help us to be happy and to return to health. Remedies made from these flowers help you to help yourself, to bring harmony, happiness and health. For more detailed instructions refer to *A Guide to the Bach Flower Remedies* by Julian Barnard. We are grateful to Julian Barnard for the following information.

DIAGNOSIS AND DOSAGE
Select from the list any remedies that feel appropriate. It is best to limit the number to no more than five or six. (The First Aid combination may count as one.)

To make a medicine strength mixture: take 2 drops from each chosen stock remedy and put into a small bottle of water, about 30ml, adding brandy if desired, as a preservative. If First Aid Remedy is chosen then 4 drops of stock are used. Dosage is then 4 drops, 4 times daily. Alternatively, for short term problems, put 2 drops of each stock remedy into a glass of water and sip at intervals until relief is obtained.

Benefit is derived from small, regular doses rather than by the volume of remedy that is taken. An inappropriate remedy will not hurt or cause adverse reaction. There is no need for fear of overdose or error – feel confident and trust yourself. Remedies may be taken direct from the stock bottle but this has no greater benefit than the diluted remedy.

FIRST AID REMEDY
Dr Bach chose five of the thirty-eight remedies as a first aid combination, naming them the *Rescue Remedy*. This may be used in any kind of emergency, trauma or in circumstances when we need immediate help, before and after moments of difficulty, for accidents and upsets of every kind.

This first aid combination is always helpful bringing calm, restoring peace and emotional balance. It will help both the people affected and those who assist or watch. It is also good for plants and animals, with the addition of other single remedies as appropriate. *Dosage:* mix the First Aid Remedy to medicine strength using 4 drops in a small bottle (30ml) of brandy and water, then take 4 drops as often as required. Alternatively put 4 drops into a glass of water and sip frequently.

THE REMEDIES
The remedies were grouped by Dr Bach under seven headings. In these brief descriptions the negative state is given first with some

positive aspects at the end *in italics*. The full description for each remedy state, as given by Dr Bach, can be found in *The Twelve Healers & Other Remedies*.

FOR FEAR:

ROCK ROSE	Panic, terror, hysteria, horror, dread; *the courage to face an emergency*.
MIMULUS	Fear of specific, known things – animals, heights, pain, etc., nervous, shy people; *bravery*.
CHERRY PLUM	Fear of losing control, doing dreaded things, desperation; *mental calm and sanity*.
ASPEN	Vague, unknown, haunting fears, trembling apprehension and premonitions; *trusting the unknown*.
RED CHESTNUT	Worry for others, anticipating misfortune, projecting anxiety; *trusting to life*.

FOR UNCERTAINTY:

CERATO	Distrust of self and intuition, easily led and misguided; *confidently seek individuality*.
SCLERANTHUS	Cannot resolve two choices, indecision, alternating; *balance and determination*.
GENTIAN	Discouragement, doubt, melancholy; *take heart and have faith*.
GORSE	No hope, accept chronic illness or difficulty, pointless to try; *the sunshine of renewed hope*.
HORNBEAM	Weary and can't cope, temporary fatigue; *strengthens and supports*.
WILD OAT	Lack of direction, unfulfilled, drifting; *becoming definite and purposeful*.

INSUFFICIENT INTEREST IN PRESENT CIRCUMSTANCES:

CLEMATIS	Dreamers, drowsy, absent-minded; *brings down to earth*.
HONEYSUCKLE	Living in memories; *involved in present*.
WILD ROSE	Lack of interest, resignation, no love or point in life; *spirit of joy and adventure*.
OLIVE	Exhausted, no more strength, need physical and mental renewal; *rested and supported*.
WHITE CHESTNUT	Unresolved, circling thoughts, mental turmoil; *a calm, clear mind*.
MUSTARD	Gloom and despair suddenly cloud us, for no apparent reason; *clarity*.
CHESTNUT BUD	Failing to learn from life, repeating mistakes, lack of observation; *learning from experience*.

FOR LONELINESS:

WATER VIOLET	Withdrawn, aloof, proud, self-reliant, quiet grief; *peaceful and calm, wise in service*.
IMPATIENS	Irritated by constraints, quick, tense, impatient; *gentle and forgiving*.
HEATHER	Longing for company, talkative, overconcern with self; *tranquillity and kinship with all life*.

OVERSENSITIVE TO IDEAS AND INFLUENCES:

AGRIMONY	Anxiety and worry hidden by a carefree mask, apparently jovial but in agony; *steadfast peace*.
CENTAURY	Kind, quiet, gentle, anxious to serve, weak, dominated; *an active and positive worker*.

WALNUT   Protection from outside influences, for change and the stages of development; *the link breaker*.

HOLLY   Jealousy, envy, revenge, anger, suspicion; *the conquest of all will be through love*.

DESPONDENCY AND DESPAIR:
LARCH   Expect failure, lack confidence and will to succeed; *self-confident, try anything*.

PINE   Self-critical, self-reproach, assuming blame, apologetic; *relieves a sense of guilt*.

ELM   Capable people, with responsibility, who falter, temporarily overwhelmed; *the strength to perform duty*.

SWEET CHESTNUT   Unendurable anguish, desolation and despair; *a light shining in the darkness*.

STAR OF BETHLEHEM   For consolation and comfort in grief, distress, after a fright, a shock or accident.

WILLOW   Dissatisfied, bitter, resentful, life is unfair, unjust; *uncomplaining, acceptance*.

OAK   Persevering, despite difficulties, strong, patient, never giving in; *admitting to limitation*.

CRAB APPLE   Feeling unclean, self-disgust, small things out of proportion; *the cleansing remedy*.

OVERCARE FOR WELFARE OF OTHERS:
CHICORY   Demanding, self-pity, self-love, possessive, hurt and tearful; *love and care that gives freely to others*.

195

VERVAIN   Insistent, willful, fervent,
                         enthusiastic, stressed; *quiet and*
                         tranquillity.

VINE   Dominating, tyrant, bully, demands
                         obedience; *loving leader and teacher,*
                         setting all at liberty.

BEECH   Intolerant, critical, fussy; *seeing more*
                         good in the world.

ROCKWATER   Self-denial, stricture, rigidity, purist;
                         broad outlook, understanding.

FIRST AID REMEDY   The rescue remedy combination of
                         Dr Bach: Cherry Plum, Clematis,
                         Impatiens, Star of Bethlehem,
                         and Rock Rose. For use in any
                         emergency.

FLOWER REMEDY CREAM

This is made from the five flowers in Dr Bach's rescue remedy combination with the addition of Crab Apple for cleansing. The cream may be used freely for any external problem or injury: for bruising, irritation, bites and stings, for dry skin, spots, strains, etc. Like the remedies it helps the physical condition by helping the subtle energies of the body.

Flower Remedy Cream is made with great care from the purest natural substances using no animals products. It may be used safely and with confidence.

Health improves as our emotional state becomes more positive. 'Any disease,' said Dr. Bach, 'however serious, however long standing will be cured by restoring the patient to happiness, and the desire to carry on with his life work.' Flower remedies work 'not by attacking disease but by flooding our bodies with the beautiful vibrations of our Higher Nature'. They help to remake the contact with our true self which has become hidden by our reaction to life's difficulties.

While these remedies will not interfere with other treatments, they do not replace professional medical advice if that is appropriate. They are harmless, natural and made in the best possible conditions with love, care and attention. They can be taken in any circumstances by anyone needing help.

Materia Medica

Aconite *Aconitum napellus*

This is a homoeopathic remedy to give at the beginning of illnesses. It is good for people that are generally healthy and robust, and then suddenly fall ill. It can be given after a fright, shock or chill, or where there is a rapid onset of symptoms. Use it as a remedy when treating children. *Mental and emotional indications*: Include restlessness and over-sensitivity. Often highly-strung, excitable, with great anxiety and fear. There is a fear of death, crowds, crossing streets and the future. They can be impatient and frantic from intensity of pain, moods are fitful – laughing, giggling one minute, sad and fearful the next. It is a remedy to give after disasters, such as earthquakes, to deal with the effects of shock and fright.

Physical symptoms: Marked by feverishness. Pains are sudden and sharp, sticking and tearing. Complaints about exposure to cold, dry weather or when it is windy; especially respiratory complaints and earache. *Head*: Feels heavy, hot, with a bursting headache and a burning sensation like a hot, tight band. After-effects of being in the sun too long. Fever with strong headaches, encephalitis. The senses are very acute, sensitivity to noise, smell and light. There is an anxious expression on the face. The face alternates between being red or pale. *Eyes*: Conjunctivitis, especially after exposure to cold winds, making the eyes inflamed. Photophobia. Loss of sight after shock. *Cough*: Comes on after a chill. Hoarse, dry, croupy and painful or barking. It gets worse from breathing in, in the evening and from drinking. The cough is relieved by lying on the back.

Stomach: Gastritis, especially when brought on by drinking cold water after being overheated. Thirsty, especially on waking in the morning, pains in abdomen which extend to the chest. It is a good remedy to give where there is retention of urine after fright, for example in new-born babies. Use when urination is difficult, red, hot, scanty and painful and has blood in it, and there can also be blood in the stool. *Women's complaints*: Good for sudden inflammation of the ovaries when the period is suppressed. Fear of dying during labour. *Heart problems*: Includes the tendency to high blood pressure. Hard, full pulse, use at the beginning of acute heart attack symptoms.

In the same way that you can use Ferrum Phos, use Aconite for the onset of sore throats and chills, and where there is a burning thirst for water. Give Aconite to children who wake up screaming in terror. Use for bringing down high temperatures. During fevers one cheek is warm the other is pale, there is restlessness and a desire to toss off the bed covers which then makes them chilly. Hot and cold in waves. The child is normally robust and healthy. It is also very good to give for cramps in children. This remedy is good where there is fear accompanying any symptoms, fear of death, nightmares that wake you up. *Modalities*: Symptoms get worse from fright, shock, being chilled, a cold, dry wind in the evening, at night, at midnight. They improve in the open air, from rest, from warmth and from sweating.

Agnus Castus *Vitex agnus castus*

See Vitex.

Agrimony *Agrimonia eupatoria*

This is mainly a liver and digestive herb. It has stimulating, toning, healing and astringent qualities. By improving the functioning of the liver and the outflow of gastric juices, Agrimony will assist digestion. It is a good tonic herb and will help to assimilate nutrients. This makes it particularly useful in convalescence and for children. It will help general weakness and is a gentle-acting herb (unlike Balmony or Boldo). Since it is also healing and astringent, it is good for peptic ulcers, ulcerative colitis or mucous colitis. It can be combined with Marigold, Bistort or Cranesbill. Agrimony will help stop fluid loss with nervous diarrhoea.

Agrimony also helps tone the bladder and can be used if there is incontinence or nervous cystitis. Where urgency and frequency of urination has become a nervous habit, Agrimony can be used to retrain the body to heal itself, by toning the muscles and the mucous lining of the urethra. It is also slightly expectorant and is mainly appropriate for coughs where there is a tendency to hold the ribs to prevent aching. Agrimony can be used as an oil (see pages 186–7 on macerating oils) or in an ointment. It can also be made into a poultice to help draw thorns and splinters, and as it has mild blood-cleansing properties, it can be combined with Nettles for a spring tonic.

SUGGESTED DOSAGE Take 30g(1oz) to 570ml(1 pint) of boiling water and drink a cup 3 times daily, or take 2ml of tincture in water 3 times daily.

Alfalfa (Lucerne) *Medicago sativa*

This herb is very rich in vitamins and minerals. It is good to use for convalescence, diabetics or for people who need help to gain weight. It will help to increase breast milk. It contains iron and therefore can be combined in mixtures for anaemia. It also has oestrogenic properties which make it an excellent herb for menopausal women. There is some discussion as to whether taking extra calcium is helpful for women suffering from osteoporosis or for preventing the onset of osteoporosis, but Alfalfa may help as it contains calcium and has an effect on the parathyroids which regulate calcium metabolism. Alfalfa sprouts are a good addition to any diet, or the dried herb can be made into an infusion.

SUGGESTED DOSAGE Infuse 1 tspful to a cup of boiling water and take 3 times a day.

Allium Cepa *Allium Cepa*

This homoeopathic remedy has no marked mental indications. It is used to treat excess secretions of the mucous membranes in the nose, eyes, larynx, etc. It is good where there is burning in the nose, throat and mouth. *Colds*: This remedy treats symptoms which include mucus streaming from the nose and eyes, with frequent sneezing and profuse acrid, burning discharge from the nose, that excoriates lips and nose. Profuse, bland lachrymation (this is the opposite in Euphrasia). The person feels hot and thirsty. Symptoms get worse indoors, in the evenings and in a warm room. The symptoms improve in the open air. *Laryngitis*: The larynx tickles, the throat feels hoarse and raw and the pain extends to the ears. There is a sensation of a lump in the throat. Coughing seems to tear the larynx (you need to hold the throat when coughing). *Cough*: This is incessant, hacking, tickling which is worse in cold air. There is a desire to suppress the cough because it is so troublesome.

Allium Cepa can be used to treat hayfever if the symptoms already mentioned fit. They get worse from warmth. *Modalities*: Symptoms get worse in a warm room and from wet feet. They improve from cool, open air, motion and from bathing.

Aloe Vera *Liliacea*

This is an easy plant to grow and keep in your kitchen. You can break off one of the succulent stems and use it for treating burns and insect bites. Apply to sunburnt skin to bring relief. Taken internally, Aloe Vera is healing and cleansing to the gut.

It is definitely preferable to use the fresh plant, as Aloe Vera is generally dehydrated at source and then reconstituted and preserved.

SUGGESTED DOSAGE Take 5ml of the juice or gel 3 times a day, but this will vary according to the dilution.

Alumina *Alumina*

This homoeopathic remedy will be indicated by an overall dryness, debility and lack of reaction. There will be sluggishness and exhaustion. It is a good remedy for old people and long-term chronic complaints, e.g. constipation. The appearance may be thin, withered, wrinkled and old looking. *Mental and emotional indications*: Marked by confusion, irritability, obstinacy and absent-mindedness, with poor concentration and memory. There will be dullness, a feeling of sluggishness and aversion to work. Alumina can help more serious states of mental confusion when everything seems unreal and there is a marked fear of insanity or suicide, even to the point where the person cannot look at a knife without fearing the desire to kill themselves or others. Time seems to pass slowly and although appearing to be in a state of haste, things are actually done slowly. There may be disturbance in co-ordination or mistakes in speech.

The Alumina type will feel guilty, as though they have committed a crime.

Physical symptoms: Marked by a dryness of all mucous membranes, except in the genitals. *Abdomen*: Constipation is marked by a lack of desire, as though the rectum is paralysed, and there is a need to strain even though the stools are soft or lumpy and covered with mucus. There may be a craving for indigestible things such as chalk, charcoal or soil. There is a need to sit down all the time due to weakness in the legs. *Women's complaints*: Periods which are early, pale, short and scanty will leave the woman feeling physically and mentally exhausted. Leucorrhoea during the daytime can be very profuse and burning, and is better after washing with cold water. The vulva may be sore and itchy. *Skin*: Complaints are dry, rough, burning, itchy and accompanied by a desire to scratch until blood is drawn (similar to Sulphur).

It is always best to avoid using aluminium pans, especially when cooking eggs, or for fruit or making tea. Although people use less aluminium at home, it is still widely used in restaurants, hospitals, etc. If you feel you are having to eat a lot of food cooked in aluminium, it may be worth considering taking the occasional dose of this remedy to allay any of the above symptoms. It is also used in anti-perspirants, so choose a deodorant which is not an anti-perspirant, or check to see if it contains aluminium. *Modalities*: Symptoms get worse in winter, warm rooms, when eating potatoes and while talking. They get better in damp air and with cold washing.

Angelica Root *Angelica archangelica*

This herb is both a stimulant and a tonic, it gives an instant lift. It acts particularly on the respiratory and nervous systems. It can be used for lung infections and inflammations, especially those which cause nervous and physical exhaustion with depression. It is really good for coughs, colds, bronchitis, asthma and TB. It is a herb that raises your confidence and creates a sense of well-being. Angelica Root is an aromatic bitter herb which has an effect on the liver, and in turn this assists digestion. In small doses (less than 5ml per week), Angelica Root can decrease gastric acidity, which makes it very good if you have ulcers. In larger doses it will increase the appetite so it is good for anorexics and convalescents. It is contra-indicated in diabetes as it increases the sugar level in urine.

SUGGESTED DOSAGE Decoct 30g (1oz) of the root to 570ml (1 pint) of water and take 2–3 tbsp 3 times a day, or take 1–2ml of tincture diluted in water 3 times a day.

Aniseed *Pimpinella anisum*

The main actions of this herb are on the stomach, the intestines and the lungs. It is known to increase the action of the tiny cilia in the lungs and this makes it an excellent expectorant. It is anti-spasmodic and it is wonderful for children's coughs. It is also soothing on the gut, making it helpful for colic and wind. It is particularly appropriate where indigestion is caused by nervous tension, and it will also help with palpitations or a racing heart. Aniseed is a herb that will help with milk production in nursing mothers. It can be mixed with Chamomile and honey and made into a tea for children, as it is calming for teething, digestion and respiratory problems, including whooping cough.

SUGGESTED DOSAGE Use 1 tspful per cup of boiling water and drink 3 times a day, or 1ml tincture mixed with water 3 times daily. Halve the quantities for children and give ¼ for babies.

ANISEED OIL
This can be used for very similar conditions to the herb, but because of its high concentration and higher level of toxicity do not use more than 1 drop of oil in a saucerful of base oil. Massage into the chest or belly. Combine with Chamomile oil to increase its calming and sedative effects.

Ant Crude *Antimonium Crudum*

The keynote of this homoeopathic remedy is overindulgence. It is primarily a gastric remedy and is good for children and for old people. *Mental and emotional indications*: Ant Crude will suit a person who is greedy, gluttonous and fat, with a dislike of life. They feel weary of living but are sentimental and love moonlight, twilight or soft lighting. The child is fretful and cries when touched or looked at, they are angry when they get attention and get weepy from touch, coughing or during sleep. An indication of Ant Crude is becoming sulky, snappy and resentful if the person is disturbed. There is varying delirium during a fever and a vicious temper when they feel sick and want to be left alone. They blame other people for their troubles, although very often problems are caused through their own indulgences.

Physical symptoms: There is a bitter taste in the mouth, also vomiting and belching. A key symptom for this remedy is a thickly-coated white tongue. There can be a violent thirst accompanying diarrhoea and liquid stools. Also, detached gums that bleed, toothache, cracks in the corner of the mouth and nostrils, redness of the eyelids, split or deformed nails, corns and rheumatoid arthritis. Ant crude is a good remedy for pimples, vesicles, pustules and scaly, pustular eruptions that are itchy and burning and become worse at night. It is useful for chickenpox and measles as long as they are accompanied by the general and emotional symptoms of this remedy. Other symptoms are: callouses, brittle hair and hair loss. *Modalities*: Symptoms get worse with cold bathing, from damp, water, heat of summer and over-eating. They improve in the open air, with rest and from moist warmth.

Ant Tart *Antimonium tartaricum*

This is a good homoeopathic remedy for acute heart cases where there's heart failure, or for extreme cases of pneumonia and bronchitis where the skin has become blue, pale and sweaty. *Mental and emotional indications*: Ant Tart is a remedy for a worn out, exhausted body, and any mental symptoms reflect this; there is apathy, great sleepiness or sleeplessness, drowsiness, a bad temper, and irritability, especially when being touched or looked at.

Physical symptoms: They feel the cold but dislike stuffiness, thirstlessness. *Cough*: One of the keynotes of this remedy is coarse rattling in the chest. It is good to give in cases of whooping cough, asthma, pneumonia and bronchitis. The rattling is accompanied by a feeling of oppression and suffocation and it is more comfortable to sit up. There may be intense nausea which is relieved after vomiting. It is a good remedy for old people who have no reactive power, when their chests are full of rattles and wheezes, the lungs have filled up and there is no power to raise phlegm. It is also a good children's remedy for coughs when the child is angry and for nursing babies who let go of the nipple and cry, reaching for breath. The child feels better if he is carried around or is upright.

Head: Ant Tart is a 'last gasp' remedy (also see Carbo Veg) where the face is pale, sickly drawn, with sunken eyes and dark rings around them. Lips are pale and shrivelled. Nostrils dilate and flap. There is a death-like face with coldness and cold sweat. *Skin*: It is a good remedy for pustular eruptions such as chickenpox, herpes, impetigo and spots that are slow to come out with accompanying chest complaints. *Abdomen*: Symptoms include frequent stools, diarrhoea with mucus, summer diarrhoea. Violent pain in the lumbar-sacral region, the slightest movement causes cold, clammy sweating. *Modalities*: Symptoms get worse in a warm room, from warm clothing and warm weather, from anger and lying down. They improve with expectoration.

Apis   *Apis Mellifica*

This homoeopathic remedy will suit the type of person that is busy, active and industrious. *Mental and emotional indications*: They can be spiteful, rather excitable, jealous and fidgety, they always appear restless and possibly clumsy, awkward and prone to dropping things. Often they are absent-minded and indifferent or apathetic. Apis can treat ailments after anger, jealousy, grief or fright. The Apis-type person is often hard to please or irritable, and is said to demonstrate 'foolish, childish behaviour'. This may come from the person being very changeable and tearful, with no obvious cause, and prone to tantrums or shrieking or screaming suddenly, even when asleep.

Physical symptoms: The main physical characteristic for which this remedy is used is oedema or watery swellings. This remedy is made from a bee-sting so the symptoms will be red, swollen, hot and sensitive to touch. The pains are stinging and pricking, with a dry, burning heat (compare with Belladonna). There can be swellings under the eyes and in the hands and feet. Symptoms will be mainly right-sided and there will be thirstlessness. It is also excellent where there is anaphylactic shock (allergic reaction) to the sting. *Women's complaints*: Features of Apis also include ovarian cysts, stinging pains in the ovaries and burning in the breasts. There may be a tendency to miscarry in the first months of pregnancy. It will be good for oedema in pregnancy, and for cystitis where the urine is scanty, perhaps bloody, almost suppressed and accompanied by a frequent desire to urinate. The passing of urine may be helped by pressing on the area of the bladder. It may also be good for urine retention in new-born babies (see also Aconite). *Modalities*: Symptoms get worse from heat, touch and after sleep. They get better from cold, cold air and cold applications.

Arg Nit *Argentum nitricum*

This is a great homoeopathic remedy for fears. It is the 'What if . . . ?' remedy. *Mental and emotional indications*: The Arg Nit type will object to any suggestion through fear, this is especially true of children. They fear open and confined spaces or heights, or they have anticipatory fear. The nervous system is taut. They are highly-strung individuals who are impulsive, hurried and jumpy. They are always early because they are afraid of being late, they are always in a rush and they will be hot and flustered. Also, they are full of suspicions that things are going to happen to them and that people are out to get them: they always check that doors are locked. These fearful people often manage to just avoid dangerous things, like stepping into a deep hole. They will make certain that they sit at the end of a row of people. They will not travel on the subway because they suspect that they will be robbed; and they are fearful of undertaking anything. They walk and eat fast, and play mental games and build up fantasies about 'What if . . .?' They are obsessive and talk easily. They get frightened of flying and crossing bridges. Excessive mental exertion causes headaches, and if they are overtired they become trembly and paralysed. This remedy has been useful for multiple sclerosis sufferers; it can also help premature ejaculation due to excitement, and speech impediment.

Arg Nit is very good to take for anticipatory ordeals such as exams, a driving test or public speaking (the person will very likely get diarrhoea before the event). As a constitutional type, an Arg Nit person will probably be thin, wiry and look prematurely old, having lived on their nerves and emotions. They worry about their health and desire fresh air, cold food and drinks. *Physical symptoms*: They crave sweets and sugar, although sugar tends to bring about diarrhoea. They like salt and strong cheeses – there is flatulence after eating. Complaints are caused or made worse by eating. There is a strong sense of nausea which will lead to vomiting. In children and babies, it may be the remedy for discharges from the eyes. Pains are splinter-like, cutting, tearing and get worse from lying on the right side. *Modalities*: Symptoms get worse with emotion, anxiety, from sugar and lying on the right side. They improve from the cool and open air.

Arnica *Arnica montana*

This homoeopathic remedy must form part of any first aid kit. It is used for throbbing, burning and stitching pains, but the underlying or main sensation is one of being bruised. It can be used for physical trauma or accidents, where there is extensive bruising and shock to the system as in car, head or sports injuries, surgical operations, dental extractions and childbirth. It can also be used where there is over-exertion. Arnica works by removing any shock caused by physical trauma; the complaints may heal in themselves but a feeling remains of not being quite well. Arnica will heal on all levels, but where complaints are caused by emotional trauma other remedies are probably more appropriate.

In the general symptom picture there is great oversensitivity to pain or discomfort, for example the bed feels too hard making the person feel restless, and there is a fear of being touched or approached. The face may be red-hot but the body is cool and the extremities cold. *Mental and emotional indications*: The Arnica-type person may say there is nothing wrong and believe that they are well; they will be anxious and apprehensive about the future, and will talk slowly, often making mistakes when speaking and using wrong words. One symptom of Arnica is that a person may come out of a state of unconsciousness or delirium to answer a question and then return back.

Physical symptoms: Include burping where there is a taste of rotten eggs, and also a similar-smelling flatulence. *Women's complaints*: It is the first remedy to consider for a threatened miscarriage after an injury or fall, and it is often the only remedy routinely given during and after labour. It can help where there is soreness in the body and uterus during pregnancy (see also Bellis Perennis) and for varicose veins in pregnancy, but there must be the accompanying bruised sensation. Arnica can be used for postpartum haemorrhage and for afterpains, and in some cases of septicaemia; also in mastitis where the nipples are bruised and sore. *Modalities*: Symptoms get worse from injury and touch; they get better from lying with the head low.

Use: 6C for over-exertion, bruising, etc., and repeat as necessary; 30C for more serious injuries, and, for example, in labour and childbirth, take 2 times a day for 3 days; 200C for injuries to the head or before and after operations, etc., take 1 or 2 doses. Externally Arnica ointment and tincture can be applied locally for stiffness and bruising etc., but be careful not to use on any open cuts or wounds.

Arsenicum Album   *Arsenicum album*

This remedy can be used where there is a picture of restlessness, due to anxiety which is on both physical and emotional levels. *Mental and emotional indications*: The Arsenicum-type person will want to change position constantly, and will be anxious about death, being alone, the future and disease, and will weary easily. They may suffer from weakness and prostration which is out of proportion to the illness, and which can come on suddenly. They may be afraid that they will not recover. Arsenicum is usually seen as a 'selfish' remedy, where there is a need to be in control, and the person is demanding and fastidious, critical and suspicious, peevish, rude and irritable.

Physical symptoms: Marked by burning pains which are better from heat, but the head is better from being cold. There are headaches which can be severe and burn and throb generally over the left eye. It is one of the most widely used remedies for food poisoning or digestive disturbances after eating ice-cream, fruit or bad meat. There is vomiting and diarrhoea which will be burning, smelly and watery, and followed by weakness. All discharges are burning and excoriating, with a rotten, putrid smell. Piles burn but are better from warmth. *Women's complaints*: Burning pains in the ovaries, and there may be leucorrhoea which is also burning and excoriating. There may be retention of urine after childbirth. *Skin*: Symptoms include a scaly and wrinkled appearance, and feels like parchment. Arsenicum will be marked by periodicity, for example headaches will occur at regular intervals. *Modalities*: Symptoms become worse between midnight and 3 a.m., in the cold, with ice-cold foods and drinks. They improve with heat.

Aurum   *Aurum metallicum*

This homoeopathic remedy is good for depression, destruction of tissue, memory weakness, restlessness and headaches. It is made from gold, and symbolically it can be said to be good when the light has gone out of a person's life. *Mental and emotional indications*: There is blackness and loss of the love of living, they feel weary and a desire to die. Suicide is a real possibility. There is no enjoyment of anything or anyone – work, family, and so on. They are pessimistic and gloomy, they feel thwarted. It is a self-centred remedy, full of self-condemnation and guilt. They feel unworthy and that they have neglected their responsibilities, they feel that they have failed to do what they should have done. Aurum could be appropriate for someone whose business has failed. They sit and brood. They feel much worse at night, becoming worse during the evening, dwelling on their failings. Pains come on during the night-time and drive them to despair. They may improve during the day and stop being broody by becoming angry or even violent. They are very impatient. These states can come on from prolonged physical pain, worry, too much responsibility or loss of property or a business. They can hold everything together intellectually and keep up appearances, but the will goes, and they can shock everyone with their collapse.

Physical symptoms: Aurum is good for heart disease. It is the remedy to use when there is a weight on the chest as if the heart has stopped, if it feels as though the heart is giving a large thump; or there are violent beatings, palpitations, breathlessness on exertion and watery swellings of the lower limbs and ankles. Also, waves of violent heat and flushes as if the blood is bursting out of the veins, with rushes of blood in the head. The liver feels large, hard and inflamed. There are bone pains, which are aching, boring pains going down long bones, especially those in the legs. Joints are affected, the cartilage around the joints swells and becomes painful, especially at night and prevents sleep or wakes the person up. This leads to depression. Pain will make mild depression severe. There is a fear of death; a destruction of bones in the ears and nose; ulcers in the mouth and throat and on skin which is near to bones. Headaches are really bad with a tearing pressure, throbbing and rushes of blood to the head. Complaints that can be helped by this remedy also include swollen testes and prolapse of the uterus. *Modalities*: Symptoms get worse at night, in the cold air, from mental exertion, from resting and in the winter. They improve from warmth, movement and walking and in the summer.

Avens Sativa *Avens sativa*

See Oats.

Avens *Geum urbanum*

This herb used to be known as a 'heal all', now it is mainly used to strengthen the respiratory and digestive systems, and to help the skin fight off infections. It is appropriate to use where oily, spotty skin is connected with poor digestion, and where there are frequent colds and flus that settle in the chest. It is an aromatic bitter which stimulates the liver and calms indigestion, and the toning action helps stop diarrhoea and mucous colitis. It will generally get rid of phlegm and help with headaches, especially those where the forehead feels tight. It can help you to recover from weakness and exhaustion, and is good for convalescents.

SUGGESTED DOSAGE Take 1 tspful of herb to a cup of boiling water 3 times daily, or with a tincture take 1 ml in water 3 times daily.

Balm (Lemon Balm) *Melissa officinalis*

This is a mild herb but an effective tonic. It acts as a tranquillizer of the nervous system, and is especially good where anxiety is the cause of insomnia (here Scullcap can be added). Balm is used to help where there are functional disorders of the gut and heart. It is an anti-viral herb and can be used to treat herpes simplex. Use as a tea internally, and apply locally as a wash. Balm is refreshing and uplifting to the mind and is excellent for mentally tired and depressed people. Combine with a little Rosemary in a tea in these cases. It has anti-spasmodic actions on the gut and is good combined with Chamomile to help stop nausea and flatulence. Combine with Hawthorn for nervous palpitations. Balm is pleasant to drink and perfectly safe during pregnancy.

SUGGESTED DOSAGE Take 1 tspful per cup 3 times daily or as often as required, or take 1–2 ml of tincture 3 times daily.

MELISSA OIL *Melissa Officinialis*
It is very difficult to obtain pure Melissa oil because almost none is produced commercially. Most oils called Melissa are in fact a lemon oil which is further distilled with Balm. This is due to the fact that it requires approximately 500kg (½ ton) of dried herbs to produce 100g (3½ oz) of oil. If it is available you can expect to pay at least as much as for Rose oil. Use it for similar complaints as you would the herb. A massage using 1 drop of Melissa oil and 1 of Rose or Lavender in Almond or Grapeseed, is very uplifting if you are feeling nervous, depressed or anxious, and especially before bedtime. The oil

may work well for pre-menstrual tension and menopausal symptoms: combine with Chamomile and Rose oil. It may also be very good for headaches, and it makes a pleasant massage for children and babies.

Balmony *Chelone glabra*

This herb tones the liver and stimulates the production of bile. It is good for nausea and biliousness, and where the gall bladder is inflamed. It can be used for jaundice, and being a laxative, for constipation.

SUGGESTED DOSAGE Take 1 tspful of herb in a cup of boiling water 3 times daily, or 1ml of tincture in water 3 times daily.

Barberry Bark *Berberis vulgaris*

Used as a homoeopathic remedy Berberis affects the urinary organs, liver and gall bladder. General symptoms of Berberis are pains that are radiating, shooting, sticking and burning, and that change locality and character. There are gurgling or bubbling sensations, and symptoms alternate, e.g thirst with thirstlessness. *Physical symptoms*: It is very good to use for renal and gallstone colic, the main characteristic being that the pain radiates in all directions. The person looks generally distressed, pale and sickly.

Abdomen: Use for nephritis, cystitis and soreness in the lumber region and kidneys, where there is a need to step carefully as any pressure or jolting is intolerable. Also, take Berberis for burning, sticking pains in the kidneys; bubbling sensations, pain in the bladder, frequent urination, a burning urethra when not urinating or renal colic; pains that are more common on the left side; pains that start in the kidney region or along the course of the urethra and radiate out; and pains that go up to the kidneys and down to the bladder. There can be an urge to urinate and this is accompanied by pain on urination in the groin and thighs. The urine usually contains a sort of mucousy, grey deposit or a sandy, reddish sediment. It is dirty looking but not offensive or bloody. Berberis is an excellent remedy for kidney stones and gallstone colic, and for sticking pains that get worse from pressure. *Modalities*: Symptoms get worse with motion.

USING THE HERB

The herb Barberry Bark is a good tonic for the congested liver. It is stronger than Balmony to use for weak, debilitated people. It is especially useful when there is also irritability and constipation. It is helpful to give for piles which are caused by poor liver function. This herb has a direct action on the spleen. It is good to use where there are protozoan infections of the gut. **Caution**: Barberry Bark is contra-indicated in pregnancy as it stimulates the uterus to contract.

SUGGESTED DOSAGE Infuse 1 tspful of herb per cup of boiling water and drink three times a day, or dilute 1–2ml of tincture in water and take three times a day.

Basil Oil   *Ocymum basilium*

The oil usually available is distilled from *Ocymum basilicum* or Sweet Basil Oil. It is a wonderful reviving oil and also has a relaxing effect on the nervous system. It is an excellent nerve tonic because it is restorative, uplifting and strengthening. It can relieve brain fag, nervousness, anxiety, depression, tension headaches and nervous insomnia. Basil is a useful oil for the digestive system – it helps indigestion and nervous dyspepsia. It will stimulate the appetite, and being antiseptic will help intestinal infections. It can also promote sweating, so it can be used to help bring down a fever, and because it is anti-spasmodic it will assist respiratory conditions such as whooping cough, asthma and bronchitis. Basil Oil can also help stimulate the menses and generally help tone the female reproductive system. This oil should not be used for prolonged periods of time, as it can become an irritant.

Primarily, Basil Oil is good for the person who is worn out and debilitated, either from illness or overwork. It can be combined with a wide range of other oils, for example: with Fennel for the digestion; with Rosemary, Melissa or Bergamot for overwork; with Eucalyptus for sinus problems; and with Bergamot, Geranium or Neroli for anxiety. These are just a few suggestions. It is worth experimenting to find out which combinations you find effective and prefer. Use 2–3 drops of Basil Oil in a saucer of base massage oil.

Belladonna *Belladonna*

This can be an excellent homoeopathic remedy for children and children's diseases. Belladonna is for people who are generally healthy and have vitality; it is a strong, robust remedy for when symptoms suddenly appear. *Physical symptoms*: These will be marked by redness, burning heat and brilliant eyes, with dilated pupils; there may be a wild expression. Pains are throbbing with a hot head and cold hands and feet. There can be a high fever which is accompanied by a rapid, full pulse; the tongue and throat can be bright red. There is a need for cold drinks. As the fever gets higher it can develop into delirium, with biting, spitting, tearing at bed clothes, trying to escape, laughing and talking. The senses can become very acute.

The violence and suddenness of the onset of any complaint is one of the main identifying aspects of Belladonna. It is excellent for turmoil in the brain, for example with strange delusions. Pains are violent and throbbing; there is sensitivity to draughts. Periods can be early, profuse, with hot, bright red blood, and painful, often accompanied by a throbbing headache. This can be relieved by moving the head backwards. There may be mastitis with bright red patches on the breast, accompanied by a fever. Belladonna is the main remedy for bright red skin complaints and for sunstroke. *Modalities*: Symptoms get worse from sun, draughts, touch, motion, noise and light.

Bellis Perennis *Bellis perennis*

See Daisy.

Benzoin *Styrax benzoin*

This is a brown, sweet-tasting resin. It is used where there is stagnation and lack of flow: it helps movement to occur. One of the main areas of action with Benzoin is on the lungs. It helps the person to expel tar and mucus. It has a strong anti-bacterial action and is a good expectorant. It can be used for colds and fevers, particularly to warm the person when they are feeling chilled. It is helpful in the treatment of urinary tract and bladder infections. Benzoin is an important oil in the treatment of cystitis. It can help treat arthritis when there is stiffness and where the pain is worse from cold. Benzoin is appropriate for those people who have a weak appetite and where there is a slow, sluggish digestion with poor absorption. Its antiseptic properties will help to clear sluggish, blocked, congested skin, e.g. acne. For circulation problems this oil is useful when the feet are cold and clammy. Benzoin has a rich, vanilla-like odour and is very useful to combine with the lighter oils. It is said to have a base note and is useful as a fixative in perfumery. Combines very well with Rose or Sandalwood and Lemon. It is difficult to use Benzoin unless it is in tincture form or diluted with a solvent; it is possible to partly dissolve it by warming some of the sticky resin in a base oil, but you will probably find that it will not completely dissolve.

Berberis   *Berberis vulgaris*

See Barberry Bark.

Bergamot Oil   *Citrus bergamia*

This is a light, green, floral smelling oil which calms the nervous system, and is pleasant as a reviver or freshener in the bath after work and before you go out again in the evening. It can be used as an antidepressant and is good to combine in a massage oil when you are feeling low and debilitated. It is good to use in the winter when there is less sunlight. Bergamot contains coumarin which makes it very photosensitive and so it must never be used directly on the skin or in a massage oil before exposure to strong sunlight. It is an anti-spasmodic oil and it can be used for problems in the digestive system, especially where there is colic, flatulence and indigestion. Its antiseptic qualities make it suitable for urinary infections, e.g. cystitis, where there is heat and inflammation. It can be used for skin complaints such as acne, herpes and psoriasis, and it is also an insect repellent either for mosquitos, or as a parasiticide for scabies and lice. Use in a compress to help draw-out thorns and boils. Bergamot is a very good oil to combine with others. For cuts and wounds combine with Lavender, for indigestion combine with Chamomile and Melissa, for cystitis Eucalyptus and Juniper, and for bad breath combine with Lavender and Myrrh. Use 2–3 drops of Bergamot oil in a saucer with base massage oil.

213

Beth Root   *Trillium pendulum*

This herb is good for heavy periods, breakthrough bleeding and irregular periods during the menopause. It can also help leucorrhoea. Use when there is too much fluid loss in the reproductive area. Beth Root contains precursors of the female sex hormones which not only make it a good uterine tonic, but it has an oxytocic effect in that it will act like oxytocin, which is the hormone released during labour. This helps the uterus to contract and also has an effect on letting down breast milk. This is a gentle, easy herb which would be good to include in mixtures for gentle effects.

SUGGESTED DOSAGE ½ – 1 ml (12–25 drops), 3 times a day or 1 teaspoon decocted 3 times a day.

Black Cohosh   *Cimicifuga racemosa*

This herb must not be given during pregnancy. It is classified as an emmenogogue which is a herb that tones the womb and reproductive organs, brings on a period or triggers labour. It is an anti-spasmodic herb and has alterative and sedative properties. As it contains oestrogenic substances, this herb is particularly useful for conditions where there is an oestrogen deficiency. It is suitable for women who have been diagnosed as having low oestrogen levels, especially when they are feeling weak and tense. It is good for helping with any menstrual and menopausal upsets and irregularities. Because of the anti-spasmodic and sedative properties of Black Cohosh it is an excellent herb to use for PMT, pains and bloating and any accompanying emotional symptoms. Its alterative properties help with skin complaints, spots or acne that occur on a cyclical basis. Consider combining this herb with Vitex.

Black Cohosh will give strength to weakened contractions during labour by stimulating the uterus to contract, but the effect will be modified due to its anti-spasmodic properties. It can also help the womb to involute after giving birth, and will soften any afterbirth pains. Here this herb could be usefully combined with Raspberry Leaf or Blue Cohosh. It can be used for rheumatism, and being anti-inflammatory and sedative will help with swelling and pains. It will relax the arteries and help strengthen the heart beat, relaxing the pulse. In this way, it would relieve the strain placed on the heart during labour and birth. It has also been known to help with tinnitus (often due to blood congestion or pressure in the head). As a sedative and anti-spasmodic, it can be used to help with nervous asthma or stress-related indigestion and colitis.

Black Cohosh has a wide range of actions and can be included in many combinations. It can be given regularly three times a day over a period of time, or, for example, every half-hour throughout labour if necessary.

SUGGESTED DOSAGE Use 10–30 drops of tincture diluted in water, or ½–1 tspful of root decocted to a cup of water.

Blackcurrant Leaves   *Ribes nigrum*

One of the constituents of Blackcurrant Leaves is rutin. This has a strengthening, nourishing effect on the blood vessels, and makes it a good herb to use for the hot flushes of menopause. It is also cooling for fevers and helps rheumatism, and it is a very cleansing herb with diuretic properties that aid the elimination of uric acid and clear toxins from joints. It helps restore the appetite which makes it good to give to anorexics.

SUGGESTED DOSAGE Infuse 1 tspful of herb to a cup of boiling water and drink 3 times daily.

Black Haw   *Virburnam prunifolium*

See Crampbark.

Black Pepper Oil   *Piper nigrum*

Pepper is one of the most important and oldest spices. It has been valued for centuries. Both Black and White Pepper come from the same plant, a climbing or trailing vine. Black Pepper is the dried, whole unripe fruit, whereas the white pepper is the ripe fruit from which the dark hull has been removed. The oil is obtained by steam distillation. Therapeutically, Black Pepper is hot and drying, and can be used for any cold and weak condition where energy reserves have been depleted. It is a strongly stimulating oil and can be used in cases of shock. It can have a marked effect on a sluggish digestive

215

system, and can be used in cases of constipation, indigestion, flatulence, dyspepsia and lack of tone in the gut. It stimulates the circulatory system which makes it a good, warming addition in a massage oil for cold hands and feet or where there is rheumatism or sprain. Its muscle toning and stimulating properties suggest that it should be considered where there is paralysis and wasting. It also has a stimulating effect on the lymphatic system. **Important**: This oil must be tested on a small part of the body before overall use in a massage oil, as it can irritate the skin. Use 1–2 drops in a saucerful of base oil for a warming massage.

Bladderwrack   *Fucus vesiculosis*

This is popular to help cleanse the blood and assist in the eliminative process. It has diuretic and slightly laxative properties. Bladderwrack contains iodine and through this has a regulating effect on the thyroid. It is especially good for an under-active thyroid but can also be used for over-activity. Use for a generally sluggish metabolism, obesity and constipation, and also where bloating and fluid retention occur before a period. It is good for skin diseases, in particular those that are flaky, e.g. psoriasis, eczema, dandruff and acne. Use to help with lymphatic swellings and rheumatism, arthritis and gout. It is helpful to make a seaweed bath with an infusion of 25g (1oz) of herb in boiling water added to your bath or footbath to relieve hot, swollen joints. Seaweed also makes a final rinse for the hair. It is cleansing, rich in minerals and nutritious and helps to keep the skin and hair healthy.

SUGGESTED DOSAGE Take ½ tspful of dried Bladderwrack in a cup of boiling water 3 times daily, or 1ml tincture diluted in water 3 times daily. It may be preferable to take Bladderwrack in capsules or tablets. Take 2, 3 times a day before meals.

Blue Cohosh   *Caulophyllum thalictroides*

As a homoeopathic remedy, Caulophyllum is used for weakness in the reproductive system of women. *Physical symptoms*: It is an excellent uterine tonic for exhausted women, and it helps improve uterine tone so that it is a remedy for where there is a risk of miscarriage in the early weeks of pregnancy. *Periods*: There are labour-like pains that fly about or drawing-like pains in the legs, feet and toes; also cramping pains that are violent with little flow. Periods are too early or late. Leucorrhoea is acrid and profuse especially in young girls. *Labour*: Caulophyllum is indicated during labour when contractions are irregular and fly about not doing the job efficiently, and the cervix is not dilating. Or when contractions disappear due to exhaustion during a long labour. It is a good remedy for: labour pains that are erratic, short, irregular and spasmodic; rigidity of the cervix, when pain is like pricking needles in the cervix; ineffective uterine spasms and very painful contractions; when the woman is irritable and fretful. Use for prolonged and profuse after-pains and lochia.

USING THE HERB
The main actions of the herb Blue Cohosh are as a uterine tonic, emmenogogue (see Black Cohosh), anti-spasmodic and anti-rheumatic. It is not advisable to give this herb routinely during pregnancy as it will help bring on a period, and is therefore good for suppressed or delayed menstruation. It could be included in a mixture for a generally late cycle, as a uterine tonic and to tone up the generative area. It can be good for painful periods or where the uterus is inflamed (through infection, injury, e.g. a fall, or being punched or kicked). It will tone up the uterus and so could be taken in the last six weeks of pregnancy to prepare it for labour, making delivery easier and shorter. It will soothe any irritability of the uterus where a woman is prone to go into early labour or suffer from false labour pains. As with Black Cohosh, this herb can be taken for weak or irregular contractions in labour as it is good for an over-contracted uterus. It will make the contractions less painful and more productive. In similar ways, it will help with afterbirth pains. It is good for the pain of rheumatism, especially in the small joints, e.g. fingers and wrists.

SUGGESTED DOSAGE Use ½–1 ml of tincture diluted in water 3 times daily, or infuse ½–1 tspful of herb in a cup of water 3 times daily.

Blue Flag *Iris versicolor*

This is a bitter herb because it is the root that is used. It is good for digestive and liver problems, for migraines that are exacerbated by digestive upsets and for those people that cannot eat cheese, chocolate or rich foods. If Blue flag is taken over a period of time it can help people to become less prone to these foods. It is good for headaches with sickness or nausea. This herb has been used for morning sickness (the gentler herbs suggested for this are probably better to use, as this is a strong herb and must be used carefully). It is useful for skin problems, such as acne etc., which are caused by a poor sluggish digestion.

SUGGESTED DOSAGE Use 5–10 drops of tincture in water every 3–4 hours. Or use 30g (1oz) of herb to 1 pint of water, decocted, and take a dessertspoonful every 3–4 hours.

Bogbean *Menyanthes trifoliata*

Bogbean is mostly used for rheumatoid arthritis, osteo-arthritis and rheumatism when they get worse from cold and damp. It is also good for migraines and trigeminal neuralgia when affected by damp and cold. It will aid digestion by stimulating the production of digestive juices. It also has a stimulating action on the bile flow and stimulates the colon. This makes it slightly laxative and helps to eliminate waste products. It can be used for wet oozing skin disorders. Bogbean is contra-indicated in diarrhoea and colitis.

SUGGESTED DOSAGE To make an infusion, use 1 tspful of herb to a cup of boiling water and take 3 times daily, or 1ml of tincture diluted in water, taken 3 times daily.

Boldo *Peumus boldus*

This is a gentle, calming, sedative herb that is good for a congested liver where the symptoms are emotional irritability and liverishness. Boldo can be used to help tension, insomnia and nervous cystitis (where you get up in the night to pee). It is especially indicated if there is a sensation of fullness and soreness on the right side which gets worse after eating. It is an antiseptic herb and is soothing on the digestive and urinary tract.

SUGGESTED DOSAGE Take 1 tspful of herb to a cup of boiling water 3 times daily, or 1ml of tincture diluted in water 3 times daily.

Boneset *Eupatorium perfoliatum*

The general picture of the homoeopathic remedy Eupatorium Perf is a bruised feeling all over the body, as if the bones are broken. The person moans with pain and has violent aches in the bones. It is a remedy that is often used for flu. *Head*: Symptoms include sore, throbbing pain; it is better for vomiting. *Eyes*: Sore, aching, yellow eyeballs with a headache. *Nose*: There is coryza (nasal catarrh) with sneezing and aches around the face. *Respiratory symptoms*: Hoarseness which is worse in the morning, a cough with soreness of the chest and a desire to hold the chest. Hands and knees feel better from resting. *Mouth*: Yellow tongue, bitter taste and cracks on the corner of the mouth. *Fever*: There is thirst or nausea, then a violent, aching chill which begins in the small of the back. Also, bitter vomiting after a chill or during heat. There is burning heat. Sweat relieves all symptoms except headache. Sweat is scanty. There is an insatiable thirst, before and during a chill and fever. *Modalities*: Symptoms get worse in the cold air, during menstruation, with motion, from coughing, the sight or smell of food and lying on the affected part. They get better with vomiting bile, from conversation, with sweating and lying on the face.

USING THE HERB

The herb Boneset is known particularly for relieving symptoms of the respiratory system. It is particularly good where there are colds or flu and a feverish condition, with aching legs (joint and muscle pains), etc. It helps to lower fevers and clear mucus. It has a slight laxative effect so that it would be good if there is constipation accompanying flu symptoms. It can be combined very well with Elderflower and Yarrow.

SUGGESTED DOSAGE Infuse ½–1 tspful of herb in a cup of boiling water. Take 3 times daily or as appropriate.

Borage   *Borago officinalis*

This herb is said to give courage and gladden the heart. It will help lift a depressed state. It is an adrenal tonic and is good to give to people who are weak or run-down, or have recently been on a course of steriods or cortisone. It is an excellent herb to take if you are under stress. It has diuretic actions, and as well as being anti-inflammatory and cleansing, Borage will help lower a temperature so it is useful for lung complaints, e.g. pleurisy, bronchitis and TB. It can be used for night sweats, skin complaints (especially those caused by stress) and also as a galactogogue (promotes milk production in nursing mothers). It can also be combined in mixtures for rheumatism.

SUGGESTED DOSAGE To make an infusion use 1–2 tspfuls of herb per cup of boiling water, or use 1 ml of tincture diluted in water, and take either 3 times daily.

Borax   *Borax veneta*

Mental and emotional indications: The main features of this remedy are anxiety, especially around downward motion, and fear of going downhill, downstairs, being put down or being swung in babies. There is an oversensitivity to noise and a tendency to become excessively startled – they are frightened of sudden or unusual sounds, such as coughs, sneezes and fireworks. It has been an effective remedy when given to very nervous animals. It is good for babies who cry out in their sleep as if they are frightened of a dream, or those who cling to the side of a cot because they are afraid of falling. Babies who fit this remedy picture often cry or scream before passing a stool, urinating or whilst nursing. They are fidgety, the skin is often unhealthy and the hair gets matted at the back of the head. They may have ingrowing eyelashes.

Physical symptoms: Include injuries that suppurate and are slow to heal, the nose can be red, shiny and the nostrils may get inflamed and crusty. There may be ulceration and thrush of the mucous membranes and mouth ulcers may bleed while eating or when touched. The person feels worse from eating sour or salty food. In babies, thrush in the mouth is hot and tender and will make it difficult to suck. There can be soreness in the vagina, accompanied by itching, and hot smarting pains; the vulva may be itchy. Leucorrhoea appears like uncooked eggwhite and is excoriating. There can be erosion of the cervix. Periods can be too early, profuse or accompanied by colic, which can be griping and nauseous. If the symptom picture fits, Borax may help conception, which is often prevented by the acrid leucorrhoea. *Modalities*: Symptoms get worse from downward motion, sudden noise, damp and cold; they get better from pressure.

Bryonia *Bryonia alba*

This is one of the main homoeopathic remedies which is excellent for a wide variety of symptoms. If the person being treated fits into the picture of Natrum Mur when they are well but suffers from the acute symptoms of Bryonia, it is likely that this remedy will work. *Mental and emotional indications*: In general, people needing Bryonia will be upset by the slightest disturbance, they suffer from extreme irritability and anger and want to be left alone with no interference. They are anxious about the future and have no sense of security. They are confused and can become delirious. They may also be quietly morose, with great fear of poverty and uncertainty. The confusion will become worse when they are talked to or moved, even when sitting up or walking.

Physical symptoms: Will come on slowly, unlike with Aconite or Belladonna. The person will want rest, quiet and no attention. Complaints are more often right-sided, although not always, and can come on when the weather changes after summer, or after getting cold. Discharges are suppressed, but the pains are usually intense – stitching or bursting. These seem better when lying on the painful side and with pressure. The main physical symptom which can be relieved by Bryonia is the excessive dryness of the mucous membranes of the whole body: stools are dry, lips are parched and the cough is dry, hard and racking, with very little expectoration. The urine is dark and scanty. There is a thirst for large quantities of liquid, but only infrequently. *Head*: There is dizziness or fainting on rising, and a headache that is bursting. There is a bursting pain when the person stoops or coughs. They can wake with a headache that gets worse during the day – often this is a pain behind the eyes. The headache is similar to that in the Natrum Mur picture.

Abdomen: Where there is constipation the stools are large, hard, crumbling and dry, as if burnt. Or there may be 'summer diarrhoea', which comes on from being chilled after overheating: the stools are like dirty water. *Women's complaints*: Periods may be replaced by

221

frequent nose-bleeds, or they may be early and profuse or suppressed altogether. There may be sticking pains in the ovaries, and a headache may come on before the period starts. Breasts may be swollen and sore during periods; Bryonia is good for mastitis where there are sticking pains in the breasts.

This remedy can be used for a number of chest complaints – coughs, bronchitis, pneumonia, etc. – where the pains are acute and sticking and get worse by breathing deeply. There may be pains in the joints which can be swollen, hot and red. Also, the face may be dark red and bloated, with dry lips. *Modalities*: Symptoms are worse from motion, sitting up, stooping, coughing, exertion, deep breathing, getting hot, touch and anxiety. They get better from pressure, lying on a painful part, coolness and open air.

Buchu *Barosma betulina*

This is an antiseptic herb that is good for general inflammation and infection, particularly in the lower urinary tract, the bladder and the urethra. It soothes the mucous membranes and can be used to help relieve cystitis and urethritis.

SUGGESTED DOSAGE Use 1 tspful of herb and infuse in a cup of boiling water, or dilute ½–1ml of tincture in water and take 3 times daily.

Buckthorn, Cascara Sagrada *and* Senna *Rhamnus cathartica, Rhammus purshiana* and *Cassia angustifolia* (*Cassia senna*)

These three herbs can be dealt with together because all of them can be used for treating different degrees of constipation. **Senna**, the strongest laxative, can be given as a single treatment; use the leaves if possible as they are less griping. If the constipation is chronic, use Senna as part of a mixture to help the gut as well. **Cascara** is less strong than Senna and has a more toning action on the gut. **Buckthorn** has a weaker action than the other two. It can be added to mixtures for skin problems accompanying constipation. Where there is severe constipation these three herbs can be combined; as the condition improves cut out Senna, then Cascara. It may be appropriate to consider other herbs, such as Liquorice, Fennel and Crampbark. Children who need a laxative can be given Buckthorn.

It is not a good idea to take laxatives over a long period of time. Eventually they will weaken the walls of the gut and will not encourage the body to function correctly. Only give laxatives at night. They will take 8–12 hours to work. They contain anthroquinones which are absorbed through the gut into the circulation, and then stimulate peristalsis through the gut wall.

SUGGESTED DOSAGE With these herbs, make a decoction using 30g (1oz) of herb to 570ml (1 pint) of water, and drink ½–1 wine glassful at night.

Burdock   *Arctium lappa*

Both the root and leaves are used and both are anti-microbial, although the root is considered to be more powerful. It is most commonly used for skin diseases, either acne, dry, scaly skin conditions or for pustular yellow heads. Burdock acts strongly by pushing the toxins out onto the skin surface, but you can give it as a diuretic with Dandelion or Celery Seed to help flush out toxins from the liver and kidneys. Likewise, it will be good for rheumatism and gout, as it helps to cleanse joints. Burdock reputedly lowers blood sugar levels, making it useful for diabetes.

SUGGESTED DOSAGE Use 15g (½oz) decocted in 570ml (1 pint) of water, and drink a ½ cup 3 times daily, or in a tincture use 10 drops in water 3 times daily. It is recommended that you do not use more than 15ml (½oz) per week. For measles, make a decoction of root (30g/1oz to 570ml/1 pint); take a tbsp every 2 hours to heal eruptions and also lift the spirits.

Caladium   *Caladium seguinum*

This homoeopathic remedy is very good for mosquito and insect bites that burn and itch intensely. There can be nervous excitability and great sensitivity to noise; intense itching of the genitals, with burning; and dryness in areas which are usually moist. There may be a red, dry stripe down the centre of the tongue which gets wider

223

towards the tip. The person is usually thirstless and wants to lie down and not move. This remedy will modify the craving for tobacco. *Modalities:* Symptoms get worse from movement, sudden noises, tobacco and sexual excess; they improve with cold air, short sleeps and sweating.

Calc Carb *Calcarea carbonica*

Children: This can be an excellent homoeopathic remedy for children. Babies are fat and flabby and chilly. The sweat and stools smell sour. They vomit milk and there is a loss of appetite. They often have large heads and the fontanelle stays open. The glands in the neck, as well as the parotid and maxillary glands, can be hard and swollen. They can be slow to teethe and experience pain during this time. They can have pot bellies. They are placid and not usually active. As these babies grows up they are seen to be stubborn, they frequently get colds, are often overweight and tend to whine and grumble. They generally have strong constitutions and sweat readily. They tire easily and get red, sweaty and breathless with slight exertion. They have cold, clammy, sweaty feet. Calc Carb is a remedy for chilly people. Children are worse from heat and push away bed covers, but as they get older they get chillier and may wear socks in bed until the feet get too hot and they take them off. Diarrhoea is pale and may alternate with constipation. They feel better when they are constipated. At school, the Calc Carb child will be a 'plodder' because although the thinking processes are good they are slow. They are hard working and organised but can overdo their concentration and then lose interest. They may have nightmares and wake up screaming and are afraid of the dark.

Adults also tend to have big heads, faces are often lined and they have scraggy necks. They also tend to be flabby and are known for being stubborn and obstinate with good stamina and a strong spirit. They may have a strong sex drive. *Mental and emotional indications*: They are thorough and methodical people, often pale, breathless and anaemic. They may be mentally sluggish but very sensitive to injustice. They get peevish and are slow to respond, generally depressed. Their mental grasp tends to get slower as they get older, they take longer to understand and pause before answering. They tend to get anxious about the future and their own health, as they get tired the anxiety increases. There is an aversion to work, a fear of infection and they are afraid for their health, particularly for their heart, and for their sanity. They are worried about others seeing them and despair of recovery. There is a fear of death and thoughts of ill-health dominate their lives but they very rarely admit it. Their thoughts churn around constantly. An indication of Calc Carb is a clammy handshake.

Physical symptoms: These include eruptions behind the ears that form cracks which go over the lower lobes of the ears. Brittle nails. A tendency for headaches which come on after exertion but get better from lying on the left side. There may be vertigo on descending stairs and severe vertigo on suddenly turning the head. They get headaches if they do not eat. There is a continual feeling of emptiness which gets better from eating. Calc Carb may be a good remedy to use for those who catch colds easily or suffer from chronic catarrh where the mucus goes down the back of the throat. It is also good for all kinds of arthritic conditions which get better in dry heat and worse in the cold and damp. The sluggishness in the circulation leads to chilblains, varicose veins and then leg ulcers. Breasts may get swollen and painful before a period with accompanying constipation. Periods are often early, painful and heavy. It is a good remedy to consider for uterine fibroids. Individuals that fit the Calc Carb picture are often prone to strong sexual impulses.

An indication in children for this remedy is their desire to eat indigestible things, such as coal and chalk; adults like a lot of salt. Calc Carb symptoms can arise after vaccinations – it may be worth checking this when you are considering this remedy. *Modalities:* Symptoms get worse from exertion (both physical and mental), cold air, bathing, cooling, dentition and pressure of clothes. They get better in dry weather and after breakfast.

Calc Fluor *Calcarea fluorica*

This is one of the main homoeopathic remedies for pregnancy. It has no strong mental or emotional indications. It is used to improve elasticity in the skin, veins or glands. As a tissue salt, it is connected with the astrological sign of Cancer. *Physical symptoms*: It is good for glands that become swollen and for strong, hard swellings, such as swollen tonsils. It can be used for hard nodes in the breast. It is one of the best remedies to help distended varicose veins, inflamed skin and stretch marks in pregnancy. It can really help if it is used on a regular basis. It is also good for piles during pregnancy. Calc Fluor can be used during a diet or fast to help the elasticity of the skin when excess weight is lost too quickly. *Teeth*: It is used for enamel deficiency; it can be taken with Calc Phos, and as a course of 6X, night and morning for a fortnight, to children with forming teeth. Give this twice a year. *Modalities*: Symptoms become worse at the beginning of motion, from cold and damp; they become better from continued motion.

Calc Phos   *Calcarea phosphorica*

This is a biochemic tissue salt and a homoeopathic remedy. As a tissue salt, Calc Phos is linked to the astrological sign of Capricorn. Calcium phosphate is an essential part of good nutrition and proper growth. It is found in blood plasma and corpuscles, saliva, gastric juices, bones, connective tissue and teeth. The main functions of Calc Phos include: giving solidity to bones, promoting cell growth, assisting digestion and assimilation, and as a good tonic for debility and after illness. It is useful in the treatment of anaemia, especially in conjuction with Ferr Phos, when it accompanies constitutional treatment. Calc Phos is particularly appropriate for young people with anaemia who are rapidly growing, or for heavy periods. It is good for women who have lost a lot of body fluids, e.g. from excessive leucorrhoea or night sweats. Give for bone diseases, osteoporosis or brittle bones. Calc Phos would be a good supporting remedy with Symphytum for the non-union of fractures. It will help speed up the healing process. It is very good for slow-growing, slow-teething children, or for those with rickets. Give for growing pains in children and adolescents. It is also useful to take for brain fag, and for a tired mind after too much studying.

Mental and emotional indications: These are influenced by overall mental weakness – an inability to sustain any mental effort, impaired memory, confusion, prostration of the mind from over-talking, or a dullness and sluggishness that is made worse by mental exertion. The Calc Phos type is discontented, displeased, dissatisfied and complaining. There is a nervous restlessness, with sighing and a desire to get away or travel, a feeling of wanting to be on the move and an irritability which gets worse when tired.

Physical symptoms: This picture of Calc Phos starts with the head. It can be used for headaches of school children brought on by over-study or anaemia. They seem nervous and restless, the head feels cold to touch and the vertex of the head is cold or sore. The headache is worse in cold air and draughts, but better with bathing.

Teeth: It is an excellent remedy to give for painful, difficult, slow teething, or for teeth which are soft and decay easily and the gums are pale, painful and inflamed. *Throat*: Symptoms include a sore, aching throat, swollen glands, radiating pain on swallowing and chronic enlargement of tonsils. It is a good remedy for bronchitis where there is inflammation of the middle ear, the glands are swollen and the ear aches. *Respiratory symptoms:* There is tendency to catch colds easily and often from becoming chilled. Coughs will have yellow expectoration.

Abdomen: Calc Phos can be used for digestive problems marked by heartburn, flatulence and colic. There can be a large appetite, particularly for salted or strong-tasting foods. The abdomen can be flabby, and stools hot, watery, offensive and spluttering. Diarrhoea gets worse in the summer and with fruit. It can also be used for diarrhoea that accompanies teething. *Women's complaints*: Give to girls with amenorrhoea where their menses started early (around 10 or 11 years). Give for menstruation that occurs during lactation or for labour-like pains before or during periods. The pains get worse as a result of a change of weather and improve when the flow starts. Menses are often excessive. There can be weariness during pregnancy and breasts can be sore. Give for anaemia after heavy periods, or weakness after prolonged breastfeeding. Calc Phos can help with prolapse after weakness.

Often symptoms in the Calc Phos picture are: a stiff neck which comes on after being in a draught; rheumatism caused by cold weather; and cramps, spasms and numbness. A person who suits Calc Phos may have cold hands and feet, poor circulation and be prone to moaning and groaning in their sleep. *Modalities:* Symptoms get worse on exposure to weather changes, and from draughts, colds, during melting snow, teething, loss of fluids, mental exertion and puberty. They improve in the summer, when the weather is warm and dry, and from lying down.

Calc Sulph   *Calcarea sulphurica*

As a tissue salt or homoeopathic remedy, this mineral acts on the connective tissue. It is a cleanser, it heals wounds, purifies the blood and is good for conditions that arise from impurities in the bloodstream, e.g. acne, catarrh and gumboils. As a tissue salt, this remedy is associated with the astrological sign of Scorpio. *Physical symptoms*: It will help conditions that tend to suppurate and where

227

there is thick, yellow, lumpy or blood-streaked pus. It is good for painless abcesses about the anus area, which can be pusy, watery or recurrent. Use to treat old, oozing ulcers where the pus is thin and watery, or for purulent discharges that will not heal. Calc Sulph is very good for adolescent acne or for pimples, particularly on the face and shoulders. Calc Sulph covers other symptoms such as burning, itching soles of the feet, excessive sensitivity of the nerves and when the temperament is on edge. It helps to clear out worn out blood cells. If Calc Sulph is given to someone with catarrh, the condition will seem to continue for a while, but it will help eliminate it completely in the end. *Modalities*: Symptoms get worse from draughts, touch, the cold, wet, working in water, such as washing up, and the heat of a room. They improve in the open air, from eating and heat when applied locally.

Calendula   *Calendula officinalis*

See Marigold.

Cantharis   *Cantharis vesicatoria*

General: This remedy affects the urinary and sexual organs. It is good to use when violent, painful inflammation causes frenzy and delirium, where pain has a rapid and intense onset. *Mental and emotional indications*: Irritability and anger which gets worse with pain. There may be a general oversensitivity, anxiousness, and restlessness. Liable to contradict attempts to do things but cannot accomplish them. *Physical symptoms*: These types tend to be very pale during bouts of pain but become flushed in between. *Pains* are cutting, biting, smarting, burning. They cause great mental excitement. There is oversensitivity in all parts of the body. There is burning in the body, both internal and external, and this leads to extreme weakness.

Head: Feels heavy. *Stomach*: Burning, there is a thirst but aversion to fluids; retching or vomiting. *Abdomen*: Burning pain throughout the digestive tract, shreddy stools that burn. *Urinary*: The urinary and generative organs are in a state of irritation and sensitivity. The kidney area is very sensitive to the slightest touch. Urine is burning, scalding, with constant urges. This is intolerable from the cutting, burning pains which get worse before and after urination. They are

228

accompanied by spasms and a sore, raw sensation. Urine can be bloody and burns like fire. Urine passes in drops. Cantharis is the most frequently indicated remedy for cystitis; it is also good for rephritis and renal colic. *Skin*: Burns and scalds, before or just after blisters form. *Modalities*: Symptoms get worse on urinating, sound of water and cold. They improve with warmth, rest and rubbing.

Carbo Veg   *Carbo vegetabilis*

This is a life-saver remedy. It can be used after a haemorrhage where there are cold sweats, cold feet, cold breath, a thready, weak pulse, a need for cold air, and a blueness in the face. It can be used for a newborn in this state – in this case use a single 200C potency. Carbo Veg can be used after an exhausting illness, and it is good for children who have never totally recovered from measles, whooping cough or a loss of body fluids. It is a remedy for people who are greatly debilitated, weak in a state of collapse and are without vitality. *Mental and emotional indications*: The Carbo Veg type of person is fat, chilly, sluggish and flatulent. There is a weakness of memory, a slow grasp of things, confusion, irritability, anxiousness or indifference.

Physical symptoms: There can be persistent nosebleeds and offensive discharges. The digestive symptoms include flatulence, bloated rumblings, indigestion, a distended stomach, which is worse from lying down but improved by burping, and there is excessive gas in the stomach and intestines. Although women's problems are not central to this remedy, it does cover periods that are profuse and accompanied by colicky pains, and green leucorrhoea.

Cardamon   *Elattaria cardamomum*

This herb is used mainly to aid digestion, although it does have a slight action on the lungs. It is a good herb to give to people who are feeling weak or to convalescents, and it will help increase the appetite. It is anti-spasmodic which makes it useful for any griping or cramping pains. It is also antiseptic and is good for putrefaction. Cardamon has a toning action on the nervous system. It will bring relief to headaches, especially those of a digestive origin. Cardamon seeds are a valuable spice and can be combined in a wide variety of foods and drinks. The seeds can also be chewed as a breath freshener.

SUGGESTED DOSAGE Use 2–4 crushed pods and seeds per cup of boiling water.

CARDAMON OIL This is distilled from the seeds and is a fragrant, spicy oil which is used mainly for digestive complaints or where a nervous condition affects the digestion. Dilute in a base oil and massage gently into the stomach area for flatulence or griping pains. Here it can be combined with Chamomile Oil or Aniseed Oil.

Cascara Sagrada *Rhamnus purshianus*

See Buckthorn.

Catnip *Nepeta cataria*

This remedy is particularly appropriate to give to young children with colds and flu. It helps chills and stomach upsets with diarrhoea. Being an anti-spasmodic herb, it will help colicky cramps and it is also known to have an effect on the respiratory system. It is good to give children with bronchitis and it can be combined with Aniseed for this. Catnip also has sedative properties, this makes it a relaxing herb.

SUGGESTED DOSAGE Infuse ½–1 tspful of herb per cup of boiling water. Drink 3 times a day.

Caulophyllum *Caulophyllum thalictroides*

See Blue Cohosh.

Causticum *Causticum*

Mental and emotional indications: This homoeopathic remedy suits the person who has a defeatist outlook, with feelings of hopelessness or a sense of impending disaster. They can be pessimistic, apprehensive, weepy and despair of any chance of recovery. They are afraid that something will happen, of the dark and twilight. They can be irritable, distrustful and absent-minded, they can sit quietly in a room paying no attention. They are sympathetic and easily upset by other people's suffering and get very concerned and worried about their own family and loved ones. They have a very low sexual drive. Ailments come on from grief, loss of sleep and anger. They are chilly people, with tears near to the surface; they often have a sallow, sickly look.

Physical symptoms: Causticum can really help where there is weakness or paralysis. It can be very good for multiple sclerosis, neuralgia, rheumatoid conditions and one-sided paralysis arising from exposure, e.g. from a car window being left open. There can be burning sensations, and vertigo, with a tendency to fall forwards or sideways which gets worse from lying down, stooping or during a period. There can be a sensation of space between the brain and the skull, and also paralysis of single areas, such as the face, voice, eyelids, throat or limbs. Causticum is a remedy for conditions that occur after cold winds. *Eyes*: Water in the open air, vision can become dim through paralysis in the optic nerve, there can be drooping eyelids, cataracts or tiny warts on the upper lids. *Respiratory symptoms*: There may be a loss of voice or a burning hoarseness in the morning, with rawness in the throat. There is an inability to raise phlegm, as it slips back. The expectoration can taste greasy. The chest is full of mucus. Involuntary urination when coughing. A hollow tickling cough brought on by cold air that improves by drinking cold water. *Stomach*: The person likes stimulants, e.g. coffee, tea, spicy food, etc, and can sit down to a meal feeling hungry but then the actual smell of food is upsetting. They can feel ravenous but then a little food makes them feel full. There's a desire for salt.

Abdomen: There can be paralysis in the rectum and constipation with no urge to pass a stool even when soft. There may be burning, stinging piles which get worse when touched or washed. Causticum is a remedy that is often given for cystitis. It is appropriate when symptoms are brought on by a cold or chill. There is only a small amount of urine passed, sometimes only after a long wait. There's involuntary urination on sneezing, laughing, coughing or sudden movement. It is a very good remedy to give after operations if a shooting pain occurs in the rectum when the person cannot urinate. *Skin*: It is a remedy for warts that bleed easily on the hands, nose, face and eyelids. It is excellent to give for second or third degree

231

burns, for burning pains and to help relieve continuing discomfort even after initial healing.

Causticum can be given for rheumatism which gets worse in the cold, dry weather and better from damp conditions. *Modalities*: Symptoms are made worse by cold, dry air and winds, in the evening, twilight and darkness, during extremes of temperature, changes of weather and between 2–4 a.m. They improve from damp, rainy, moist conditions, cold drinks, washing, the warmth of bed and gentle motion. This remedy is inimicable with Phosphorous: this means they do not work well together.

Cayenne *Capsicum minimum*

This is a very warming herb. It stimulates the circulation and it is very good where the hands and feet are often cold or where there is low blood pressure. It is good to take for colds and flu, and is generally stimulating for cold, apathetic, depressed states. This herb is said to increase the adrenal-cortico activity and corticosteroid production. It is possible that the implication of this is that it is immune-boosting, like Ginger. It will help with cases of flatulence and increase the appetite. It can also promote fertility in women where there are problems due to low body temperature: Cayenne increases the body temperature which allows ovulation to occur.

SUGGESTED DOSAGE Use only a small pinch, ⅛ – ¼ tspful, in a cup of boiling water and drink 3 times daily, or if the tincture is preferred, use 5–10 drops diluted in water, and take 3 times daily.

Celery Seed *Apium graveolens*

Celery Seed acts in 3 main areas: it is an alterative, a diuretic and a digestive herb. But it can be used as an uplifting nerve tonic which is especially good where anxiety and depression lead to insomnia. It is appropriately used where a nervous state accompanies at least one of these areas. As an alterative, Celery Seed affects the blood and cleanses the skin. It is good especially when the skin is itchy, as in urticaria or psoriasis, or if there is heat, as in acne. As a diuretic, it helps remove the uric acids from the blood and joints, and it is a good herb to use for gout, arthritis or gravel in the kidneys. Celery Seed helps the digestion, stimulates the appetite, calms the gut and lowers blood sugar. It also increases the flow of breast milk.

Important: Celery Seed is not appropriate to use where there is inflammation or infection, as in nephritis, for which it is contra-indicated. Also, it must not be used during pregnancy, as in the last 3 months it will make the full uterus contract, causing early labour. The plant, however, is perfectly safe to eat and it is mildly cleansing and diuretic.

SUGGESTED DOSAGE Take ½ tspful of seeds infused in a cup of boiling water 3 times daily, or 10–30 drops of tincture 3 times daily.

Chamomilla *Matricaria chamomilla*

See Chamomile.

Chamomile *Matricaria chamomilla*

This plant is extensively used and is a valuable remedy for a wide range of ailments. It has been used for centuries either as a herb or as an oil, and more recently as a homoeopathic remedy. It is easily cultivated and is now used widely as a tisane.

Homoeopathically, Chamomilla has a significant mental and emotional picture. *Mental and emotional indications*: The person who fits this remedy feels generally disturbed, often angry, irritable, dissatisfied, quarrelsome, excitable, nervous or obstinate. They dislike being touched, spoken to or even looked at. Children want to be carried. They may want something, then reject it, and exhibit general peevishness. Children needing Chamomilla will seem impossible. They will be oversensitive to pain so that it seems unbearable. Chamomilla treats ailments arising from anger, excitement or abuse of stimulants.

Physical symptoms: Marked by one cheek that is red and hot while the other is pale and cold, and great sensitivity to the open and to wind, which can lead to earache. Stools are green, like watery chopped spinach, with hot, offensive, sulphurous smells. Teething babies will often have hot, strong-smelling discharges. *Women's complaints*: Periods are excessive with dark clots, accompanied by

233

irritability, restlessness and nervousness. There may also be cramping pains in the uterus, which arise after being angry or before and during a period. Chamomilla is an excellent remedy to give in labour when pains are excessive and spasmodic. It is very good for the transition stage and at any time when the woman becomes abusive or extreme. During labour, give 200C and repeat as necessary. It is also good for afterpains. It is indicated for inflamed nipples which have become very tender and make breastfeeding painful. *Teeth*: Chamomilla is well known as a teething remedy. It is appropriate when one cheek is red or there is a spot on the cheek, and the child is restless and frantic. There may also be diarrhoea, which is often green. It is also a good remedy for toothache, which is worse from heat, hot food or hot drinks.

It can be used for insomnia that is caused by anger, stimulants or pain. There may also be crying or weeping during sleep. It is good for babies who suffer from colic at around 3 months old, and want to be carried. This may be accompanied by green stools. *Modalities*: Symptoms become worse from anger, teething, at night-time, from coffee, cold/damp air, wind, touch and being looked at; they improve by being carried, sweating and cold applications.

USING THE HERB
The fresh Chamomile plant contains matricine which turns to chamazulene when heated (the blueness in the oil is azulene). This is antiseptic. Although herbalists use Chamomile for its antiseptic, anti-spasmodic, anti-inflammatory, analgesic, carminative and vulnerary actions, it is also a herb that makes a pleasant drink known for its relaxing effects. In a medicinal dosage, it can be used for anxiety and tension which lead to insomnia or migraines. It contains bitters and is very good as a digestive as it has an anti-inflammatory, analgesic and calming effect on the system. It is especially good for indigestion and gastritis. Externally, it can be used as a mouthwash to help mouth infections or gingivitis. Use as an eyewash to soothe sore, puffy, sticky eyes. It can also be used to heal burns and wounds.

Chamomile is an emmenagogue and can help with painful periods, and together with its anti-spasmodic properties, it will help where there are spasms or colic. It is believed to increase the leucocyte count, so that it helps to combat infection. Chamomile tea is excellent to give to children; it can be sweetened with honey and given to help teething and digestive problems, especially when the child is fretting or sleepless.

SUGGESTED DOSAGE Use 1–2 tspfuls of herb per cup of boiling water 3 times daily, or take 2–4ml of tincture in water 3 times daily. For external use, make a stronger infusion using 4 tspfuls per cup of boiling water and strain well.

CHAMOMILE OIL *Matricaria chamomilla*
The Chamomile Oil used in aromatherapy is generally blue, due to the high content of azulene in it. It is viscous and its fragrance is even more concentrated and overpowering than the herb. It must be well diluted. When the oil becomes greenish and then brown oxidation has taken place. It can still be used but this is a sign that it is from a previous year's crop. As the healing properties of azulene are now attracting the interest of scientists, Chamomile is at last receiving medical recognition, even though it has been used for centuries.

One of the best ways of using Chamomile Oil is by putting 5–7 drops into a bath; in the evening, it will calm and relax you for sleep, but it will also help heal urinary or gynaecological infections or pains, e.g. cystitis, pre-menstrual tensions or vaginal pruritis. Using Chamomile Oil for massage can also prove very effective: rub gently on swollen joints or on the small of the back for menstrual cramps. For an all-purpose massage, it combines well with Lavender or Rose, especially where a soothing, sedating massage is required. Use 2–3 drops in a saucer of base oil for general massage. Chamomile Oil is probably the easiest form of Chamomile to include in an ointment base if desired (see page 184–8 for recipe). It can be one of the most effective ways of helping eczema and other skin conditions. It is very widely used in cosmetics for this reason.

Chickweed *Stellaria media*

This is a cooling and moistening herb which can be used internally and externally, and is appropriate particularly for the lungs, skin and joints. It is good for lung diseases, lung complaints, where there is hot, yellow phlegm, a loose cough or a very dry, hacking, hard cough. For these conditions it is useful to mix Chickweed with Borage and Elderflower. It is also very helpful for dry, cracked skin, as with eczema and psoriasis: for this, combine with Elderflower and Chamomile. It is a slightly diuretic herb which makes it cleansing of the whole system, and it is therefore helpful for rheumatism where the joints are hot and tender. Chickweed calms the heart, it can be given where there are palpitations, especially when these come on during tiredness. It is a very useful herb and known mostly as an external skin remedy. It can be put into ointments or made into strong infusions to be added to the bath.

SUGGESTED DOSAGE To make an infusion use 1 tspful of herb to a cup of boiling water.

China   *Chinchona officinalis*

This is a very good homoeopathic remedy for any weakness and debilitation which has developed after loss of vital fluids, such as blood, sweat and mucus. It is used to deal with the effects of long-term heavy discharges or recurrent fevers, such as malaria. It can be given after a long period of heavy, sweaty flu. *Mental and emotional indications*: Marked by touchiness, a tendency to over-react when stimulated, being nervous and excitable. China is indicated for artistic people who are refined and have a sense of beauty. They feel and think intensely and can be oversensitive to noise, colour and sound. They tend to be withdrawn and do not talk much, they are able to spot phoney sympathy. They have a very good imagination and they escape through their own fantasies. They find communication difficult so they try and avoid it and prefer to remain silent, or they are sarcastic and hurtful. Their feelings can be very strong, but they cannot talk and look at the person at the same time. They consider themselves ill-used, although they are very loyal. They tend to be opinionated, passively aggressive and self-sufficient. They do not appear to need approval, and tend to dislike parties. They may be afraid of animals, especially dogs.

Physical symptoms: China is a good remedy for exhaustion, especially nervous exhaustion where the nerves are on edge. It is good for nerve-based pains, such as neuralgia and sciatica which are worse when touched but better from firm pressure. *Digestion*: There is often a history of wasting and weight loss as a result of illness through poor digestion. There can be gallstones and gallstone colic. Also, bloating and fermentation which does not improve for passing wind. There is a desire to loosen clothing. There is very little appetite but after a mouthful of food they feel hungry, or there can be a sensation of fullness when only a little food has been eaten (compare with Lycopodium). There is a bitter taste to everything, even water. Symptoms get worse after meat or fish. There is swelling of the legs and the abdomen. There can be sleeplessness, but when they wake up it is as if they are still dreaming. *Chills*: May lead to a fever which causes heavy sweating. The person will feel thirsty when they are sweating, but not in the initial fever stage. There can be chilliness after flu, with weakness. The tongue is flabby and yellow-coated. Stools may be undigested and watery, but painless.

This is a good remedy to give to people who are anaemic and weak, especially those who have had a haemorrhage. *Abdomen*: It is good after operations if there are pains caused by wind. Use China when the abdomen is very distended and wind is stuck, with a sense of painful bloating. These symptoms improve with movement. It is good for colic which feels much worse through doubling-up, or for gas in the stomach that is accompanied by bitter or sour risings. Loud belching will not relieve any symptoms. *Modalities*: Symptoms get worse from losing vital fluids, from touch and from eating fruits. They improve with pressure from the hands.

Cina   *Artemisia maritima*

This is a good children's homoeopathic remedy. *Mental and emotional indications*: Marked by the child's apparent indifference to or dislike of being cuddled. They complain and are discontent and cross. They seem very touchy, are inclined to hit out and disinclined to play. They cannot bear being looked at or approached, although they may want to be carried. They want things but then reject them when they get them.

Physical symptoms: The face is pale and sickly with bluish-white around the mouth, dark rings around the eyes and dilated pupils. There is a marked tendency to pick the nose until it bleeds. The nose will itch and the child will rub its nose constantly. Cina is an excellent remedy for threadworms. There is a ravenous appetite and hunger soon after a meal, and a constant craving for sweets and bread. The child may develop a distended, hard abdomen and have twisting pains which are better with pressure, or there may be cutting, pinching pains from the worms, with an itchy anus. When a child has worms, it is good to give the remedy in 200C. Give one at night-time and one the following morning. (See pages 190–1 on homoeopathic dosage.) *Sleep*: Will be restless and there may be night terrors or crying out. The child may grind its teeth during sleep. *Modalities*: Symptoms are made worse by being touched or looked at, during sleep and appear to be worse at full moon. They improve with lying on the abdomen.

NATURAL HEALING FOR WOMEN

Citrus Oils

Information on Lemon Oil can be found under its own heading. Grapefruit Oil (Citrus paradisi), Sweet Orange Oil (Citrus auranticum) and Mandarin Oil (Citrus reticulata) are dealt together under Grapefruit Oil as they mainly act on the liver and gall bladder.

Clary Sage Oil *Salvia sclarea*

This oil gently stimulates and strengthens one's vitality as well as having a sedating effect. It is an excellent oil for treating disorders of the nervous system as it is sedating, anti-convulsive and regenerating. It is useful during convalescence, and in all forms of mental and physical debility, where the person has become weakened and depressed. It is appropriate in the treatment of postnatal depression and when recuperating from a breakdown. Clary Sage strengthens the kidneys and digestive system, and is particularly good for the female reproductive system. It strengthens a weak uterus, and is good for absent, scant or painful menses. It will also be helpful for asthma and cramps, and it lowers the blood pressure. Often Clary Sage can be used instead of Sage; it combines well with Jasmine, Geranium, Basil, Lavender, etc. Use 2–3 drops in a saucerful of base-massage oil.

Cleavers *Galium aperine*

The primary actions of this herb are on the lymphatic system and as a diuretic. It works by helping the lymph to flow and thereby draining the lymph nodes and stimulating the kidneys. Being a lymph-cleansing herb, this makes it good for skin problems where the circulation is sluggish and the skin looks lifeless and dirty. It is good for swollen glands – when the lymph glands are inflamed combine with Echinacea and Marigold. Take for ulcers and tumours, and combined with Nettles, it can be very effective as a spring tonic, or to accompany a cleansing diet. It can be taken internally or used externally as a poultice.

SUGGESTED DOSAGE Use 1–2 tspfuls of herb to 1 cup of boiling water, or 1–2 tspfuls of tincture in water, and drink 3 times daily.

Cloves   *Eugenia caryophyllata*

This is a pungent, aromatic and warming herb which calms the digestive tract, it will soothe wind and allay nausea. It will help stop putrefaction in the gut, and is also beneficial for the lungs. It is a good herb for people who feel cold and are prone to colds; it can be included in a mixture for children who are cold, weak and nauseous. Cloves can be used in cooking to add a spicy, warm flavour, or in a tea (see Ginger). It can be simmered in wine and it is refreshing and relaxing. The herb is also antiseptic and analgesic; it can be used locally on swellings and for pain in the gums and teeth. Because it can irritate or burn the skin, it may be preferable to put a Clove inside a ball of Marshmallow herb, soaked in water, to put next to the infected area.

SUGGESTED DOSAGE Use 2–3 Clove buds to a cup of boiling water.

CLOVE OIL
Use Clove Oil sparingly – only 0.5–1 per cent diluted in either a base oil or in combination with other oils: It can easily dominate any mixture. Combine with Eucalyptus, Lavender and Bergamot for a room spray: this is an excellent air freshener and the antiseptic properties will be good where there is sickness or a bad smell in a room. Use 2–3 drops of Clove Oil combined with 5–6 drops of Rosemary oil, in a warm bath for a soak that is stimulating and helpful for sluggishness, dullness or confusion. **Important**: This oil can cause irritation to the skin so before including it in an oil for massage test a small area of skin.

The oil can be used as an insect repellent and parasiticide. Mix with Lavender, Eucalyptus or Cedarwood and use in a base oil or in a room spray. To eliminate cat fleas, moths or mosquitos, we have used a Pyrethrum herb infusion with a couple of drops of Clove Oil as a spray, with effective results. It can also be used in a mixture to eliminate head lice (see Rosemary Oil). Clove Oil has a 'base' note, it is often used in perfumery to help hold a fragrance together.

Coccus Cacti   *Coccus cacti*

This is a good homoeopathic remedy to use where the bronchial tubes are full of mucus. *Physical symptoms*: There may be rawness of the air passages, or a sensation of a crumb or lump behind the larynx which causes coughing, and there is a desire to swallow constantly. *Coughs*: This remedy can be given for whooping cough. A child can be seized by violent fits of coughing ending in vomiting, or where clear, ropey mucus hangs in strings from the mouth. Attacks of coughing will come on at night-time with tickling in the larynx. This remedy can be considered for an early morning cough which starts off being dry and barking, and then brings up stringy mucus. Expectoration can be stringy, yellow or reddish. It is viscous and sour-tasting. The cough tends to come on more in a warm atmosphere and gets better in a cold room. *Modalities*: Symptoms get worse periodically, from heat, lying down, waking up, irritation of the throat, the slightest exertion, brushing teeth and rinsing the mouth. They improve in cold rooms, from washing in cold water, cold drinks and walking.

Coffea (Coffee) *Coffea canda*

Coffea is a homoeopathic remedy for insomnia that is caused by over-stimulation. If you are familiar with the effects of a strong cup of coffee, recognising the symptoms of Coffea should not be too difficult. There is a sense of exhilaration and excitement: the mind is restless, full of ideas and plans, the memory is alive, and so on. The symptoms can be brought on by the shock of good or exciting news. These types find it impossible to sleep. There is insomnia from sudden emotion – the person is wide awake and the body is overactive.

If you've been using homoeopathic remedies and you feel you have got in a muddle – you have tried too many different types and your body does not know how to react – then a couple of strong cups of coffee will probably antidote the previous couple of months' treatment.

Colocynthis *Citrullus colycynthis*

The main action of this homoeopathic remedy is on the abdominal area. It is excellent when ailments come on after anger, frustration, grief, humiliation or embarrassment; all these states are accompanied by a sense of indignation. *Mental and emotional indications*: Marked by restlessness and nervousness, and crying out from intense pain. There is a strong dislike of being questioned or being interfered with.

Physical symptoms: This remedy can work very well for abdominal pain which causes the person to double up. It is often indicated for babies with colic when they pull their legs up and the pains seem cutting and griping. An adult will clutch the area of pain or apply hard pressure to bring relief. It is good for colic which comes on after anger and is accompanied by vomiting or diarrhoea. Colocynthus is a good remedy for period pains where there are severe cramping pains in the uterus, and the menstrual flow is either early or suppressed. It is relieved by warmth (see also Mag Phos). Pains may be accompanied by dizziness when the head is turned to the left. Colocynthus can be used for sciatica where there are cramping pains in the hip; these are improved by lying on the painful side and by heat, and are made worse by movement. *Modalities*: Symptoms are worse from emotional states, especially anger, and at night. They improve with hard pressure, doubling up, heat and rest.

Coltsfoot *Tussilago farfara*

This is a popular herb to use for coughs, and to combine with other herbs into a syrup. The flowers and the leaves are used. It has anti-inflammatory, anti-spasmodic and expectorant actions. It is a very good respiratory tonic and can be used to relieve chronic lung conditions, for example emphysema and asthma, or to help coughs, e.g. a smoker's cough, nervous cough or dry cough in old people. It helps strengthen the lungs. It combines with Thyme, Plantain and Elecampane to help keep infections away and to reduce or prevent mucus from forming, as in asthma.

SUGGESTED DOSAGE: Infuse ½ tspful of herb in a cup of boiling water and drink 3 times a day, or with a tincture dilute 1ml in water and take 3 times a day.

Comfrey *Symphytum officinale*

As a homoeopathic remedy, Symphytum is one of the main remedies to treat broken bones and to use in cases when fractures do not mend. It will help accelerate the union. It is a great remedy to give for wounds which penetrate the periosteum (the membrane that covers the surface of the bones) and for damaged sinews, tendons, cartilages and joints. It is also one of the best remedies for eye injuries, especially when the injury has been caused by a blow or knock or there is damage to the eyeball from a blunt instrument. *Modalities*: Symptoms are worse from being touched.

USING THE HERB

Both the leaves and the roots of Comfrey can be used. This well-known herb contains allantoin which makes it excellent for healing, and it is one of the few plants that contains Vitamin B12. The main actions are as a demulcent, astringent and expectorant. Comfrey can be used internally to heal gut problems, stomach ulcers and lung complaints where there is bleeding. It helps the capillary action in the lungs. The demulcent and expectorant actions can help respiratory problems by soothing and healing irritations in the tract, and it can be taken to heal damaged connective tissue in the body. But Comfrey can also be applied externally, either as a poultice, tincture or macerated oil, to heal fractures, sprains, strains, pulled muscles or back strain. It promotes or regulates the overgrowth of skin tissue, so it can be used very effectively for psoriasis and skin ulcers, and to help clear bruises and heal scar tissue. It helps relieve inflammation caused by gout and rheumatic joints.

Comfrey promotes rapid healing. It is best to use it on shallow rather than deep wounds, as the surface tissue may heal more quickly than the tissue below. This herb contains pyrrozolidine alkaloids which in very large doses can cause liver damage. It has been given in large doses to certain animals which then grew liver tumours, but taken in a normal, general dose this herb is a very effective healer.

SUGGESTED DOSAGE Infuse 1 tspful of dried herb in a cup of boiling water, or 1ml tincture in water, 3 times daily. With a poultice it is probably best to use the powdered root. See the section on macerated oils on how to make the oil (pages 186–7).

Cornsilk *Zea mays*

This herb contains allantoin which is healing and anti-inflammatory, especially on the urinary tract. Cornsilk also contains three indigestible sugars and they act as an osmotic diuretic. It is a demulcent herb which makes it soothing for all urinary conditions: it is good for cystitis and any inflammations, for example nephritis. The silica in it helps to give tone to the bladder and the prostrate gland. It is an excellent herb to help treat frequency of urination and prostatitis.

SUGGESTED DOSAGE Infuse 1–2 tspfuls of herb per cup of boiling water and drink 3 times daily, or use 1–2ml of tincture diluted in water and take 3 times a day.

Couchgrass   *Agropyrum repens*

Couchgrass is a diuretic herb. It is rich in silica, as is Cornsilk, and can be used similar in ways (see above). It is useful for infections such as prostatitis, and also helps tone the bladder. It soothes cystitis and is good to combine with Marshmallow herb, especially when the urine is dark and gritty. Couchgrass can be added to skin-cleansing mixtures as it helps eliminate toxins from the blood.

SUGGESTED DOSAGE It is necessary to make a decoction as it is the rhizome of the plant that is used. Use ½–1 tspful per cup of water, bring to the boil and allow to simmer for a few minutes before cooling and drinking; this can be taken 3 times a day. With a tincture, dilute ½–1ml in some water and take 3 times a day.

Crampbark *and* Black Haw   *Viburnum opulus* and *Viburnum prunifolium*

These two herbs have very similar actions. The main difference being that Black Haw is more specifically indicated for treating female pelvic organs, although Crampbark can also be used in the same way. They were both traditionally used by the Native Americans; Black Haw being a favourite for women's complaints. They contain a bitter glycoside, viburnin and also valerianic acid. The latter contributes to the herbs' relaxing properties and together they help to release tension in the smooth muscle (see Vitex for explanation).

These herbs can be taken for painful periods or dysmenorrhoea. They can relieve any tension and will be particularly helpful for women who work under pressure and tend to get cramping and much pain during periods. Also, for those who are run down and have scanty, pale periods, especially resulting from stress and irritability. Combined with False Unicorn Root, these herbs will help threatened miscarriages. They will help with labour contractions that are too strong, particularly when they are associated with tension, resistance and fear. Also, combine with Valerian for general stress and anxiety, cramping of tendons, spasms and nervous asthma. It is best to take these herbs on a regular basis and continue for the duration of three cycles for menstrual problems.

SUGGESTED DOSAGE Take 1–2ml of tincture, diluted, 3–4 times a day. Depending on the severity of the painful periods or dysmenorrhoea, take 3–5ml of diluted tincture every 20–30 mins.

Crataegus   *Crataegus monogyna*

See Hawthorn.

Cypress Oil   *Cypressa sempervirens*

This is one of the best oils for the circulation, it is astringent and refreshing. It will be useful whenever there are relaxed veins, e.g. varicose veins and broken capillaries, and it is one of the main essential oils for treating haemorrhoids. It can be combined with Ginger and massaged on the hands and feet to treat circulatory disorders, especially chilblains. Its astringent properties make Cypress an important remedy for the treatment of excessive discharges, hot and burning diarrhoea, frequent urination, and most forms of haemorrhage, including nosebleeds. It has a toning effect on uterine and pelvic tissues and can be used to treat heavy, prolonged and inter-menstrual discharges. It can also help with any menopausal problems.

Cypress is a good oil to use on its own or combined with other oils, for treating oily, loose or wrinkled skin. It also checks perspiration, so that it is good to add to foot baths to deal with smelly feet. It has a strong anti-spasmodic effect and can be used for the treatment of any spasmodic cough, asthma and whooping cough. It combines well with Lavender, and a good recipe for varicose veins consists of 3 drops of Lavender, 3 drops of Cypress, 1 drop of Ginger and 1 drop of Rosemary, combined in a saucerful of base-massage oil.

Daisy   *Bellis perennis*

This homoeopathic remedy is a kindred one to Arnica, Hypericum and Calendula. It is chiefly used for the effects of accidents, sprains and bruises. It is good to use where muscles have become sore and bruised after heavy work. It can be especially effective for elderly people, for those who have difficulty getting well or suffer from drinking cold drinks after being overheated. *Physical symptoms*: Use Bellis Perennis for injuries to the back or slipped discs, after major surgical operations, injuries or blows to the breasts and where tumours develop from injuries.

The indication for this remedy is tiredness; the patient wants to lie down. The joints and muscles feel sore. There are pains down the thighs and the wrists feel contracted, as if held by elastic bands. This remedy is good to use during pregnancy where there is difficulty in walking and the uterus can feel sore and squeezed. Waking up early can be an indication of Bellis Perennis, but it is also known that giving this remedy in the evening can cause waking at 3 a.m. It is therefore a good idea to give it during the day. *Modalities*: Symptoms feel worse from touch, cold bathing, cold drinks, becoming chilled after being hot, hot baths, a warm bed and surgical operations. They improve from continued motion and cold applications.

USING THE HERB
As a herb the daisy can be made into an infusion or combined with other herbs, to use after childbirth to help restore muscle tone or after a blow to the pelvic area. It is good to use where there is menstrual flooding. It is a cleansing, uplifting, freshening herb to use. It would be worth adding to a cleansing, restorative bath after being abused, or bruising to the generative area.

SUGGESTED DOSAGE Use 1 tspful of herb to 1 cup of boiling water. Use 30g (1oz) placed in a muslin bag in a hot bath of running water.

Damiana   *Turnera difusa*

This herb can be used as a general tonic, it is good for low spirits and sluggishness. It has a strengthening action on the genito-urinary tract, and its mild antiseptic properties keep the tract in good order. It also has a strengthening effect on the nervous system, and it is

245

thymoleptic (lifts moods). Together these actions make it a possible aphrodisiac, especially for men – being weak and depressed can undermine the libido and this herb should lift spirits and relieve depression.

SUGGESTED DOSAGE Take 1ml of tincture diluted in water 3 times a day, or infuse the herbs in a cup of boiling water and take 3 times a day.

Dandelion   *Taraxacum officinale*

The root, leaves or flowers can be used and all are rich in vitamins and minerals. The main vitamins are A, B, and C (carotene). It contains up to 5 per cent potassium, and a bitter glycoside, taraxacin, which is found in the leaves in the spring and in the root in the early autumn. This will increase bile production fourfold. Dandelion also contains tannins – one of which, Inulin, increases by 40 per cent in the root in autumn. There are enzymes in the whole plant that activate kidney and liver secretions and functioning. The leaves are reputedly more diuretic and the root has a stronger action on the liver, but both parts of the Dandelion have properties in both areas. Most diuretics cause the body to lose potassium but because of the high content of the mineral in Dandelion, this does not happen. It is especially useful where there is oedema (fluid retention), a heart problem or bloating from pre-menstrual tension. Dandelion does not seem to have a diuretic action on healthy people.

Dandelion stimulates the general metabolism, aids cell respiration and is particularly good as a spring tonic. It can be put in a mixture for all liver and gall bladder disorders. It will help with sluggish digestion, digestive headaches, piles, constipation and acne (where the liver is involved). It is good for diabetes, because it helps the pancreas to work more efficiently, and for rheumatoid arthritis, gout and kidney disorders. Dandelion can be used for mastitis – combine with Poke Root and Marigold.

SUGGESTED DOSAGE Use 1 tspful decocted in a cup of boiling water 3 times daily; as a tincture, use 1ml in water 3 times daily. It is worth remembering that once the root has been roasted into 'coffee', its effects are greatly weakened.

Dill *Anethum graveolens*

This has similar properties to Aniseed and Fennel, and it combines well with both. It aids digestion and is particularly good to give to babies with colic. It is also very useful for flatulence. It stimulates the production of milk in nursing mothers, and the seeds can be chewed to freshen the breath.

SUGGESTED DOSAGE Infuse ½–1 tspful in a cup of boiling water and take 3 times a day. For a baby, make very weak tea using ¼ tspful of seeds to 60–120ml (2–4fl oz) of water and give in a bottle.

Drosera *Drosera rotundifolia*

Physical symptoms: This is a good homoeopathic remedy for whooping cough or other violent, rapid coughs. Several coughs may follow, one from another, which end up with a whooping noise as the person runs out of breath and tries to inhale. The person may rest for a few minutes and then the cough will start up again. It can be deep, barking, choking and incessant. It can end up with gagging, choking and vomiting. Food will be vomited. The child holds the stomach as it hurts so much from coughing. There may be a red, congested face from the effort of coughing. They feel exhausted. Tickling in the throat can promote the cough. Although the cough may not be very noticeable during the day, as soon as the head touches the pillow at bedtime it can become constant, with gagging and vomiting. *Modalities*: Symptoms get worse at midnight, from lying down, getting warm in bed, singing, drinking and laughing.

Echinacea (Purple Coneflower) *Echinacea angustifolia* or *Echinacea purpurea*

In order to understand the value of Echinacea it is probably worth explaining how it works. Cells are 'glued' together with the help of hyaluronic acid. The cocci bacteria, such as in staphylococci and Streptococci, produce hyaluronidase which dissolves the 'glue', thus allowing the bacteria to infiltrate the cell membrane or cell wall. Echinacea has an active constituent which neutralises the hyaluronidase and stops the bacteria from spreading, leaving the white blood corpuscles to deal with the infection locally. Cell membranes have receptor sites to which viruses attach themselves and gain control. Echinacea has molecules which block the receptor sites so that viruses cannot become attached. It can be used prophylactically, for example use Echinacea where it is thought that an infection caused by an injury may spread. It will also increase the activity of the immune system by activating the coding of T-cells.

Echinacea is also anti-fungal. Take for thrush, ringworm and athlete's foot. Its main uses are for pustular infections of the skin or elsewhere. It can also be used for viral infections, both as a preventative measure and as a cure. It is worth bearing in mind that although Echinacea can be used for a whole range of complaints and ailments, it is better to take the specific remedy. For example, it may help colds and flu, but Elderflower, Peppermint or Yarrow may be more appropriate.

SUGGESTED DOSAGE Simmer 30g (1oz) to 570ml (1 pint) of water for 20 mins for a decoction and drink a cup 3 times a day, or take 1ml of the tincture in water 3 times a day; with an acute infection, take every 2–3 hours.

Elderflower *Sambucus nigra*

Elderflower is a really lovely herb to use. It is known mainly as a pleasant drink which comes in the form of either a tisane or, traditionally, a country wine or champagne. It is one of the main diaphoretic herbs (encourages perspiration and elimination of toxins). It is also anti-catarrhal and diuretic. It acts on the skin, lungs and the kidneys. It is excellent to use for colds and flus: combine with Peppermint and Yarrow for a pleasant and effective mixture. It helps strengthen the chest against infection. It can be used for coughs and catarrh of the upper respiratory tract. Use also where there is deafness caused by catarrh. Being a diaphoretic herb, it can be given for eruptive fevers, especially where the lungs are involved, for example in measles or chickenpox when the infection affects the chest. An Elderflower infusion or using Elderflower water is very soothing on the skin. It can help calm inflammation. It contains rutin which strengthens the capillaries. Elderberries are nutritious and are a laxative; these are best infused and drunk when they are hot.

SUGGESTED DOSAGE Infuse 1 tspful of the herb per cup of boiling water, or take 1–2ml of tincture in hot water. Take either every 2–4 hours.

Elecampane   *Inula helenium*

This has antiseptic, anti-spasmodic and expectorant properties. It is also bitter, and because of the helenin in the essential oil contained in the plant, it has a strong anthelminthic action (kills parasites). It is an excellent herb to take for chronic lung conditions where there is weakness and lack of appetite. Use for asthma and whooping cough. It is a refreshing herb and a good tonic and can be given to children. It is said to have an effect on the mental state by encouraging a feeling of positiveness and receptiveness.

SUGGESTED DOSAGE Take 1–2ml of tincture diluted in water 3 times daily. A decoction can be made by using 1 tspful of the root to a cup of water, brought to the boil and simmered for a few minutes. Drink 3 times daily.

Equisetum   *Equisetum arvense*

See Horsetail.

Eucalyptus Oil   *Eucalyptus globulus* and *Eucalyptus citriodora*

This oil is widely produced. The most popular variety used is *Eucalyptus globulus*. It has a notable reputation for being strongly antibiotic and it is also said to strengthen the immune system. It is good to use on the chest and ribs where there is white phlegm and the person is feeling cold or chilly. It can be used in a steam inhalation for coughs and colds, it is a good expectorant and is excellent for helping all conditions of the respiratory tract. Use for rheumatism where symptoms are worse from cold, damp conditions, or for cystitis brought on by a chill. Eucalyptus is a very drying oil and is good to combine with Fennel for digestive infections, or with Aniseed for coughs, etc. If you wish to use Eucalyptus as a massage oil it is probably best to try *Eucalyptus citriodora*, a variety which has a slightly less cooling action than *globulus* but has more anti-spasmodic properties. This oil has a lemony smell but is strong and must be used sparingly. Use 1 drop in a mixture. Either oil is good to use in a room spray as a disinfectant.

Eupatorium Perf *Eupatorium perfoliatum*

See Boneset.

Euphrasia *Euphrasia officinalis*

See Eyebright.

Eyebright *Euphrasia officinalis*

Euphrasia is the main homoeopathic remedy for the eyes. *Physical symptoms*: Include a redness of the eyeball, with a marked sensitivity to light, and profuse watering from eyes and nose. The secretion from the eyes is acrid and burning but it is bland from the nose. The eyes may water constantly, the margins of the lids can be red, swollen and burning and feel as though there is a hair in the eye, and there is a constant need to wipe them. They may burn, smart and feel itchy. This can be accompanied by a dimness of vision and a sense of contraction in the eyelids, or twitching.

Euphrasia is good for tired eyes, where they feel as though there is something in them or there is in fact something there. Take for conjunctivitis and for the first stage of measles. Also, for hayfever where there is a lot of sneezing and tears. Use for colds where the eyes are very watery and the nose is streaming. Euphrasia is also excellent for sticky eyes where there is a thick, yellow, acrid discharge. Use for cases of whooping cough when there are excessive tears accompanying the cough during the day-time. The picture for Euphrasia is similar to Pulsatilla for eye conditions. The headache is bursting, there is catarrh and discharge from the eyes and nose. There can be very painful periods which only last one hour per day.

USING THE HERB

Herbalists use Eyebright either internally or externally. It can work as a tea to help strengthen eye muscles; it can also work on the eyes generally, as well as on the upper respiratory tract. It is good for congested catarrhal conditions and is an antiseptic for glue ear (deafness), sinusitis, hayfever and runny colds. Externally, use as an eyewash for its antiseptic, soothing and healing properties.

SUGGESTED DOSAGE Use 1ml of tincture diluted in water, or 1 tspful of herb infused in 1 cup of boiling water. For external use, 2–3 drops of tincture in an egg cup of freshly boiled cool water.

False Unicorn Root *Chamaelirium luteum*

This has an oestrogenic effect (Vitex being progesteronal). It is often given in combination with Vitex and is good for all weaknesses of the uterus. It is good for prolapses and discharges, particularly for cold, white discharges. It is also good for weak ligaments and dragging pains. It is safe to use in pregnancy and is good for morning sickness and for threatened miscarriage. It is a uterine tonic and can be taken for growing pains in pregnancy, and can be combined with Raspberry Leaf. False Unicorn Root is a balancer of the uterus lining, the endometrium, so it may be helpful for women who suffer from infertility that is caused by weakness of the womb or endometriosis. It can also be given for infertility that is caused by anovulation. Tired, debilitated women with backache or who feel fed up or gloomy will benefit from this herb.

SUGGESTED DOSAGE Take 1ml (25 drops) of tincture in water 1–3 times a day. If you are using this as a herb, which is hard and woody, make a decoction by using 30g (1oz) to 570ml (1 pint) of water and take a tbsp per day.

Fennel Seeds *Foeniculum vulgare*

This is an excellent calming and anti-spasmodic herb for the digestive system. It helps expel wind from the gut (carminative) and is a mild laxative. It is good for constipation that is caused by tension and

251

is milder than Crampbark. It is often used in combination with Crampbark and Liquorice. It has mild diuretic properties. Make up a pleasant mixture to ease spasms in the intestinal tract consisting of: equal parts of Aniseed, Orange Peel, Chamomile and Fennel Seeds. Use 1 tspful of mixture per cup of boiling water and drink after meals. An infusion could be used in a foot bath for hot swollen ankles and feet. Fennel is also an expectorant, although it is milder than Aniseed; it can be combined in a mixture for coughs.

A tea made up of the herb is excellent for nursing mothers and helps milk production; it can also help with colic in babies (give a very weak infusion). Chewing Fennel Seeds after a meal aids digestion and before a meal reduces the appetite. They can also be chewed to freshen the breath. An infusion of Fennel Seeds can be used as an eyewash to help conjunctivitis.

SUGGESTED DOSAGE Use 1 tspful of crushed seeds to a cup of boiling water and infuse for 10 mins. Take 3 times daily.

FENNEL OIL *Foeniculum dulce*
This oil can be taken for slow digestion and constipation, or where there is swelling in the stomach or abdomen. It can be combined with Aniseed or Chamomile, diluted in a base oil, and massaged gently into the lower abdomen. A few drops can be added to a bath or foot bath for any swollen, bloated conditions; or combine with Cypress, Juniper and Lavender in a base oil and massage into rheumatic joints.

Fenugreek *Trigonella foenum graecum*

This herb contains steroidal saponins, including diosgenin. It can be used mainly to increase milk production and is reputed to increase breast development. It is a bitter and can aid digestion and absorption. It will strengthen the body and can help if you need to put on weight. It is useful for convalescents and diabetics. You can use Fenugreek as a poultice to heal boils, cuts and fistulas.

SUGGESTED DOSAGE Use 1 tspful per cup of boiling water and drink 3 times daily, or with a tincture take 1–2ml in water 3 times daily.

Ferrum Phos   *Ferrum phosphate*

This is a homoeopathic tissue salt found in the blood which carries oxygen to all parts of the body. It is a very useful remedy for the first stage of an illness, before any discharge starts. It is good for anaemia, inflammation and fever. *Mental and emotional indications*: These people are talkative, excited and oversensitive, with alternating moods. There is weakness of memory, forgetfulness and anxiety about the future. Loss of courage and hope. Sadness, listlessness and depression.

Physical symptoms: The person feels much better with sleep. *Head*: This is the remedy when the head feels dull and heavy on the top, with pains which feel as if a nail is being driven in on one side. Hammering pains that are worse on the right side and feel better with nosebleeds and cold pressure. Ferrum Phos is good for children's headaches when they also have red eyes and a red face. *Eyes*: These are inflamed, red and with a burning sensation, as if there is dust under the eyelid. *Ears*: The remedy is good for the first stage of an ear infection, inflamed ears, radiating pains, and pulsating, chronic catarrh of the middle ear.

Nose: Take Ferrum Phos for the first stage of all colds. It is good for the person who catches colds easily and has nosebleeds, especially for children when the blood is bright red. There is congestion of the mucous membrane similar to Aconite. *Throat*: This is sore, dry, red, inflamed with much pain; an ulcerated throat. *Digestion*: There is vomiting of bright red blood or undigested food, and the stomach aches. Ferrum Phos can be a good remedy for haemorrhoids that are inflamed and bleeding bright red blood. *Respiratory symptoms*: It is good for the first stage of all inflammatory respiratory conditions: bronchitis, painful tickly cough, hard, dry cough with soreness in the lungs, croup, loss of voice with hoarseness. *Women's complaints*: Take for profuse periods that are painful with bright red blood, and for anaemia (combine with Calc Phos for this).

Use Ferrum Phos for fevers where the face is flushed and the skin is hot and dry. There is a quick, full pulse, they are thirsty and there is pain and redness. It is also good for haemorrhages from any part of the body when the blood is bright red. Other symptoms of Ferrum Phos are right-sided shoulder pains, a bruised soreness of the chest, shoulders and surrounding muscles. It is better to give this remedy in the morning. *Modalities*: Symptoms get worse at night, especially between 4–6 a.m., from suppressed sweat, from touch and movement. They

253

improve with cold applications, from lying down and from bleeding.

Feverfew *Chrysanthemum parthenium*

This is a popular remedy for migraines. It can be effective for those that are associated with digestion or caused by foods that upset the system. It is an anti-inflammatory herb and is good for arthritis or an aching face. It can help with dizziness, tinnitus, painful and sluggish periods and hot flushes. It is also an anti-spasmodic and can be taken for wheezy coughs. This herb is an emmenogogue and therefore contra-indicated in pregnancy. Use Feverfew in an infusion as chewing the leaves can cause mouth ulcers. It is perhaps worth pointing out that Feverfew appears to work symptomatically, so that symptoms tend to return although they may be relieved for the duration of the pain or discomfort.

SUGGESTED DOSAGE Infuse 1 tpsful of the herb in one cup of boiling water and drink 3 times daily, or dilute 1ml of tincture in water and take 3 times daily.

Figwort *Scrophularia nodosa*

This is primarily a lymphatic and liver cleanser. It has the effect of cleaning the whole system which makes it very good for hot, itchy skin complaints. It has laxative and diuretic properties as well. Figwort is contra-indicated in tachycardia (where the heart beat is rapid).

SUGGESTED DOSAGE Infuse 1 tspful of herb to a cup of boiling water and drink 3 times a day, or take 1ml of tincture diluted in water 3 times a day.

Frankincense *Boswellia thurifera*

See Olibanum.

Fringetree Bark *Chionanthus virginica*

This herb has a stimulating effect on the liver, it increases the bile production and helps the gall bladder to store and secrete it. This means that Fringetree Bark can help where digestion of fats is a problem. It is a laxative herb, especially where there is nausea and biliousness accompanying constipation. It is a good general tonic for liverish people, and is a specific for inflammation of the gall bladder and for gallstones. It is a good herb to use to help with skin problems where there is poor liver function.

SUGGESTED DOSAGE Take ½–2 ml of tincture in water 3 times daily.

Fumitory *Fumaria officinalis*

This herb specifically helps relax spasms of the bile duct and colic of the gall bladder. It has a cleansing action on the liver, and is good for skin problems, such as eczema and acne, when the condition is related to a poorly-functioning liver.

SUGGESTED DOSAGE Infuse ½ tspful of herb to a cup of boiling water and drink 3 times daily, or dilute 10 drops of tincture in water and take 3 times daily.

Garlic *Allium sativum*

This is one of the most well-known and well-used medicinal herbs. It must have a strong, pungent odour to be effective. It is known to become inactive with charcoal. Garlic is highly antiseptic and anti-viral: these properties, together with its anti-spasmodic and diaphoretic (induces sweating) actions, make it excellent for lung infections and any spasmodic complaint of the lungs – coughs, whooping cough, asthma, etc. It also helps colds and catarrhal conditions. It is a cholagogue (increases flow of bile into the duodenum) so that it helps to tone the gut. It is especially good for elderly people with a sluggish digestion, and it will actively deter amoebic dysentery. It is a highly effective detoxifying agent and acts to prevent lead poisoning.

Use Garlic for rheumatic complaints. It also protects the arteries against the build up of fats (atheroma) and also arteriosclerosis. It helps to lower blood pressure and prevents high cholesterol levels. Use Garlic crushed and diluted for wounds to fight infection. Apparently this was very successful during the 1914–18 war. It is also anti-fungal so it can be used on ringworm or athlete's foot, or for parasites such as scabies. Apply daily on acute infections for the duration of the problem. Where there is a chronic condition, Garlic should be taken internally every day. Some people believe it is very beneficial to place a clove of Garlic in the anus. It certainly deters worms but remember to leave the skin of the clove on otherwise it will burn you. If you need an example of how what goes onto the skin goes into the body, rub a crushed clove of Garlic onto the sole of your foot – within 20 minutes you can smell it on your breath.

SUGGESTED DOSAGE Take 1–3 fresh cloves daily or take fresh juice or Garlic capsules.

Gelsemium   *Gelsemium*

The keynote of this homoeopathic remedy is weakness. Everything is depressed, there is physical weakness, a lack of vitality and the mind is constantly cloudy, unable to think or fix its attention. There is weakness in reaction to stimuli, the person is inclined to be hysterical, confused, dazed, apathetic, slow to answer and brooding. It is an anticipatory remedy which is good for stage fright when the legs tremble and feel like jelly, or when the knees go weak in labour. It can be used for fear that has a particular past association and creates trembling. *Mental and emotional indications*: The person is pathetic in their weakness. They are easily influenced, e.g by the weather or passive sympathy. They do not want to do anything about their state. They get tired very easily. Worry can bring on extreme weakness and so can drugs, flu or colds.

Physical symptoms: These are felt especially in the legs. The central nervous system is affected. The person will tremble, and experience spasms and use the wrong words. *Head*: The eyelids feel heavy, vision becomes blurred and there are headaches which feel better after urinating. The headaches are associated with catarrh, periods or emotional upsets. They are mostly at the back of the head but then they move forward to over the eyes. The tongue feels thirsty and dirty, there are irregular heart beats, palpitations and feelings that the heart will stop if they keep still. *Flu*: Gelsemium is the number one flu remedy when there is a hot, flushed face and a heavy feeling. The onset is slow and accompanied by severe aching pains. There is stiffness in the cervical region of the neck, aching in all the muscles and shivers run up and down the spine. Also this is a remedy for those who have never fully recovered from a bout of flu. *Modalities*: Symptoms get worse with emotional stress, shock, dread, ordeals, in humid, cold, damp weather and in the heat of the sun. They improve with alcohol, shaking, sweating and urination.

Geranium Oil *Pelargonium graveolens*

This sweet-smelling oil has a cooling, moistening, regulating effect. It is beneficial for the nervous system and is particularly appropriate for restlessness, hot flushes and states of anxiety. It can be well combined with Bergamot, Melissa or Rose. It has a calming and cooling effect on the heart which make it useful in the treatment of tachycardia, palpitations and panic attacks. It will be particularly good for those who wake in the night feeling hot, clammy and having palpitations. The oil is a good tonic for the liver and kidneys, and it also has a stimulating effect on the lymph system. It helps prevent the build up of cellulite, and is generally a very good oil for skin care because it is anti-inflammatory. It is good for dry skin and eczema, but it is also slightly astringent and can be used to restore the balance in skin which over-produces sebum. Geranium Oil has analgesic and haemostatic (stops bleeding) properties and it is good to combine in a wash, either for the skin or mouth.

Geranium Oil is a hormone-balancing oil with oestrogenic properties. Use during the menopause and for PMT. It combines well with Rose, or can be used as a replacement. Geranium Oil is a valuable oil to use in massage-oil blends: suggestions are Lavender, citrus oils, Juniper, Rosemary. Use 2–3 drops in a saucerful of base-massage oil.

Ginger *Zingiber officinale*

This is a warming, stimulating herb which is especially good for the circulation in the hands and feet: it helps treat deadness, cramping and chilblains. It warms the digestive system, although the extra heat may be difficult for someone who has an irritable stomach and suffers from acid or heartburn. Ginger will help to calm wind and is good for nausea, especially in pregnancy and travel sickness. It is a diaphoretic herb (induces sweating) and can be used for colds and fevers. It is also toning and it builds up resistance. The Chinese regularly use Ginger in cooking.

SUGGESTED DOSAGE For nausea take 2–3 drops of tincture in water when needed; to improve circulation take 15g (½oz) to 570ml (1 pint) of water and drink 3 times daily, or in tincture form use 10ml per week diluted in water. A very warming and delicious tea can be made by boiling Ginger, Cinnamon and Cloves for a few minutes, then using the water to make tea as usual. For a cold, add some crushed Ginger to lemon and honey for a very pleasant and helpful drink.

GINGER OIL
This warming oil can be used for the same symptoms as the herb; it can be diluted in a base oil and massaged over the kidney area and spinal column to help weak and cold people. It is especially good in winter and can be massaged into the extremities to help circulation. Combine with other oils such as Lavender or Juniper for stiffness, sprains and rheumatic pains. A few drops of Ginger Oil in the bath, with extra crushed Ginger root, is very warming.

Glonoine *Glonoine*

The keynote of this homoeopathic remedy is quick, violent and bursting pain. *Physical symptoms*: It acts on the circulation and is good to give for violent pulsations and a sense of the blood rushing upwards. It is an effective remedy for sunstroke. *Head*: Feels enormous, as if the skull is too small for the brain. There are waves of bursting, throbbing, pounding, pulsating pain, as if blood were rushing to the head. The terrible pain gets worse in the sun, and improves with vomiting. The pain will tend to increase and decrease as the sun moves higher and lower in the sky. The person holds their head, the throbbing pain sychronises with the pulse, the head throbs with every movement, the veins of the temple are swollen. There is complete intolerance of heat near the head. This remedy can be given for headaches which occur before or after the period or take the place of the period. There may be violent palpitations and throbbing in the

258

ears. It is a remedy to give for nosebleeds that are the result of the heat of the sun. The face may look flushed and hot, or blueish, with the jaws clenched. There may be nausea and vomiting. *Modalities*: Symptoms get worse from heat, movement, jarring and suppressed menses; they improve in the open air, when lifting the head up and cold applications.

Golden Rod   *Solidago virgaurea*

This plant has beautiful yellow flowers, it is appropriate that it can be used to relieve all cold conditions. It is good for people who feel the cold and get colds and flu easily, or are prone to phlegmy conditions, have poor digestion and often suffer from wind. It can also help with cystitis, especially when it occurs as a result of being worn out and run down.

SUGGESTED DOSAGE Infuse 1 tspful of herb with a cup of boiling water and take 3 times a day, or 1 tspful of tincture diluted in water 3 times daily.

Golden Seal   *Hydrastis canadensis*

This herb is powerfully anti-microbial and antiseptic. Its main action is through its alkaloids and there are three main ones: hydrastin, berberine and canadin. There is also a trace of volatile oil. Its cooling and astringent action makes it good for hot, yellow conditions. It acts as a uterine tonic by increasing circulation to the uterus, and can be given for heavy periods, with Shepherd's Purse, for its toning action. Golden Seal stimulates the uterus to contract, so it can be given to encourage labour, but obviously it must not be taken during pregnancy. It is also good for thick, yellow, burning leucorrhoea. It is a good herb for piles and varicose veins, especially where they are inflamed or bleeding. It can be used for catarrhal or infected conditions of the respiratory tract, such as bronchitis or sinusitis, or where there is inflammation. Combine with Echinacea, Plantain and Eyebright for this.

Golden Seal is a bitter herb and therefore it stimulates the liver and digestive system. It is a good herb for jaundice or a swollen liver, e.g. hepatitis. It can be used for loss of appetite, indigestion

259

and constipation. It is a laxative but can also be used for watery, mucousy diarrhoea. It is known to help peptic ulcers or where the mucous lining of the gut needs toning. This is a harsh herb and needs to be used with caution. It also raises blood pressure, so do not use it where there is a history of high blood pressure. Externally, Golden Seal can be made into a very effective lotion: use for ringworm, oozing eczema or any infected skin condition. Do not use on dry skin conditions because of its drying properties.

SUGGESTED DOSAGE Use 10–30 drops of tincture in water 3 times a day or drink ½–1 tspful of powdered root in a cup of hot water, left to infuse for 10–15 mins, 3 times a day.

Grapefruit Oil, Sweet Orange Oil *and* Mandarin Oil *Citrus paradisi, Citrus auranticum* and *Citrus reticulata*

These three oils mainly act on the liver and gall bladder. They are useful when the liver is sluggish and this leads to feelings of discomfort on the right side, where there is nausea and a bitter taste in the mouth. They work on the stomach and can be massaged onto the area for belching, a swollen stomach or where the digestion is slow and there are burning sensations. **Sweet Orange Oil** works on the intestines, it helps with bloating in the lower abdomen and can be combined with Fennel for colic and constipation. **Mandarin Oil** has a warming action on the intestine, and because it is more astringent, it is better for diarrhoea. It can also be used as an expectorant and it is good for coughs. It has a sedating effect and can help aid sleep if there is restlessness. **Grapefruit Oil** is a more cooling oil and is good to use when there are liverish complaints, headaches, constipation and bad temper. It is an oil to try for hangovers: combine with Rose, Geranium or Rosewood. It can also be helpful for the respiratory tract or can help strengthen immunity against colds and flu. To use these oils, put 2–3 drops in a saucerful of base-massage oil.

Graphites *Graphites*

Mental and emotional indications: The mental characteristics of this homoeopathic remedy are marked by sadness and despondency.

There is an overall fearful foreboding that something terrible will happen. The person is constantly miserable and very easily discouraged and dejected. They lack vitality and are timid, shy and cautious, with a constant desire to grieve. Their sadness may increase when they listen to music.

Physical symptoms: Marked by a chilliness (great sensitivity to draughts); Graphites types are often obese and flabby (associated with constipation) and have delayed periods and unhealthy skin and nails. The head feels numb and heavy, as if cobwebs are over the face, and the skin of the forehead is drawn into folds. *Skin*: The skin is dry and parchment-like. Every injury suppurates. Eruptions are found between the toes and fingers, on the scalp and behind the ears, on the nipples, labia and in and around the anus. Eruptions contain a sticky, honey-like fluid that exudes from cracks and fissures which are extremely sensitive. Eczema is found on the scalp, face, eyelids and in the folds of the skin. The moist eruptions are covered with scales or crusts. They appear particularly during menstruation.

Women's complaints: The picture for periods is similar to that of Pulsatilla – they are late, scanty and accompanied by feelings of weakness and fainting. Leucorrhoea is excoriating and gushing. There may be period pains. *Abdomen*: There is dyspepsia, a bloated abdomen, lots of wind, the mouth tastes like rotten eggs. Also, excessive hunger, pains in the stomach which feel better from eating; there is desire for cold food and an aversion to salt, sweet food or fish. A general sourness: vomit, sweat and stools smell sour. Constipation with large stools joined together by mucus, when passed the anus becomes fissured. There can be numbness in the extremities. *Modalities*: Symptoms get worse in the cold, in light, during and after periods, from suppressions, at night, from hot drinks and from listening to music. They improve with walking in the open air, from hot drinks (especially milk) and touch.

Gravel Root   *Eupatorium purpureum*

This herb is mainly used for its diuretic and nervine properties. It has an effect on the kidneys and urinary tract, and it helps to calm spasm and pain. It is good to take for kidney stones and cystitis, and through its diuretic and cleansing properties, it is good for gout and rheumatism. Gravel Root combines well with Couchgrass, Marshmallow and Cornsilk.

SUGGESTED DOSAGE Use 1–2ml tincture diluted in water 3 times daily, or decoct 30g (1oz) in 570ml (1 pint) of water and take a wine glassful 3 times a day.

Hawthorn *Crataegus monogyna*

This herb is mainly used by the homoeopath as a mother tincture. Therefore its uses are described under the herbal classifications. For the herbalist, this is one of the most valuable herbs for the heart. It is an excellent general tonic which protects all the blood vessels of the heart and general circulation, as well as those servicing the lungs and kidneys. Hawthorn can be used for any condition that affects the heart, such as emphysema, chronic bronchitis or chronic kidney disease. It affects the action of the heart by increasing the strength of its muscle contraction. This enables the heart to beat slower, which means that the heart rate is reduced. It has the effect of dilating the coronary arteries which supply the heart muscle with blood, this oxygenates the heart which make the process more effective. Therefore, it is good for conditions like angina.

The flowering tops are thought to act more on increasing circulation to the heart, and the berries are used more to help lower blood pressure. It is good to combine both the tops and the berries, except in cases where there is low blood pressure when it is better to use the tops on their own. Hawthorn can be used for heart spasms caused by emotional trauma or grief, etc., and it is also good for hot flushes during the menopause because it helps to regulate the circulation, especially if there is depression or anxiety. It can be helpful for tinnitus, caused by poor circulation or high blood pressure.

SUGGESTED DOSAGE Decoct 6–10 berries per cup of water, or infuse 1 tspful of tops per cup of boiling water. Take twice a day. For a tincture, take 1ml diluted in water 2 times a day.

Heartsease *Viola tricolor*

This is a soothing herb, the main action is on the lung, skin and bladder. It is good for cystitis and can be a soothing expectorant on the lungs, making it good for whooping cough and bronchitis. Heartsease is good as a syrup. For the skin, it is a softening yet drying herb. It can be used for eczema, nappy rash, cradle cap and impetigo. It can be taken internally or used as a wash.

SUGGESTED DOSAGE Infuse 1 tspful of herb to a cup of boiling water, or use 1ml of tincture diluted in water. Take either 3 times a day.

Hepar Sulph   *Hepar sulphuris calcareum*

This is one of the main homoeopathic remedies. It is identified by extreme sensitivity on both physical and emotional levels, even to the point of fainting, and any pains which are sharp and splinter-like. *Mental and emotional indications*: The person who fits the general mental picture of Hepar Sulph is dissatisfied and argumentative, prone to fits of anger, easily annoyed and irritated by the slightest things. They take offence easily and tend to talk quickly. They are unreasonably anxious, and fearful of their own health. Their quick, impulsive behaviour can become extreme, even leading them to arson, suicide or murder.

Constitutionally Hepar Sulph often suits someone who tends to be sluggish. *Physical symptoms*: It can be used for people who tend to be extremely chilly, who catch colds easily and often wear coats, even when the weather is hot. One of the most identifying symptoms of this remedy is that all injuries will suppurate, even scratches, and discharges are profuse and smell offensive, like old cheese. The person will sweat a lot but this does not bring any relief, they are reluctant to uncover themselves through fear of getting cold. The sweat, too, is very sour-smelling. Inflamed glands and suppurating skin abscesses are other important symptoms. Hepar Sulph is an excellent remedy for swellings that have become very painful and splinter-like. It will help to open up an abscess and to drain it. It is excellent for ulcers and boils, and any injury that heals slowly and is red, painful and forms pus. *Throat*: Symptoms include swollen tonsils and glands of the neck. The throat seems as though it is being pierced by a fishbone or a splinter, and the pain extends to the ears when yawning or swallowing.

Colds and catarrh: Symptoms include pain at the base of the nose, sneezing in a cold wind and a running nose. Coughs rattle in the chest with loose mucus, which is difficult to get up and is then thick and yellow. The cough will be barking or choking and get tighter in the cold air. The child will cry before coughing. The cough will get worse in the wind or cold air and when any part of the body is uncovered. *Ears*: Hepar sulph can be very good for earache when there are splinter-like pains, when the eardrum is perforated or for mastoid disease. *Women's complaints*: This remedy covers profuse leucorrhoea, which smells sour or of old cheese, and abscesses on the labia which can be very painful. Someone in need of Hepar Sulph will like sour things, such as vinegar. Refer to the section on homoeopathic dosage (pages 190–1) for the suggested dosage. *Modalities*: Symptoms get worse in the cold, wind, air, draughts, from being uncovered and from touch. They improve from heat, warm wraps and hot applications.

Holy Thistle   *Carduus benedictus*

This is a bitter herb with bacteriostatic properties for the *Streptococcus faecalis* and *Staphylococcus aureus*. Its main action stimulates the digestive juices and flow of bile. It is very good to give to cold, weak people who have a poor digestion, no appetite and are prone to stomach infections. It can be given to people with poor memories, chronic colds, low blood pressure and who often feel faint. As with all bitters, it is contra-indicated for those people that have ulcers and sensitivity in the stomach.

SUGGESTED DOSAGE Infuse 1 tspful of herb with a cup of boiling water and take 3 times daily, or use 1ml of tincture and take 3 times a day.

Hops   *Humulus lupulus*

This is a herb that contains two bitters which become isovalerianic acid when stored. This means that Hops become more sedating when they are stored and are less so if fresh (although if they are very old they are probably inactive). The herb's primary use is for stomach disorders. They are good for colitis and for a nervous stomach, and also useful when nervous disorders affect the appetite as they help the gut to assimilate food and the body to put on weight. They can also be used for gut infections as they have anti-bacterial properties. For this, combine with Calendula, Chamomile or Myrrh. Hops are good for pustular skin diseases, weeping eczema, acne or impetigo (in the days when hops were picked by hand to make beer, they frequently gave young girls skin problems and there was also a tendency for them to menstruate very early).

Hops are an emmenogogue, this means that they are contra-indicated in pregnancy. They are also said to be an aphrodisiac for men. They are mildly sedative and can be used in cases of insomnia, but care needs to be taken because they can depress the spirits and a person's vitality. They are therefore contra-indicated in cases of depression. Hop pillows can be used to help sleep, but again, it is advisable to make certain that the insomnia is due to nervousness and not to depression.

SUGGESTED DOSAGE Infuse 2 tspfuls of herb to a cup of boiling water and drink 3 times a day, or use 10–20 drops of tincture diluted in water and take 3 times a day.

Horsechestnut *Aesculus hippocastanum*

The Horsechestnuts themselves are used and they are a good circulatory tonic and astringent. It has the effect of lowering the blood pressure as it causes the excretion of sodium. It is therefore contra-indicated if there is kidney disease. It lowers blood cholesterol, it is an anti-coagulent so it is also contra-indicated if the person is on anti-coagulants. Horsechestnut strengthens the cell membranes of the red blood cells, but does not affect the iron content. It strengthens and tones the lining of the veins which makes it an excellent herb to give where there are varicose veins or piles.

SUGGESTED DOSAGE Take 1–2ml of tincture, 3 times a day.

Horsetail *Equisetum arvense*

As a homoeopathic remedy, Equisetum is good for urinary complaints. It is helpful where there is a dull pain in the kidney area with the desire to urinate, and where pain is not improved by urinating. There can be bloated feelings and distention in the bladder, and large quantities of urine, which is light-coloured but does not bring any relief to the pain which occurs at the end of urination. There can be a sensation of burning in the urethra, with sharp cutting pains. There can also be a strong need to urinate but only a small amount is passed. There may be mucus in the urine. It is a good remedy to give for habitual enuresis in children (bedwetting), or where there is dribbling in old people. Give in tincture form when it is indicated for children. Refer to the section on homoeopathic dosage (pages 190–1) for other cases. *Modalities*: Symptoms get worse at the end of urination, from pressure, motion and sitting down. They improve with lying down and in the afternoon.

USING THE HERB
As a herb Horsetail has wide-ranging actions. It contains saponins which make it diuretic, and silica which makes it good for the connective tissues of the body, especially in the lungs and urinary tract. It is also said to raise the white blood cell count. It is good to use where the lung tissue is damaged, as in emphysema and TB, and to strengthen the tone of the bladder. This helps where there is frequency and urgency of urination. It is especially good for women who have just given birth and leak urine when sneezing or laughing, also for pelvic cramps, period pains or very heavy menstrual bleeding. Use where there is blood in the urine. Horsetail helps to strengthen weak joints. It can be used in rheumatoid arthritis and osteo-arthritis. It is good for fractures, and can be made into a strong infusion for hand and foot baths to strengthen the connective tissue. It combines well with Comfrey, and it will also help diarrhoea. Use an infusion of Horsetail as a hair-rinse for split-ends. It can also be taken internally for weak and brittle nails.

SUGGESTED DOSAGE Use 1 tspful per cup of boiling water and drink 3 times a day, or 1ml of tincture diluted in water 3 times a day.

Hypericum *Hypericum perforatum*

See St John's Wort.

Hyssop *Hyssopus officinalis*

Traditionally this herb was taken as a general tonic and was put into most mixtures as a means of blending the rest together. It was specifically used for the nerves as it is a good tonic and strengthener. It is an expectorant, anti-spasmodic, sedative and diaphoretic, which makes it good for coughs, hay fever and bronchial infections. It combines well with Horehound for colds and flu. As a nervine, it is well used as a calming herb, it helps allay anxiety. It was also included in poultices to heal cuts and it was taken for the *petit mal* of epilepsy.

SUGGESTED DOSAGE Use ½ tspful of herb to 1 cup of boiling water, or 30 drops of tincture diluted in water; take 3 times a day.

Ignatia *Ignatia amara*

This is one of the best homoeopathic remedies for grief, and for ailments that have come on as a result of grief, for example from disappointed love, where the grief is silent and the mood is changeable. There is instability. Ignatia is good for ailments that come on after humiliation, sadness or depression. It is good for complaints following a fright. *Mental and emotional indications*: The person may be averse to company or consolation and be unable to talk to anyone. They may not be able to stop themselves from crying. They may be hysterical, alternating with fainting and periods of introspection. Sighing is an important keynote of this remedy, although it is not always obvious. The person who fits this remedy will appear reasonable, though sensitive and prone to romanticism, also refined, easily offended and finds it difficult to take the slightest criticism. Failings will make them feel angry with themselves. They tend to be over-sensitive to pain. Ignatia is for those who live on their emotions. They suffer from guilt, are conscientious and highly responsive.

Ignatia is usually a remedy for women. These women fight for a cause and are able to completely devote themselves to that cause, but over a period of time they begin to feel let down and this leads to disappointment. Romanticism often conflicts with the hard realities of life for them. They try not to let others see that they are sensitive. There is disappointment which leads to remorse.

Cramp is another keynote for this remedy – it may occur in any part of the body and also reflects the mind and emotions. The mind becomes dazed after a shock and is not able to focus clearly. On the emotional level, there may be an inability to speak or cry (can only sigh). On the physical level, cramp particularly affects the throat, stomach and solar plexus. There is oppression in the chest, with spasms and trembling.

Ignatia is the remedy to give after the news of the death of a loved one. They will not be able to believe what has happened. They want to cry but they cannot, they feel shocked and cramped on all levels. Ignatia is a very good remedy for loss generally, for example after hysterectomy, rape, miscarriage or after any major disappointment. The Ignatia-type woman tends to fall in love with unobtainable men and this pattern may be repeated. There is a tendency to become infatuated even after meeting casually (e.g. at a bus stop). They believe that a relationship is ideal. When it ends the disappointment is very strong and they will vow never to fall in love again. They will want to go a long way away and hide. They go to where the lover may be. They lose interest in their appearance and femininity. There are suicidal desires but there is no reality to them. If Ignatia is given for emotional trauma or delayed shock, it is likely that the person will release all the grief that has got stuck. This release may occur even if the remedy is taken several months later and the sense of loss is unexpressed, or has manifested itself on the physical level (for example, as headaches, stomach cramps, comfort eating or irregular periods).

Ignatia is a remedy of contradictions. They may experience roaring in the ears but be better for hearing music, they may have piles which feel better when walking or a sore throat which gets better with eating food. There may be an empty feeling in the stomach which does not improve with eating, a cough might get worse from coughing. There may be spasmodic laughter when feeling sad, or sexual desire at the same time as being impotent. When they are chilled they may feel thirsty, but have no thirst during a fever. The mental conditions can change rapidly, swinging from one extreme to another. These contradictions leave the individual feeling mentally and physically exhausted. The main fears that they have are of burglaries and robbers, of being frightened, not sleeping and dying during the night.

Physical symptoms: Include a white-coated tongue, a weak trembling voice, spasms and violent yawning. It may be noticeable that there is a tendency to bite the side of the tongue or cheek when speaking. Limbs may jerk during sleep, accompanied by cries and whimpering. There is restriction in the throat which feels as if there is a plug in it. There is a desire for acid, sour, raw, indigestible food. There is either a desire for or an aversion to fruit, smoking and coffee. The abdomen will feel full, the stools may be soft and they are difficult to pass. The skin can be very sensitive with itching and nettle rash-type eruptions all over the body. This remedy should be compared with Staphisagria. *Modalities*: Symptoms get worse from grief, shock, worry, loss, being touched, coffee, tobacco and alcohol. They improve from swallowing, eating and lying on the painful side of the body.

Ipecac *Ipecacuanha*

One of the best guides to the use of this homoeopathic remedy is nausea which is not improved after vomiting. *Mental and emotional indications:* These are marked by anger and indignation, a rather contemptuous, impatient state where ailments come about as a result.

Physical symptoms: The face may be pale and with a blueness around the eyes and lips. The nausea and vomiting is accompanied by profuse saliva and a clean tongue. It is a very good remedy to use for morning sickness in pregnancy where there is constant nausea and burping. The stomach can feel as if it is hanging down and there is a desire for food or drink. There may also be the following symptoms: diarrhoea and colic with nausea, cutting pains around the navel, stools coloured grass-green, fermented or slimy and bloody lumps of mucus in the stools.

Respiratory symptoms: Ipecac is also a very effective remedy for coughs which are dry and spasmodic (as in asthma). There can be difficulty in breathing which gets worse with exertion or anxiety. There may also be rattling mucus in the chest, especially when breathing in, but no expectoration. It can be used for whooping cough where there is retching, the child may go rigid and the face may turn red or even blue, and any vomiting may contain mucus. Ipecac can be used for haemorrhaging, where the blood is bright red, gushing and accompanied by nausea (see also Phosphorus, which is accompanied by more fear), for uterine haemorrhage that occurs during or after labour and when blood is either gushing or in a steady flow. Breathing may be partially suppressed and there are sticking pains from the navel area to the uterus. A woman in need of Ipecac may have periods that are typically profuse, bright red and clotted. *Modalities*: Symptoms get worse from warmth, overeating or rich foods and damp. They improve in the open air and with rest.

Jamaican Dogwood *Piscidia erythrina*

This herb is an effective sedative. It is a specific for headaches and can be used to treat neuralgia and pains in the ovary and uterus. It is a good remedy to take for insomnia, especially when it is caused by neuralgia or there is tension and it is difficult to unwind and relax. This is a powerful remedy and must be taken with caution: it can cause gastritis and nausea.

SUGGESTED DOSAGE Take 1ml of tincture diluted in water 3 times a day.

Jasmine *Jasminum officinale*

This is not available as an oil but as an absolute or concrete extracted by means of solvents. Jasmine is one of the most uplifting of all the 'oils', its beautiful, heavy, sweet, fragrance has an effect on the emotions, it is both refreshing and soothing and promotes a state of relaxed awareness. Jasmine will be most effective where there is a clear link between psychological stress and physical discomfort. It is useful where there are symptoms of contraction, tension and blockage as it is an antidepressive and anti-spasmodic oil. It will help build self-confidence. For women, it is lovely to include a few drops of Jasmine in a massage oil during labour: it will help speed up the contractions. It is excellent for both men and women as it is one of the classic aphrodisiacs in that it helps treat both impotence and frigidity. It can help all kinds of depression, including postnatal depression. It is also good to use for menstrual discomfort and cramps. Generally, a little Jasmine (as it is so expensive) can be blended with oils such as Lavender, Sandalwood and Rosewood to create a calming and delightful massage for emotionally overwrought people.

Juniper Oil *Juniperus communis*

The main action of this oil is on the kidneys and urinary system. It is one of the most important remedies for the treatment of cystitis, especially when it gets worse in cold weather, although care must be taken not to use it if there is acute inflammation in the kidneys. Juniper Oil will help to eliminate uric acid and other toxins that a cold, sluggish system may fail to excrete efficiently. It is a very good cleansing and purifying oil. It can be combined with Cypress Oil to assist this process of detoxifying, e.g. for cellulite or water retention. It is also one of the main oils for the treatment of rheumatism and arthritis, especially for people who get worse in cold, damp weather.

It can be used for unhealthy skin and sores that do not heal, and for acne. It can also stimulate a cold, sluggish digestion and improve the appetite.

Juniper oil can be used or combined with other oils to tone and cleanse the whole body. Use 2–3 drops in a saucerful of base massage oil. The berries may be made into an infusion and drunk 2–3 times a day for the same conditions, but should be used with caution with diabetes as Juniper lowers the blood sugar.

Kali Bich *Kali bichromicum*

A significant indication of this homoeopathic remedy is ulcers, with thick, stringy discharges. *Mental and emotional indications*: These are not marked but Kali Bich people seem to be indifferent and possibly lazy. They dislike people and avoid them wherever possible. They feel worse after mental work.

Physical symptoms: Pain in the Kali Bich picture is in specific, localised spots on the body. *Headaches*: Preceded by blindness, but the sight returns as the pain gets worse. They are localised in one spot such as sinus headaches. The pains shift quickly around the body, e.g. from rheumatism to a stomach complaint. The stomach feels full immediately after eating. *Catarrh*: Kali Bich is an excellent remedy to give for chronic post-nasal catarrh, for stuffed-up feelings and pressure at the root of the nose. Discharges are thick, stringy, yellow or green and acrid, and they leave the skin surface raw. Other symptoms include a swollen uvula, an ulcerated septum in the nose and a dry throat with abscesses. *Cough*: This is deep, croupy, dry and hacking, with a pain that goes through to the back and shoulders. It is difficult to expectorate; mucous is white, tough and stringy. *Modalities*: Symptoms get worse from alcohol, from 2–4a.m., in the morning and from the cold and damp. They improve from the heat, from motion and with pressure.

Kali Carb *Kali carbonicum*

Mental and emotional indications: There is an obstinacy and a rigidity without apparent reason, these types are stuck in a rut, with a resistance to other people. *General physical symptoms*: They have a general puffiness and bags over the eyes. They feel chilly. *Pains*: Stitching, sitting pain; pains that get worse from rest or with motion;

pains from cold pressure or from lying on the affected side. Pains that affect the pleura, peridardium or joints which are sensitive to pressure and touch. There is a loss of elasticity and power in the ligaments, and around the joints which causes slackness and weakness.

This remedy can be good where there is a weakness in old people, particularly in the back area, or in women after childbearing. It is also useful to use for asthma, especially when symptoms get worse in the early morning between 2 and 4a.m. The asthma will cause the person to sit up and lean forward towards their knees. There is a sensation of no air in the chest: this feels worse when lying down, drinking, from motion or draughts. *Cough*: Gets worse at 3a.m.; asthmatic cough (which must cause bending forward). Cough with sticking pains in the chest or between breaths. Expectoration consists of small, round lumps of blood-streaked mucus or pus. This remedy can be used for pneumonia with sticking pains. *Modalities*: Symptoms get worse from cold winds and cold applications.

Kali Mur *Kali muriaticum (Potassium chloride)*

This homoeopathic tissue salt is connected with the astrological sign of Gemini, and the significant indication for its use is whiteness; it can be given for all catarrhal conditions where there are thick, white discharges. As a tissue salt, it is a cleanser and blood purifier. It is good for soft, glandular swellings. *Physical symptoms*: You can give Kali Mur for coughs that have thick, white phlegm which is hard to get up, and for loud, noisy 'stomach' coughs or those that are short and spasmodic (e.g. whooping cough). It is excellent for chronic catarrh of the middle ear (glue ear), and when the glands around the ear are swollen. It can be given for deafness that comes on after a cold or when there are noises in the ear. It is the tissue salt for the second stage of colds where the nose is blocked with thick white catarrh. It is also good for inflamed tonsils and when these have grey patches.

It can be used for loss of appetite and where rich, fatty foods cause indigestion, or for vomiting of white mucus. It can also be taken when this is a symptom in pregnancy. Another indication of Kali Mur is light-coloured stools. Skin conditions needing a course of Kali Mur are those with white, scaly flakes, and any eruptions or patches that have white discharges. It can be given for thick, white, bland leucorrhoea. *Modalities*: Symptoms get worse from fats or rich foods, open air and cold drinks. They improve with cold drinks.

Kali Phos *Kali phosphoricum (Potassium phosphate)*

This is a homoeopathic tissue salt which is a great remedy for the nerves. Potassium phosphate (Kali Phos) is a mineral found in nerve tissues, fluids of the body and in particular the brain and nerve cells. It is traditionally connected to the astrological sign of Aries. *Mental and emotional indications*: Kali Phos acts as a nerve nutrient; it is good for anxiety, nervousness, a weak memory and brain exhaustion, and when these states are made worse from mental exhaustion or hysteria. Other indications may be sadness, depression, shyness or being easily startled, either in sleep or when touched. It is indicated when the person seems wound up like a spring and suffers from physical or mental symptoms after excitement, overwork or worry.

Physical symptoms. Head: Include brain fag, lack of blood going to the head and headaches, often on the top of the head arising from overwork (it can be very good for students who study too much) and accompanied by an empty feeling in the stomach. The eyes may be affected, being weak from exhaustion; they may be drooping and hard to keep open. *Abdomen*: There may be nervous indigestion and smelly diarrhoea, which can come on after being frightened or with depression and exhaustion. There may be hunger, and a feeling of emptiness even after eating. *Respiratory symptoms*: Kali Phos can be very helpful for nervous asthma or hayfever where there is violent sneezing – this is made worse after eating and exertion, such as going up the stairs. *Sleep*: It is good for insomnia arising from brain fatigue and worry, and can be given to children who suffer from night terrors. *Women's complaints*: Women who need Kali Phos may have irregular and scanty periods. It is very good to give at frequent intervals during labour, where the contractions have become feeble and ineffectual due to nervous and physical exhaustion. It is often good to give to a person assisting the birth, where the labour is long and exhausting. *Modalities*: Symptoms are worse from even the slightest extra mental or physical burden and from tiredness or worry. They improve with sleep, eating and gentle movement.

Kali Sulph *Kali sulphuricum*

This homoeopathic tissue salt is linked with the astrological sign Virgo. The mental picture of this remedy is not particularly significant although there may be sense of a hurriedness and impatience,

273

wanting to lie down but feeling ill when you do, and fear. *Physical symptoms*: Kali Sulph is indicated by yellow or green, slimy discharges. It is a remedy for lingering disorders, such as thick catarrh that drags on after a cold. The tongue is yellow and slimy, the person may crave sweets and the anus may be itchy. Kali sulph can be combined with Ferrum Phos to carry oxygen to different parts of the body. Use for disorders of the scalp and hair, and for hair which is falling out. Nails are brittle with white spots (similar to Pulsatilla). The skin flakes, peels or erupts. Lips peel after a cold. Kali Sulph is good for the peeling stage of skin problems, e.g. with chickenpox, sunburn, etc. It is also a good intercurrent remedy in psoriasis (it helps the next remedy along). *Modalities*: Symptoms get worse with warmth, heat, in the evening and from noise. They improve in the open air.

Kola *Kola vera*

This contains a high percentage of caffeine which stimulates the central nervous system. Kola can be used in cases of diarrhoea brought on by nervousness. It is good for depression and apathy. It can help in cases where there is poor muscle tone, and loss of appetite as a result of depression or disinterest. This makes it a good herb for anorexics to take. It can be given to relieve nervous headaches and it helps to clear the head, so it is a remedy for hangovers. This is not a nutritious herb and it should not be given on a long-term basis: use it more as a short-term stimulant.

SUGGESTED DOSAGE Decoct ½–2 tspfuls of herb to a cup of water, brought to boil and simmered. This can be drunk 3 times a day. With a tincture, use 1–2 ml diluted in water and take 3 times a day.

Kreosote *Kreosotum*

This is a useful homoeopathic remedy for septic, putrid, decaying states, where there are profuse, burning discharges on any part of the body, but particularly from mucous membranes. There is a tendency to haemorrhage, and bleeding is profuse even from small wounds. *Mental and emotional indications*: Irritable states to the point of violence, wretchedness, complaining that nothing is right, everyone and everything is blamed but there is little energy and not much effort is made to improve things. Strong emotions can bring on septicaemia. These people also yawn a lot.

Physical symptoms. Women's complaints: It is a good remedy for symptoms centred around the female generative area. There is a fear of intercourse. Leucorrhoea is gushing, offensive, excoriating, causes itching and stains clothes yellow. Periods are heavy, intermittent, too early or too late, and clotted. The blood can be black, offensive and burning and can lead to soreness and swelling. There can be a sudden desire to urinate and the urine burns and smells. *Mouth and face*: There are often problems in the mouth with an increase of saliva, which makes the lips and corners of the mouth raw. The gums bleed easily and become raw, swollen and sore. There is toothache during pregnancy. Children's teeth decay when they come through. There are nosebleeds. The skin looks yellow and blotchy red. *Circulatory system*: This is poor and there is stagnation in the venous system. *Skin*: There can be puffy swellings and discolouration, ulceration and oozing blood (see also Lachesis), and burning pains.

Digestion: Kreosote is the remedy for stomach troubles which cause bad temper. There is undigested food, water tastes bitter, and there is burning pain in the stomach soon after eating, with a sense of dullness and nausea. This is made worse by eating cold food and improved by eating warm foods. Use for children who suffer from summer diarrhoea, especially if they are teething. *Modalities*: Symptoms get worse during teething, pregnancy, from rest or lying down and eating cold food. They improve with warmth and hot food.

Lac Caninum   *Lac caninum*

Mental and emotional indications: This homoeopathic remedy is marked by changeability and extremes. The person will want company or seek death, they can be excitable and angry as well as sad and depressed. Children shriek and are easily startled or can be weepy. They may be nervous, restless, sensitive, absent-minded and make mistakes in writing and speaking. They can suffer from intense despondency and depression with outbursts of rage. There is a fear of solitude or death, insanity, snakes, vermin or falling down stairs. They may think that their disease is incurable.

Physical symptoms: Symptoms are erratic. They can be on alternate sides, occurring from the left side to the right and back again, returning every few hours or days. *Throat*: Give for sore throats that are sensitive to touch, where the pain extends to the ears and is made worse by empty swallowing. There can be glistening patches of whiteness on the tongue and throat. Consider this remedy for tonsillitis or diptheria, or sore throats that begin and end with the period. The tongue is often white with bright red edges. There is a desire for milk and spices. Often there is a real hunger even after eating. A sinking faintness in the stomach may occur. *Colds*: One nostril is blocked and one is clear, and this alternates.

Women's complaints: Symptoms include periods that are too early or too profuse, the blood gushes and is bright red and stringy and it feels hot. Breasts get swollen, painful and sensitive before and during the period. Sexual organs tend to be very sensitive and are easily excited. There is flatus from the vagina. Lac Caninum helps to dry up milk during breastfeeding if this is necessary. It can also be given after a late miscarriage or the death of a baby. When the picture of Lac Caninum fits it can be given for rheumatic pains which move from one side to another. *Modalities*: Symptoms get worse from being touched, from being jarred, during menses and from cold wind and air. They improve in the open air and from cold drinks.

Lachesis *Lachesis*

This homoeopathic remedy, made from the venom of the snake, is a good remedy of the heart and circulation. Blueness is the first indication for Lachesis, whatever the complaint. *Mental and emotional indications*: These are significant for this remedy. Lachesis people are competent types – they like to be in control, they are self-sufficient. They nearly always feel worse in the morning when they wake up. They will go to sleep in the evening even if they are physically uncomfortable. In the morning the symptoms will be worse, and mentally they will feel confused and anxious. They are generally lively and talkative. They have abundant ideas and change quickly from one idea or topic to another; they have very good thinking processes but are often unable to synthesize them. They are intelligent gossips with vivid imaginations and can be clairvoyant. They are passionate people and often very sexual, tending to be possessive and have great attachment to things and people that they love. This can lead to jealousy and violence. They have strong instincts and are ambitious. They can be cold, ruthless, suspicious and critical of others, although they find it difficult to accept criticism themselves. They can frighten people with their sharp tongue and power to be manipulative or vindictive. They are also generous, vivacious, exitable, nervous people that can rapidly become stubborn, sulky or bad-tempered. They have a great fear of snakes.

Physical symptoms: A Lachesis person is easily over-stimulated and needs to seek an outlet for their energy. This can result in flushes, constipation, high blood pressure or haemorrhages. Lachesis can be used for varicose veins, palpitations and piles. These people cannot stand any pressure, particularly around the waist or throat. They cannot sleep on the left side and all complaints are left sided or go from left to right, except sciatica which is usually on the right. *Headaches*: This is the remedy when they are pulsating, throbbing, bursting, also for left-sided migraines. *Throat*: Symptoms include a sensation of a lump and tonsillitis; it is sensitive to the slightest touch, feels worse after sleep and with hot drinks, and feels better swallowing solids. *Stomach*: The person desires food containing flour, coffee, alcohol and especially red wine, which brings on headaches. There is pain in the abdomen which feels worse with tight clothing. *Respiratory symptoms*: Difficult respiration feels worse sitting bent forward; the person wakes from sleep with a sensation of choking.

Womens's complaints: There are PMT headaches before the period. Lachesis is an excellent remedy for symptoms that come on during the menopause: piles, haemorrhages, hot flushes, perspiration or burning sensation on top of the head. Lachesis can be used where there is profuse bleeding, slow oozing bleeding, a retained placenta, sepsis, gangrene of the mouth and extremities or a weak heart. *Modalities*: Symptoms tend to recur at yearly intervals and are much worse on waking in the morning. They feel worse with heat, in the summer, sun, hot winds, etc., from constriction, touch and pressure, during the menopause, from suppressed discharges, drinking alcohol and before periods. Symptoms improve in the open air, with discharges, from cold drinks and hard pressure.

Ladies' Mantle   *Alchemilla vulgaris*

This is a warming herb that is taken for cold and weak conditions. It is good for painful periods, with cramping or heavy flooding due to weakness. Use for leucorrhoea when the discharge is very white. Ladies' Mantle will generally increase the circulation to the reproductive organs which makes it have toning and nourishing effects. It will restore health to blood vessels in the uterus and to all fragile capillaries throughout the body. Take it if you bruise easily. Combine with Raspberry Leaf and Cramp Bark for uterine prolapses and hernias, as it will help the ligaments and muscles. Use to prevent miscarriage. Having astringent and anti-inflammatory properties, it helps infertility. Combine with Marshmallow and Violet Leaves to help soothe engorged breasts. It is good for mouth ulcers and as a gargle to relieve laryngitis.

SUGGESTED DOSAGE Take 1–3ml of tincture 3 times a day, or infuse 1 tspful of herb per cup of boiling water 3 times a day, if taken throughout cycle. Use more frequently if taken during the period – drink up to 6 cups a day to bring relief.

Lady's Slipper   *Cypripedium pubescens*

This herb could be seen as a female version of Valerian in that it is calming and will help allay anxiety and tension, and has a particular action on the female organs. It brings relief where problems are associated with anxiety: it can be used in pregnancy as it relaxes the uterus and can be given for threatened miscarriage. During labour it will help to relax an over-toned uterus and cervix. It is also helpful for afterbirth pains. It is probably a good herb to replace Valerian for depression accompanying PMT, and will act as a nerve tonic and ease stress headaches. Combine with Jamaican Dogwood for headaches.

SUGGESTED DOSAGE Take 1ml of tincture 3 times a day, or infuse ½ tspful per cup of boiling water.

Lavender   *Lavendula officinalis*

This beautiful fragrant herb has a wide range of uses and is dealt with more fully as an oil. As an infusion and a tea it acts the opposite way to Rosemary by taking blood away from the head. It relaxes the nervous system, making it good for pains, cramps and burns. It is an excellent antiseptic herb and is good to combine in mixtures for urinary tract infections. It is good to use an infusion as a wash for the face and hair. Combine with Chamomile, Cleavers and Rose petals in a muslin bag to put in the bath. It will have a soothing, cleansing and healing effect on very delicate skin.

SUGGESTED DOSAGE Infuse 1 tspful of herb in a cup of boiling water and drink three times a day, or dilute 1–2 ml of tincture in water and take three times a day.

LAVENDER OIL   *Lavandula hybrida*

This is one of the most versatile and valuable oils in aromatherapy. It can be used to treat any physical symptoms that are the result of stress or nervous tension. It calms cerebro-spinal activity, and may be used to treat irritability, depression, insomnia, hysteria and nervous tension. It also has mild analgesic properties which make it one of the most important oils for treating headaches and migraine. It can also be used for all forms of neuralgia and sciatica, and will work well if blended with Chamomile. The oil has a restorative, toning and calming effect on the heart so it can be used in the treatment of high blood pressure. It also helps fainting and palpitations.

Lavender is an anti-spasmodic oil and this makes it good for treating respiratory ailments such as asthma, whooping cough and other spasmodic coughs; the antiseptic properties make it particularly effective in treating flu, bronchitis and pneumonia. It is also good to use in a mouth-wash for the treatment of bad breath. Lavender has the effect of increasing gastric secretion which indicates its use for a cold, sluggish digestion. It is also an intestinal stimulant, and has a carminative action making it good for treating flatulence. The anti-spasmodic properties suggest its use for relieving stomach cramps and colic. It will be of most use when treating digestive problems of a nervous origin, e.g. diarrhoea, dyspepsia, nausea, etc. The anti-bacterial and anti-inflammatory properties of Lavender have a pronounced effect on the urinary-genital system – use it to treat cystitis, leucorrhoea and genital infections. The oil's anti-spasmodic properties make it soothing, it treats menstrual cramps and it is also indicated for scanty periods. It makes an excellent douche to help treat vaginal infections, e.g. thrush and leucorrhoea.

Lavender oil has many properties that make it good for skin conditions. It promotes scar-tissue and generates skin cells. It is a deodorant as well as being anti-inflammatory. It is used to treat all sorts of wounds and sores, e.g. abrasions, ulcers, gangrene, anal fistulas, etc. As part of the first aid kit, Lavender can be used for bruises, insect and animal bites and burns. In these cases, apply the oil undiluted. Other skin conditions that Lavender helps are eczema, acne, psoriasis, etc. It is also said to be effective against lice and scabies, and for repelling mosquitoes.

Massage the diluted oil into the scalp where hair loss is caused by a nervous condition. It can be blended with other oils to treat rheumatism and muscular pains. This is a unique oil because it is so versatile and easy to blend with other oils: almost any combination will be enlivened by the addition of a few drops of Lavender.

Ledum   *Ledum palustre*

This is a very good homoeopathic first-aid remedy for puncture wounds. These are wounds that are caused by rusty nails, wire, thorns, animal bites, insect stings, mosquito bites, splinters under the nail, etc. Ledum can be given for any shooting, pinching pains when there is a preference for cold applications rather than hot. It will help prevent sepsis, and if it is given quickly enough after an injury, it will be effective against tetanus. Ledum is particularly good for treating those puncture wounds where there is very little bleeding and the skin is cold, pale and swollen, and the pains are sticking, pricking and throbbing (compare with Hypericum). It is good for a black eye which is bloodshot and bruised and the eyelids are purple and puffy. It is noticeable that even though the damaged area can feel cold to the touch, the person will experience intolerable heat. *Modalities*: The symptoms feel worse with warmth and improve with cold air and cold bathing.

Lemon Balm   *Melissa officinalis*

See Balm.

Lemon Grass

This herb can be used for respiratory complaints – coughs, colds and fevers. It is a good digestive herb and adrenal tonic. Combine with other herbs in a mix for the bath. It is also a good herb to use in cooking.

LEMON GRASS OIL
The distilled oil has a very strong, lemony odour. It has antiseptic and anti-bacterial properties, but must be used with caution and always diluted. Only 1 or 2 drops need be added for a refreshing bath or

footbath. It can be used as an insect repellent. Add 1 or 2 drops to a flower water (Lavender preferably) and, after shaking, you can also add a drop of Lemon Grass Oil to a sun oil to deter insects.

Lemon Oil *Citrus limonum*

This is one of the most important citrus oils. It is a very good tonic for the circulatory system, it improves sluggishness and weak veins so use it for chilbains and varicose veins, etc. It is also said to help break down sclerotic deposits in the arterial system, and to reduce blood viscosity. Lemon oil is traditionally used for the treatment of broken capillaries, and because it is astringent, antiseptic and a styptic (stops bleeding), it is good for many skin problems and eruptions such as boils and ulcers. It helps to give tone to ageing skin and it will burn off verrucas and warts if it is applied undiluted. Lemon has a purifying effect. It can be used against parasitic infections which are both internal, e.g. worms, and external, e.g. scabies and lice. It is an insect repellent and will help prevent sepsis. It is good to spray Lemon Oil around the house to get rid of fleas and household insects. Valnet states in *The Practice of Aromatherapy*, that Lemon is one of the most important bactericidal oils for any infection or putrefaction.

Lemon oil is good for respiratory infections and helps to eliminate mucus. It can be used to treat colds, flu, bronchitis and asthma. It helps stimulate the production of white blood cells to strengthen the immune system. Combine with other oils for a preventative massage when there is a danger of an epidemic or contagious disease. Lemons are rich in vitamins, mineral salts and trace elements. Lemon juice with hot water or with honey is a very simple way of aiding a weak digestion and improving cold, weak conditions, whether as a result of an infection or, for example, anaemia. Blend a few drops of Lemon Oil into a massage oil and combine with oils such as Rose or Olibanum: choose the oils that are particularly appropriate. Lemon Oil is a favourite in the perfumery world as it adds a 'top note' to a fragrance. Only 1–2 drops are needed in a small dish of base oil. It is a powerful oil: try it out before using for a full massage.

Limeflower *Tilia europoa*

This is a very relaxing herb which is good for nervous excitability that causes palpitations and high blood pressure. It combines well with Hawthorn tops and Lemon Balm. It is a pleasant tea to drink and is a good evening substitute for coffee, tea or cocoa, which all contain caffeine. Give to children who are too excited to go to sleep, especially if they are unwell and irritable. It can be used in a tea mixed with Chamomile, Cowslip or Lemon Balm. It makes for a relaxing bath, use loose or in a muslin bag. Limeflower is a diaphoretic herb, and it is anti-spasmodic for the lungs. It is good for colds and flu and when asthma is brought on by a nervous state, here combine with Coltsfoot. It can be used as a wash to help clear the complexion – it may be good to combine with Elderflower and Borage for this.

SUGGESTED DOSAGE Use 1 tspful of herb to a cup of boiling water, or make an infusion of 25–50g (1–2oz) for the bath.

Liquorice *Glycyrrhiza glabra*

This herb is a well-known expectorant; it is a demulcent and also anti-inflammatory and anti-spasmodic. These actions combine to make Liquorice very good for lung infections where there is a tight cough. It will help to expectorate phlegm. Take for stomach ulcers; it contains saponins which help to form a soapy lining which protects and heals ulcers. It can be used as a mild laxative. Liquorice is good for cramps in the gut that cause constipation. It is an adrenal tonic: as well as getting the hormones to function, it has the effect of mimicking them. It is excellent for conditions which arise from stress put on the adrenal glands.

In Chinese herbalism, the root of Glycyrrhiza is known as Gan Lao: Gan means sweet, Lao means herb. It is included in most Chinese herb mixtures not only for its valuable actions but also to impart a sweetness which helps to balance sugar levels. It is known specifically to help detoxify the body – a strong infusion can be very useful to counter the effects of poisoning, whether of food or drugs. Recent research has shown that glycyrrhetic acid contained in Liquorice inhibits tumours. Liquorice can lead to a rise in blood pressure so it is best avoided where there is a history of high blood pressure. It can also lead to high potassium levels, causing water retention, if taken in high doses for a long time.

SUGGESTED DOSAGE Use ¼–½ tspful of dried, powdered herb per cup of boiling water or 10–30 drops of tincture 3 times a day.

Lycopodium *Lycopodium clavatum*

This is an important homoeopathic remedy. *Mental and emotional indications*: The Lycopodium type has a good, quick mind and is not as superficial as a Sulphur-type can be. They like to do everything properly. They are often mentally above average – typified by the studious intellectual bent over a book, ignoring the need for exercise and fresh air. They are aware of the feebleness of their bodies but they take their responsibilities very seriously even though they may have taken them on reluctantly. They are prone to being tearful. They are fearful of being alone; women can be afraid of men. They suffer from anticipatory fears – fearing oncoming occasions, such as presentations, giving a lecture, exams, etc., – although they will probably do well or even enjoy the actual event. They are fearful of their own failure as they set themselves very high standards and are haunted by thoughts of financial loss and of not being able to fulfill their responsibilities. Lycopodium types are ambitious and determined. They work hard and can appear cold, distainful and arrogant, but this often hides a sense of insecurity. They distrust themselves and others. Their fear around their own inadequacies can make them seem cowardly and they can appear rather bossy as a way of compensation. They can also be profoundly sad.

The Lycopodium type is often physically slight and rather weedy. They tend to age prematurely with wrinkles and grey hair, and the children appear 'grown up for their age'. *Physical symptoms*: One of the main physical indications for this remedy is a marked aggravation of symptoms from 4–8p.m, and a loss of energy at this time. Often these types are slow to wake in the morning. They can be irritable and intolerant of any pressure, whether emotional, mental or physical. Complaints tend to be on the right side of the body and may then move onto the left. They like warm drinks and feel worse with cold drinks or food. A Lycopodium characteristic is a movement of the nostrils during acute conditions. Symptoms come and go suddenly, pains are like lightning or flashes of heat, the right foot can be hot, the left one cold, burning pains feel better with more heat. There is a general dryness in the picture of this remedy: the vagina, skin, palm of the hands are dry, it is a dry, dusty remedy.

Abdomen and Digestion: Symptoms include flatulence which comes up and goes down, this is made much worse from cabbages and beans. Wind is a key symptom with abdominal distension. These people do not like to feel constricted and will loosen their clothing especially after eating. They get indigestion if they eat later than usual and also feel sick and faint if they wait too long for a meal. They may feel very hungry but then get full up after only a few mouthfuls. They suffer from acidity, wind and bloating, and desire warm food, drinks and sweet food. Onions disagree with them. They also suffer from sluggish bowels and a distension of the bowels and colon which feel better from warm applications. Lycopodium is a good remedy for congestion of the liver when the person is feeling liverish, irritable, peevish and angry.

They may have a tendency to high blood pressure, a chronic right-sided sore throat, fibrous tumours, arthritic inflammations, which get better from movement (see also Rhus Tox), and prostate trouble. There can be amenorrhoea, and there is a tendency for impotence which is probably more to do with overwhelming feelings of responsibility and shyness. *Modalities*: Symptoms get worse from pressure, constriction of clothes, warmth, eating and between 4–8p.m. They improve with warm drinks and food, burping and movement.

Mag Phos *Magnesia phosphorica*

This homoeopathic tissue salt is connected to the astrological sign of Leo and is an excellent anti-spasmodic remedy. It works very well in conjunction with Kali Phos for neuralgia, sciatica and any nerve pains that are sharp and shooting. *Physical symptoms*: It is good for muscular twitching, as in the eye or face, and good for any spasm, e.g. hiccups, cramp or a coughing fit. Take for any pain that is better from heat, hot drinks, a hot bath, a hot application and also pressure and rubbing; and for pains that get worse in the cold. Use Mag Phos for toothache that gets better with hot drinks, for babies and children who are teething, and where discomfort is worse from cold air. It can be used for colic which improves with bending double, burping and pressure, and for cramps after prolonged exertion. It is one of the best remedies to give for period pains which are cramping and feel better for heat and pressure. Also for cramping after-pains of labour. Mag Phos can be given in 200C for severe pain and cramps, and is best given in a little hot water.

Mandarin Oil   *Citrus reticulata*

See Grapefruit Oil.

Marigold   *Calendula officinalis*

This remedy is widely used by herbalists and homoeopaths. It is a great healer as a herb. It can be used externally and internally as a healing antiseptic in the form of a wash (made from an infusion), a tincture, which must be diluted in water, or in an ointment or cream. It is good for all wounds and helps prevent scarring from cuts, ulcers, boils, burns or after surgical operations. Marigold is a valuable aid in baby care, helping to heal nappy rash, and can be used to help heal the umbilical cord. Also it is good to use in an ointment for cracked and sore nipples. Marigold is very good to use after giving birth where there has been tearing or an episiotomy has been done. But be careful with stitches as a wound can heal too quickly with Calendula, and the stitches may be difficult to get out.

Use an infusion of Marigold with a plant spray for an area that is too sore to touch. Where there is damage to the nerve tissue it is good to combine with St John's Wort (Hypericum). These remedies, in combination, are usually known as Hypercal, which comes in tincture form. This should be an essential part of everybody's first aid kit. Marigold is also anti-viral, anti-fungal and anti-bacterial. It can be used for ringworm, athlete's foot and fungal candida.

The herbalist will recommend Marigold tea for its bitter action on the liver; this also makes it a mildly digestive herb. It has an emmenagogue effect and helps to relieve period pains; it improves the flow of the lymph and cleanses it. Here it could be combined with Cleavers to help treat swollen lymph glands. Marigold has also been taken after a mastectomy to help prevent seeding of cancer cells with some success.

Using Calendula in potency as a homoeopathic remedy will assist all healing to take place. But it is important to remember, though, if you choose to take Marigold as a tea, do not use the remedy in potency as well (see section on prescribing, pages 190–1). If you make a strong infusion by pouring water onto a mixture of Marigold and St John's Wort, sieve before adding it to a sitz bath or a bath. You could also add salt and Lavender Oil for a very healing effect after childbirth.

NATURAL HEALING FOR WOMEN

SUGGESTED DOSAGE Take 1ml tincture to a cup of water, or a couple of tspfuls of herb to a cup of boiling water. In potency, consult the section on homoeopathic prescribing.

MARIGOLD OIL   *Calendula officinalis*
This oil is rarely produced, being distilled from the *Calendula officinalis*, which is grown mainly in Europe. There is often confusion made between this oil and Tagetes Oil, which is distilled from *Tagetes glandulifera*. They are both members of the Compositae family but they are not the same plant. Marigold or Calendula Oil can be used to heal in similar ways as the herb, having powerful antiseptic actions. Dilute the oil (10 drops to 30ml of base oil, such as Almond or Olive Oil or macerated Comfrey oil) and apply to affected areas. It is not easy to obtain this oil but it is possible to macerate your own (see section on Macerated Oils pages 186–7) and this can be used as a base for ointments or massage oil.

Marjoram Oil   *Origanum marjorana*

This is a relaxing oil, it tones the circulatory system. It is useful for the treatment of high blood pressure and the narrowing of the arteries. Marjoram is an anti-spasmodic oil so it is good for treating colic, flatulence and dyspepsia. It also acts as a laxative by stimulating and strengthening intestinal peristalsis. The sedating properties of Marjoram make it of use in the treatment of anxiety, insomnia and nervous debility, and it is said to reduce the sexual impulse. It has analgesic properties so it is a remedy for headaches and migraines, and it is good to combine in the treatment of muscular aches, sprains, strains and rheumatism. It can also be massaged into the abdomen to relieve painful periods. Add 1–2 drops of Marjoram to a saucerful of base oil for massage, or use up to 5 drops in a bath.

Marshmallow   *Althea officinalis*

Either the herb or root of Marshmallow can be used, although the root is considered to be more demulcent as it contains more mucilage. It is a soothing linctus remedy for the gut or throat. Use the syrup made from the root for a scratchy throat or tickly cough. The leaves are also soothing and anti-inflammatory, and can be taken internally for lung complaints, urinary problems and skin

286

conditions. Marshmallow has an expectorant action on the lungs, as it loosens the phlegm. This makes it helpful for tight coughs or where the cough rattles but nothing can be brought up. It is also excellent for asthma where the mucus is so thick that the congestion cannot be shifted. For this, combine with Horehound and Hyssop.

Marshmallow is excellent for cystitis and nephritis, and helps with kidney stones and passing gravel. It has a soothing anti-inflammatory action on the skin, making it good for acne, eczema or any condition that is hot and itchy. Combine Marshmallow with the following, in equal parts: Coltsfoot and Elderflower for the lungs; Yarrow, Couchgrass and Lavender for the kidneys; Elderflower, Chickweed, Burdock and Dandelion for the skin.

SUGGESTED DOSAGE Use 1 tspful of herb infused in a cup of boiling water 3 times a day, or 2–5ml of tincture in water 3 times a day.

MARSHMALLOW SYRUP
Make a cold decoction by pouring cold water over 30g (1oz) of powdered root (this is preferable, but the chopped root is also fine) and leave overnight. By making this with cold water the mucilage will be extracted but the starch will remain. Strain and add 340g (¾lb) of sugar to every 570ml (pint) of the mixture (65 per cent). Stir thoroughly over a gentle heat until the sugar is dissolved and pour into sterilised bottles to within 3cm (1½") of the top. Seal, then place in a pan and pour in cold water until it reaches the base of the stopper. Bring to simmering point and simmer for 20 mins then remove bottles. If a cork is used, seal by brushing with melted candle wax when the bottles are slightly cooled. Store in a cool, dry place.

Meadowsweet *Spiraea ulmaria*

This herb contains sodium salicylate which is only converted to salicylic acid in inflamed tissues. Salicylic acid is the main constituent of aspirin but because it is converted already in aspirin it affects all the tissues. It has a pain-killing effect and is good for infections and inflammations. Salicylic acid can harm mucous membranes. Meadowsweet is specifically useful as a gentle and effective aid for nausea, heartburn and ulcers. It contains mucilage and other constituents which protect areas that are likely to be damaged, e.g. stomach ulcers, but it is particularly appropriate because of its analgesic action. It is good to give for diarrhoea, especially in children. Combine Meadowsweet with Marigold, Chamomile and Peppermint to help reduce inflammation and pain caused by rheumatism, to help reduce fevers and for colds and flu.

SUGGESTED DOSAGE Use 1–2 tspfuls per cup of boilng water, or 1ml of tincture, 3 times daily.

Melissa Oil *Melissa officinalis*

See Balm.

Merc Sol (Mercury) *Mercurius solubilis*

This homoeopathic remedy is noted mainly for the physical and general symptoms that it covers. *Mental and emotional indications*: These are difficult to spot. There is an amoral aspect to such people, they can be flighty, moving on all the time, changeable. The temperament is hurried, restless, impulsive, suspicious and mistrustful. They can be violent or quarrelsome. They have been described as having 'dirty minds'. They are easily influenced – giving you what they think you want to hear. Speech is hurried, perhaps with a stammer, they have poor memories and find it difficult to apply themselves. They complain and are volatile.

Physical symptoms: All symptoms are worse at night and then improve in the morning. These include bone pains, sweating, anxiety and fears. They are worse from the heat of the bed, but better from resting. Merc Sol is one of the first remedies to think of where any complaint is accompanied by profused night sweating that does not bring relief. Sweat, breath and discharges are all foul-smelling. There is a metallic taste in the mouth. A key note of Merc Sol is an indented tongue – it holds the shape of the teeth at the edges. There is trembling and weakness. Trembling is visible and is caused by any exertion. Weakness can lead to paralysis.

The main part of the body to be affected are the mucous membranes, glands and genitals. All discharges are profuse and with pus. Skin ulcerates and bleeds. There is profuse saliva out of the corner of the mouth, dribbling during sleep, and a heavily-coated tongue. Also, sore gums which bleed easily, can feel spongy and recede, and offensive breath. Teeth decay easily. There can be toothache, with tearing, shooting pains which feel better from the warmth of a bed. It is a good idea to check if the person has recently been to the dentist – mercury fillings can cause a reaction. Other symptoms Merc Sol covers are ulcers, and the irregular shape of the tongue, cheek, throat and gums. Also Catarrh, with sneezing, mouth ulcers and yellowy-green ulcers in the nose, and painful sore throats with foul-smelling breath. It is a good remedy to consider for measles, especially where there are complications and earaches. Merc Sol is good for ear problems in general, and where there are sharp pains or boils in the ears. It is also good for mumps with swollen glands, smelly breath and feverishness.

Abdomen: Digestion is poor, there are stomach ulcers, a swollen and sore liver, and gall bladder trouble. Merc Sol is excellent to give for dysentery, where the stool is slimy and bloody and there is also colic and faintness. There is a constant urge to pass a stool, or a sensation of not having finished (also compare Nux Vom). *Women's complaints*: Leucorrhoea is acrid, burning, itching; it causes rawness which is worse at night or with ulceration. Morning sickness with profuse salivation. Painful breasts during periods. Symptoms also include swollen joints and rheumatism, which gets worse at night accompanied by profuse, oily sweat. They desire bread and butter and fatty foods, are averse to sweet things, and very thirsty. Merc Sol and Silica are inimicable (they do not work well together). *Modalities*: Symptoms get worse at night, during wet or damp weather, from sweating, lying on the right side, in draughts from heat and from changes of temperature or weather. They improve in moderate temperatures, from rest and from intercourse.

Milkthistle   *Silybum marianum*

The primary use for this herb is to promote milk secretion. It is safe and good for nursing mothers. It is also good for the liver: it is said to help to make it work more efficiently by stabilising the liver cell membranes and stopping them from being damaged by toxins. It has a stabilising effect on alcohol so it is a herb for those who drink heavily, have gall-bladder problems or are at any stage of hepatitis.

SUGGESTED DOSAGE Infuse 1 tspful of seeds for 15 mins in a cup of boiling water and drink 3 times a day, or use 1ml or 25 drops of tincture diluted in water and take 3 times a day.

Mistletoe *Viscum album*

This plant commanded a lot of respect in pre-Christian times because it was considered to give protection. The Christmas tradition of hanging it up probably comes from this time because it was thought to bring good fortune to the home and ward off evil spirits. Traditionally, of course, it was used for healing: the dried leafy twigs are used as the berries are poisonous. It is calming and a nerve tonic for use where there is tension causing high blood pressure. It acts on the vagus nerve of the heart which helps slow the heart down, reduce blood pressure and also strengthen the capillary walls. Combine with Hawthorn for nervous heart complaints, a fast heart, palpitations and headaches, and tinnitus caused by high blood pressure. It is used for epilepsy as it helps calm the electrical activity of the brain. In some parts of Europe, extract of mistletoe is injected around the sites of malignant tumours.

SUGGESTED DOSAGE Take 15–20 drops of tincture diluted in water 3 times a day, or make an infusion of the herb using ½ tspful to a cup of boiling water and drink 3 times a day.

Motherwort *Leonurus cardiaca*

This herb is particularly good to use for disorders of the female reproductive system, especially when there is an emotional side to the problem. It is good to give young women who are emotionally tense, or when shock has resulted in amenhorrhea; also, for women with nervous palpitations, or infertility problems. It is useful for menopausal women suffering from menstrual irregularities, hot flushes, emotional upsets, tension or anxiety. It is a herb that can be drunk throughout pregnancy or during labour, to calm nervous tensions. This herb can also be used for nervous heart disorders. It will help regulate a fast pulse and lower the blood pressure.

SUGGESTED DOSAGE Use 1 tspful of herb to 1 cup of boiling water, and dilute 3 times daily. Or dilute 1ml of tincture in water and drink 3 times daily.

Mullein *Verbascum thapsus*

Both the leaves and flowers are used, but the flowers are particularly recommended. It is primarily for respiratory problems and has a high content of mucilage which gives it a demulcent action, as well as a soothing coating to the respiratory tract. It is also an expectorant, and is healing and anti-inflammatory. It will soothe and loosen a dry cough. It is good to use where there is light phlegm and soreness. Mullein flowers can be macerated in an oil, preferably olive oil, and used as an antiseptic for ear infections, an inflamed ear drum, middle-ear infections or earache. It would probably be worth considering adding 1–2 drops of essential oil of Chamomile to 10ml of Mullein oil. Mullein tea is also known to help soothe cystitis. A very good mixture for coughs is equal parts of Mullein flowers, Marshmallow and Violet leaves.

SUGGESTED DOSAGE Use by infusing 1–2 tspfuls of herb to a cup of boiling water and drink 3 times daily, or use 20 drops of tincture diluted in water and take 3 times daily.

Myrrh *Commiphora molmol*

This is a gum resin containing 17 per cent essential oil. Myrrh is astringent, expectorant, anti-catarrhal, carminative and healing. It is said to stimulate the production of white blood cells. It is highly antiseptic, and it can work on the lungs with its strengthening and toning actions. It can help chronic lung conditions particularly where there is thick white mucus. Myrrh stimulates the digestive system and helps fermentation and flatulence. Add Chamomile and Peppermint in this case. Because it is directly anti-microbial, it helps any gut infection. It is also very good for stomach flu. Myrrh is excellent to use for any infection and inflammation in the mouth and throat: use as a wash, or combine with Sage and Lavender as a gargle. Myrrh is an emmenagogue – it is best to avoid during pregnancy for anything other than a mouth wash. Use tincture of Myrrh, which can be mixed with Witchazel and Marigold for boils and cuts.

SUGGESTED DOSAGE It is possible to infuse Myrrh using 1 tspful of gum per cup of boiling water, or use 1–2 ml of tincture. Take 3 times a day. The tincture is 90 per cent alcohol; if this is unacceptable use the infusion, but the tincture is useful because you can add it to other oils before diluting in water.

MYRRH OIL   *Commiphora myrrha*
Myrrh Oil can be used in preference to the infusion or tincture in inhalations for respiratory complaints. It is also excellent to use either on its own or combined with Lavender, to treat wounds, ulcers and fungal and infected areas. The oil was traditionally used in perfumery and cosmetic preparations, and is known as a skin preserver. Compare with Frankincense, Cypress, Cedarwood and Sandalwood. A regular massage with Myrrh in a base oil, either Olive, Coconut or Almond oil, with or without additional oils, will help maintain the health and suppleness of the skin, preventing it from becoming dry and therefore tired and aged.

Nat Mur   *Natrum muriaticum*

As a tissue salt this remedy is associated with Aquarius, the astrological sign of the water carrier. It can be used where discharges are watery or like uncooked eggwhite. It is a popular tissue salt for colds, headaches, constipation, coldsores and dry skin problems.

Nat Mur is also one of the main homoeopathic remedies. *Mental and emotional indications*: These are marked by extreme sensitivity. It is a good remedy for the ill-effects of grief and love affairs, the person feels weepy but is unable to cry, then may weep without any apparent cause – often sobbing rather than crying. They do not like sympathy, they have a belief that they 'must be strong'. A Nat Mur type person does not generally like going to parties. They do expect recognition and if they do not get it, they feel resentful. They are very deliberate, self-conscious people. They can be awkward, clumsy and drop things. They remember grudges and hold grievances; they lack humour. A Nat Mur person is not particularly easy to live with due to their unstable moods and impatience. They are not the type to just drop by, they walk fast with a purpose and if they visit you it has taken a lot to get them there. They get worse from attention and superficial chat and improve greatly with talking for a long time when they will open up and feel a lot better afterwards. They appear poised but feel tremulous under the surface. They are flushed in exertion but when they spend a long time sitting they become sallow; the skin becomes greasy or gets acne.

Physical symptoms. Head: These people often wake up with a head-ache which will get worse at 11a.m. and then improve throughout the rest of the day, or it will stay over the eyes on the left side of the head. The pain is bursting, like a thousand little hammers, with flashing lights, zigzagging before the eyes; there can be migraines. Also, headaches after being in the sun which get worse from noise. Schoolchildren's headaches. The vision gives out when reading, the eyes get watery in the wind. The tongue is mapped with red and white patches and there is a sensation as if a hair is on the tongue (also Silica). The tongue is dry. *Digestion*: A Nat Mur type will tend to be slim, they emaciate easily. They experience a sinking, empty feeling from hunger at around 11a.m. or after a meal. They desire salt and fish and are averse to rich, fatty foods, bread, meat or coffee. *Women's complaints*: Periods often come late and are accompanied by a headache. There may be dryness or herpes of the genitals and a low libido in both men and women. Nat Mur can be good to give for oedema in pregnancy.

Abdomen: Urination can be difficult, especially in front of other people. Stools are dry, hard, crumbling with a sticking pain in the rectum. There can be anal herpes. *Skin*: Acne; itchy, scaly eruptions along the nape of the neck and the hairline, which becomes red. There may be cracks in the centre of the lower lip, herpes, cold sores on the lips and mouth. Urticaria becomes worse after exertion. The nails crack easily and the skin around the neck is dry. *Children*: Those that show Nat Mur symptoms can be slow to talk and walk. Fearful dreams are particularly about burglars. *Modalities*: Symptoms get worse from 9–11a.m., in the sun and heat, from sympathy, at puberty, from exertion of the eyes, talking, writing and reading. They improve in the open air, from sweating and from talking in depth.

Nat Phos *Natrum phosphoricum*

This is a biochemic tissue salt associated with the astrological sign Libra. It helps the body to break down lactic acid, the excess of which results in too much sugar, leading to acidity and sourness. Sourness is the keynote of this remedy. *Mental and emotional indications*: Marked by irritability and touchiness. There is indifference, mental and nervous weakness and these types become frightened easily (especially at night). They are frightened that something will happen, are generally apprehensive and fearful. They tend to be forgetful.

Physical symptoms. Headaches: Mainly at the front of the head, they come on from mental exertion. There is dizziness with cutting pains in the temples, feelings of pressure and headache on top of the head. The nose can be sticky with yellow, thick, offensive mucus. A child will pick her nose. *Digestive symptoms*: There is waterbrash, sour risings (described as having a coppery taste), flatulence, nausea and heartburn. Desire for strong-tasting foods like eggs, beer and fried fish, and an aversion to bread and butter. The back of the tongue is yellow. Nat Phos will tend to neutralise too much acidity and will help where there is too much uric acid or gallstones in the kidneys. Use for gout, pains in the joints, rheumatism and pains in the balls of the feet, knees and ankles. *Women's complaints*: Sour creamy leucorrhoea that is acidic and watery. Morning sickness and sour vomiting. Nat Phos is really helpful for heartburn during pregnancy. *Modalities*: Symptoms are worse from sugar, fats, in thunderstorms and from intercourse; they improve in the cold.

Nat Sulph   *Natrum sulphuricum*

This is a homoeopathic tissue salt found in the intercellular fluid of the body. The remedy aids the regulation of excretion and helps rid the body of superfluous water. Its action is opposite to that of Nat Mur which attracts water to be used: Nat Sulph attracts water to be eliminated. It has an effect on the liver and the pancreas. Keynotes for Nat Sulph are piercing pains and yellow, watery discharge from the skin or in the stools. Pus is thick and yellowy-green. *Mental and emotional indications:* A Nat Sulph person is affected by the moon, especially a full moon when they feel increasingly unbalanced because the fluid level rises up the spine and causes pressure and compression in the brain. They have vivid or frightening dreams, feel disheartened and sad, unable to talk. This can become extreme with bouts of wildness or insanity. There is a desire to jump from heights, with suicidal tendencies. They are suspicious and very sensitive, easily startled by sudden noises and generally irritable and melancholic. There may be mental problems which can be traced back to a head injury during infancy – the head has 'never been right since'. It is good to give Nat Sulph immediately to anyone suffering from a head injury.

Physical symptoms. Headaches: Violent, pulsating, worse on the top of the head, there is vertigo with gastric problems, excess bile, a brownish, green-coated tongue, a bitter taste and sick headaches with bilious diarrhoea or vomiting of bile. The scalp can feel sensitive with burning at the top of the head. Acute photophobia. The face is sallow and yellowish with biliousness. *Digestion*: Symptoms include a disordered stomach, vomiting of greenish/brown bile, sour risings, heartburn, flatulence, an engorged liver with cutting pains which get worse when lying on the left side and gallstones. Tight clothes around the waist are intolerable. Stools are loose and dark or green. There are rumbling, gurgling bowels, spluttering stools, foaming yellow diarrhoea mixed with green slime. Loose stools in the morning driving the person from bed, but afterwards they feel better in themselves. *Respiratory symptoms*: Nat Sulph can be used for asthmatic conditions which get worse in wet weather. It is good for damp, rattling mucus in the chest, such as bronchial catarrh, where there is a heavy weight on the chest and a loose cough with thick, ropey, greenish expectoration. There is soreness of the chest made worse by coughing. Breathlessness is worse in damp weather and the bronchial catarrh is worse in the early morning. The nasal discharge is thick and yellow/green.

Skin: There is a tendency for warts. Eruptions in the eyes, scalp, face and chest. Yellowy, watery secretions. Nat Sulph can be effective for ringworm and inflammation in the root of the nails. There are also stiff joints that crack with motion, and arthritis that gets worse with damp. Violent sticking pains at night. Watery swellings that are pitted. A Nat Sulph type is oversensitive to the damp but they desire ices, cold drinks, etc. *Modalities*: Symptoms get worse with damp, lying on the left side, from injuries to the head, late in the evening, from vegetables and fruit, cold foods and drink, light and music. They improve from open, warm, dry air, from breakfast and lying on the back.

Neroli Oil   *Citrus aurantium*

See Orange Blossom.

Nettles   *Urtica urens* or *Urtica dioica*

Homoeopaths use Urtica Urens as a remedy for burns, scalds and

295

stings; it can be taken to help the ill-effects of burns, stings, eating shell fish or suppressed milk in breastfeeding mothers. It can be used to treat urticaria, gout, urinary infections, rheumatism and neuritis. Symptoms are often seasonal and tend to return at the same time each year.

USING THE HERB
Urtica can be used in potency or as a tincture in diluted form. A herbalist will traditionally use Urtica dioica, but really, we feel that any good stinging nettles can be used. It is a very nutritious herb. In the spring, fresh young nettle tips can be gathered as a nourishing vegetable. Alternatively, a tea can be made from the herb and used as a blood-cleanser for anaemia; it is a good diuretic herb and, as it generally helps the metabolism, will help with weight problems. It improves pancreatic functions and it is good for diabetics. Use as a tonic for convalescents. It will also help increase resistance to allergic reactions. Nettles can help women with heavy periods or they can increase milk production.

Externally, use an infusion made from the fresh herb or the tincture. An infusion can be used for the skin, hair, to bathe puffy eyes, and for cold, swollen arthritic joints. Dilute the tincture for bathing burns, scalds, cuts (it will help stop bleeding) or any blistering skin condition, prickly heat, raised red blotches or weal-like symptoms. Pour boiling water on the tops of fresh nettles, gathered away from polluted areas, leave and then drain the liquid off. This can be kept in the fridge if necessary.

SUGGESTED DOSAGE With an infusion from the dried herb, use 1 tspful per cup of boiling water. Using a tincture, dilute 1ml in a cup of water.

Nit Ac *Nitricum acidum (Nitric acid)*

Mental and emotional indications: These are very definite for this homoeopathic remedy. It can be given to people who are prone to be very touchy, cold and often angry. They can be very easily provoked and fly into a rage over anything, and then weep. They may become so angry that they tremble, and feel hateful and vindictive. They can swear and curse and refuse consolation. They become tired of life, despondent and sad. One of the significant features of this remedy is extreme anxiety, especially over their health. They may despair of improvement and are terrified of dying, of being left alone and of the future. All these symptoms are worse in the morning.

Physical symptoms: The most noticeable physical indication is of being cold; compare with Arsenicum Album, Nux Vomica and Hepar Sulph which are the three other main remedies where this is such a significant feature. *Skin:* It can be very effective for all parts of the skin which meet with mucous membranes. The skin is dry, cracked and may ulcerate and bleed easily at the corners of the mouth, nose, vagina or anus. These areas can become red and swollen and are very sensitive. Ulcers look raw and warts can bleed. *Pain:* The pains of this remedy are pricking and sticking and appear to come and go. There may be a sensation of a tight band around the head or bones. The person in need of Nit Ac is very sensitive to pain, and this may come on during sleep and be accompanied by frightening dreams. There will be a tendency to smell foul, the urine will be very offensive and the smell will linger; feet, nasal discharges and sweat will all be offensive. *Abdomen:* There may be diarrhoea, or the passing of a stool will seem incomplete even if accompanied by straining. There may be great pain, as if the rectum is torn, which it may well be, and the pain will remain for several hours. This remedy is really effective for anal fissures. There are piles which are very painful and bleed.

Other aspects of this remedy are joints which crack. All discharges are thin, offensively acrid and either brown, green or yellowish. Nit Ac is very good for treating thin, watery, brown, smelly leucorrhoea. *Modalities:* Symptoms get worse from being touched, cold or cold air and draughts and any additional slight burden. They appear better from mild weather and gentle movement.

Nux Vomica *Nux vomica*

This is one of the main homoeopathic remedies, it works effectively for a very wide range of mental, emotional and physical symptoms. The picture of the person that suits this remedy has traditionally been seen as masculine, but it is not exclusively for men or women. In the last century, when homoeopathy first became used in its present form, Nux Vomica was seen as a remedy for those who abuse the body and mind on all levels, including the sexual one, for ailments stemming from excessive behaviour, generally male behaviour. Women were expected to be acquiescent supporters of the aggressive male role.

Mental and emotional indications: It is now perhaps one of the most appropriate remedies for the type of person who lives hard. For men and women who are seen to have a strong character, who are forceful, charismatic, work too hard and drive themselves beyond their own limitations. They become people who have 'the right impulse but the wrong expression', and through driving themselves become irritable, fault-finding, nagging and quarrelsome hypochondriacs. They can become violent, very reactive and self-willed. They may particularly dislike being questioned and having to be responsive to others. In extreme cases they can get suicidal, but they are also afraid of death.

Physical symptoms: They are people who chill easily, and are prone to ailments that come on from getting cold. These people feel worse from coffee, tobacco, alcohol, drugs, highly-spiced food (all of which they tend to crave), overeating, mental over-exertion, lack of exercise and loss of sleep. It is a good hangover remedy.

Abdomen and digestion: Symptoms which can be relieved by Nux Vomica include nausea, which comes on after eating, in the morning or from smoking, with a feeling that vomiting would ease the discomfort. There may be burping after eating, with sour and bitter risings, heartburn and a sensation of pressure in the stomach for 1 or 2 hours after eating, with a desire to loosen clothing. There may be pains that go into the back and chest, flatulent colic and bruised soreness in the abdomen. The person can feel sleepy after dinner – maybe finding it difficult to think – and also after feeling anxious or worried. Nux Vomica can be very good for nausea and vomiting in pregnancy, especially where the nausea is temporarily relieved by vomiting. There is constipation with a frequent desire to pass stools but these then recede, and may alternate with diarrhoea. There may be tendency to faint after passing a stool or vomiting. It is a good remedy for those who have used laxatives for years. Nux Vomica is good for piles that itch or bleed and get better with cool bathing. Also, for varicose veins which are black, hard and look like cords; these have probably come from sedentary habits. It is a very good remedy for hernias.

Coughs: These are marked by their violent paroxysmal nature, often accompanied by a splitting headache with the need to hold the head. It is good for whooping cough or asthma where there is a sensation as if something has torn loose in the chest. There may be a desire to eat during a coughing fit. There will be hoarseness and painful roughness in the larynx and chest. *Catarrh*: Symptoms include a nasal discharge which flows during the day and is dry at night. It is worse in a warm room and gets better in cold air. Nux Vomica is good for infants who have constant snuffles (especially if the mother is very active and stressed). It is also good for babies with an umbilical hernia.

Periods: This is the remedy to take when periods come on too early, are profuse or too long. They may be irregular and are prone to stopping and starting. Use Nux Vomica where labour pains are violent and spasmodic, and there is an urge for a bowel movement or to urinate.

People who need this remedy find sleep irresistible when they return home from work or in the early evening – they may sleep for a while or just benefit from catnaps, and then be wide awake at bedtime, unable to sleep, finally dropping off just before it is time to rise in the morning. They will awake feeling tired and weak. They may have sexual dreams or nightmares about being chased. They may also cry or talk during sleep. A Nux Vomica type of person often has strong sexual impulses. *Modalities*: Symptoms feel worse in the early morning, from the cold, in the open air, in draughts, after excesses, from pressure (physical) and any incidents however slight. They improve after free discharges.

Oats   *Avena Sativa*

Oats are one of the best herbal remedies for strengthening the nervous system. It is a nervine tonic. Oats have an antidepressant effect and can be used to treat depression, stress and nervous debility. They are particularly useful to take to help people attempting to withdraw from an addiction to alcohol, smoking, tranquillizers, drugs, etc.

As a food, oats are extremely nutritious. They are a rich source of B group vitamins, and the minerals Calcium, Iron, Phosphorous and Silica. Oats are one of the richest sources of Inositol, and this is important for the proper metabolism of fats, and for reducing blood cholesterol levels, preventing hardening of the arteries and heart disease. Regular use of oats as a food will also help to correct constipation. Eat Oats on a regular basis, preferably raw, for example, as muesli for breakfast. Oats are particularly good to take if you are overly relaxed, but they are best avoided when you are agitated and tense.

Taken as a tincture, Oats is useful in treating general debility, particularly when associated with appetite loss. It is nourishing for the nervous system. It can be used in the treatment of anorexia nervosa. Give for convalescence and exhaustion. Oats are very cleansing: if you are sensitive to soap, use oats or oatmeal in a wash.

SUGGESTED DOSAGE A drink can be made from Oats by boiling a tbsp in 285ml (½pint) of water for a few minutes and then straining off the liquid. This should be drunk once or twice a day for its nourishing effect on the nervous system. Alternatively, use the tincture for treating stress, withdrawal from addictions, debility, etc: take 10–20 drops in water, 3 times a day, for up to 3 months.

Olibanum   *Boswellia thurifera*

This sweet, spicy resin is known as Frankincense and is well known for its use as incense. The distilled oil can be used for similar purposes. It has an uplifting quality and can be used to help break habits and emotionally move forward. It is rejuvenating if you are feeling very low and it aids concentration. It is really useful for catarrhal conditions, it clears the respiratory tract and is soothing on the mucous membranes. It has a sedating and cooling effect on the lungs, and its anti-inflammatory properties make it good for chest infections. It is also good for digestive problems and urinary tract infections. Frankincense was very popular with the Ancient Egyptians for skin-care preparations. Its astringent action makes it good for ageing skin and wrinkles. Being antiseptic, it will be useful for cleaning and treating wounds and ulcers.

A few drops of this oil placed on a burner are uplifting and beneficial if you are feeling stressed, tired and overwhelmed. Otherwise, place a few drops in a saucerful of base-massage oil. Combine with Rose, Sandalwood, Lemon or other oils that seem appropriate.

Orange Blossom   *Citrus aurantium*

The main action of this herb is sedative. It is calming to the nervous system, especially where there is restlessness and insomnia. It is good for an anxious state, palpitations and nervousness. It is beneficial to the digestive system so take it for indigestion that has nervous causes, and also for headaches that are caused by nervousness. Orange Blossom is delicious as a tea or make a strong infusion to add to the bath for a calm and pleasant soak. It is also good for the skin, and is said to help where there are broken capillaries.

SUGGESTED DOSAGE To make an infusion use 1 tspful of herb to a cup of boiling water.

NEROLI OIL *Citrus aurantium*
This oil, distilled from Orange Blossom, has a delicate but powerful fragrance. It is both calming and uplifting. Its main action is on the nervous system and it is one of the most effective antidepressant oils. It is helpful for nervous exhaustion, depression and confusion. It also aids sleep and can be used for shock and hysteria. Combine with Sweet Orange for nervous digestive problems resulting in diarrhoea and dyspepsia. It is a very good oil for the skin as it has low toxicity and can help heal scar tissue and broken veins. Combine in a base oil for dry and weathered skin. Neroli combines well with Bergamot to help clear the brain. Also with many other oils to give the blend a light, sweet fragrance. 1–3 drops can be added to a small saucerful of almond oil.

Parsley *Carum petroselinum*

This herb, as we know, is widely used in cooking. The leaves, root and seed can be used. The leaves contain Vitamin C and iron; the herb is nutritious and extra amounts can be added to the diet for people who are anaemic. It stimulates the stomach juices, for this reason it is contra-indicated where there are stomach ulcers. It helps digestion, it is a carminative herb and soothes colic and flatulence. One of the main medicinal uses for Parsley is its diuretic action. Use where there are problems with fluid retention and for helping arthritis, osteo-arthritis and for the passing of urinary stones. Parsley also stimulates menstruation, making it good for dysmenorrhoea (pain during periods) and amenorrhoea (absence of periods), but it is contra-indicated during pregnancy in medicinal doses.

SUGGESTED DOSAGE Take 1 tspful to a cup of boiling water 2–3 times daily.

PARSLEY OIL *Petroselinum satirum*
The volatile oil is distilled mainly from the seeds. It contains apiol

and this is an abortifacient, so it is important not to use Parsley Oil during pregnancy. It can be used for similar reasons to the herb, but is mainly used for its diuretic value. It can be diluted (use a dilution of 0.5–1 per cent) and massaged in, or use a drop in the bath when you are feeling particularly bloated before a period.

Parsley Piert *Alchemilla arvensis*

This herb acts on the kidneys, it is a soothing diuretic and can help dissolve stones and gravel. If it is taken over a long period of time it helps to restore normal functions to the kidney and is good for oedema (water retention). Combine this herb with Pellitory-of-the-wall and Hawthorn to support the kidneys and the heart.

SUGGESTED DOSAGE Use 1 tspful of herb to a cup of boiling water and drink 3 times a day, or 2ml of tincture diluted in water 3 times daily.

Passiflora *Passiflora incarnata*

Passiflora or passionflower is a very calming herb, especially for the brain or nerves. It is useful to take where there is a build-up of energy and thought which leads to insomnia. It is an anti-spasmodic herb and can help epilepsy, and has been given to treat Parkinson's disease, neuralgia, and nerve pains generally. It is also useful for PMT and period pains. It can combine well with Scullcap, Orange Blossom and Chamomile, and can be taken when there is tension or part of the body is painful as a result of tension.

SUGGESTED DOSAGE Take 1–2 tspfuls of herb infused in a cup of boiling water and drink 3 times a day, or take 1–2ml of tincture diluted in water and drink 3 times a day.

Pellitory-Of-The-Wall *Parietaria officinalis*

This is a diuretic and soothing herb. It is very useful for dissolving stones and gravel, although it needs to be taken over several months. It is often combined with Parsley Piert. It is good for inflammation in the urinary system and can be used for cystitis.

SUGGESTED DOSAGE For an infusion use 1 tspful of herb to a cup of boiling water and drink 3 times daily, or 1ml of tincture diluted in water drunk 3 times daily.

Pennyroyal   *Mentha pulegium*

This is a diaphoretic herb (helps the body to sweat), and it is good to take for colds and flu. It is also warming and will create energy in the gut, helping with indigestion, digestive upsets and digestive-type headaches. It is often suitable to combine in flu mixtures. It will stimulate the uterus to contract and can be helpful during a lengthy labour to create movement; it will help expel the afterbirth. For these reasons it must not be taken in pregnancy. It can be useful for delayed periods in cold and weak women, but it must not be used if the delay is due to pregnancy. It cannot be used safely to bring about an abortion. The amount needed would possibly cause severe damage to the baby's nervous system and probably cause an epileptic fit in the pregnant woman. It is much safer to have a legal abortion. Using Pennyroyal as a abortifacient is an irresponsible and dangerous way of dealing with an unwanted pregnancy.

SUGGESTED DOSAGE Take 1–2ml tincture in water 3 times a day, or 1 tspful of herb infused in a cup of water 3 times a day.

Peppermint   *Mentha piperita*

The primary action of Peppermint is on the digestive system, in particular the stomach. It encourages food to be easily digested and can be used for symptoms of a sluggish digestion, e.g. indigestion and flatulence. It can also help with regurgitation, sour risings, belching and hiccups. Peppermint is a digestive antiseptic and can be used to treat gastric fevers, diarrhoea, intestinal parasites and food poisoning. It is also an anti-spasmodic herb and will relieve gastric spasms and colic. Use Peppermint for nausea caused by anything. It aids the digestion of fats by encouraging the flow of bile. In Chinese terms,

Peppermint is a very cooling herb; it will help cool and detoxify the liver.

The second main action of Peppermint is on the respiratory system. It is an expectorant and is useful for coughs which produce yellow or green mucus. Use also for colds, where it is good to combine with Elderflower and Yarrow. It can be used for its anti-spasmodic and decongesting properties for treating asthma, bronchitis and sinusitis. Peppermint is a refreshing and general tonic for the nervous system and for nervous fatigue; it is an important herb for helping migraine. Use it for feelings of faintness or hysteria, and conditions arising from tension and anxiety. It can be taken during painful periods.

SUGGESTED DOSAGE Take 1 tspful per cup of boiling water 3 times a day, or 1ml of tincture diluted in water.

PEPPERMINT OIL   *Mentha piperita*
Initially this oil feels cooling on the skin as it works by constricting the blood vessels, but then it dilates them, so encouraging circulation to the area. It is an oil which can be widely used for all the reasons mentioned for the herb. Combine with Fennel and Orange oils diluted in a base oil, and massage onto the stomach area for digestive problems. Use Peppermint Oil, diluted, as an insect repellent, parasiticide for scabies and fungicide for ringworm. Combine in a lotion to stop the itch of heat rash and add a few drops to a foot bath to relieve tired, aching, feet. You can also, of course, use Peppermint Oil for flavouring in cooking. It will always make any sweet, chocolaty, fatty or rich foods easier to digest. Remember, however, that if you are using homoeopathic medicines, Peppermint must be avoided, as it is known to be an antidote. This includes avoiding Peppermint-flavoured toothpastes.

Periwinkle   *Vinca major*

This herb contains an alkaloid called vincamine which has the effect of increasing oxygen to the brain and also the amount of oxygen the brain uses; this makes it have a refreshing effect on the brain. It is good to use when overwork causes giddiness, poor memory, headaches and general vertigo. Combine with Rosemary for this. It can be used for epilepsy, after a stroke, for arteriosclerosis, Menière's syndrome and tinnitus. Periwinkle is an astringent herb and a styptic (it clots blood). It is used for gut problems, e.g. colitis, and for heavy or irregular periods. It can even be used to help prevent nosebleeds. Traditionally, in old herbals, fresh Periwinkle was applied to limbs that were aching with cramp.

SUGGESTED DOSAGE Use 1 tspful of herb to a cup of boiling water and take 3 times a day, or 1–2ml of tincture 3 times a day.

Phosphorus   *Phosphorus*

This is a very important homoeopathic remedy. The typical Phosphorus person will often have a history of growing too quickly when young, and they can be tall and slim. *Mental and emotional indications:* Phosphorus-type people are usually full of vitality, quick moving, bright and intelligent. They are alert, they sit forward in their seats, and are expressive and sensitive to surroundings, people, noise, odours, light and atmospheres. They can be tense and restless, become fidgety, impatient, anxious and very fearful. They can have a sense of dread or feel nervous without knowing why, overshadowed by fear. Tension tends to increase in the afternoon, and symptoms are at their worst around twilight. They fear the dark, being alone, disease and death. They have an impending fear that something will happen.

They can be sensitive on the psychic level, tending to be clairvoyant, vulnerable or impressionable. They are often very sympathetic to the needs of others and will go out of their way to help. They are warm, friendly, affectionate and extrovert. They love being touched, stroked or massaged. They can get over-concerned for the welfare of others. They are easily influenced and reassured, they like sympathy themselves, and have vivid imaginations, often being artistic and musical. They are day-dreamers.

Physical symptoms: Generalised by chilliness. There is great weakness and trembling accompanying all symptoms. The circulation is unstable, and becoming easily flushed is an indication of this remedy – hot, spicy foods, temperature changes or even strong ideas will cause flushing. A Phosphorus type will become easily and quickly exhausted, they can be said to be 'running on their nerves'. They have short, intense bursts of energy and then need to rest. There may be a feeling of burning along the spine, in the feet, in between the shoulder blades, on the palms and in the chest. Phosphorus is a very good remedy for haemorrhage, postpartum haemorrhage (here is good to use 200C), where small wounds bleed easily and profusely, and when the blood is bright red, and for nosebleeds. There is a tendency to anaemia, and there can also be hair loss.

Throat symptoms: Frequent soreness, inability to talk as the larynx is so painful, swollen tonsils, voice loss. *Head symptoms*: Throbbing violent headache with hunger or preceded by hunger, or mental exertion. Violent, neuralgic pains darting and shooting. Symptoms get worse from light, heat, motion and lying down. They improve from cold and rest. *Coughs*: A dry, tickling, hard, racking cough which is exhausting and accompanied by a bursting headache (see Belladonna and Nux Vom). A tightness of the chest which is improved with pressure. There is trembling with the cough. Expectoration is yellow, bloody, rusty-coloured and salty. The cough gets worse from laughing, talking, eating, lying on the left side, from the open air and going from warm to cold or vice versa (see also Rumex). Coughs are often brought on by a cold going down to the chest, leading to bronchitis and pneumonia.

Stomach: Symptoms include a liking for chocolate, spicy food, fish, salt and ice cream. A thirst for cold drinks which, during illness, are vomited up once they get warm in the stomach. There is post-operative vomiting. The remedy can be indicated for nausea after anaesthesia. Also, ravenous hunger, burning in stomach, stomach ulcers, an empty, hollow feeling and waterbrash. *Abdomen*: Stools are slender, tough, dry and there may be bleeding from the rectum. There is profuse, exhausting diarrhoea, like water. It pours out but is painless, it can come on after a fright or nervousness. There can be an involuntary stool, with weakness afterwards. Haemorrhoids which bleed. *Women's complaints*: Periods of bright red blood may be frequent, scanty, can go on too long or there may be bleeding in between periods, amenorrhoea. Uterine polyps, fibroids. Leucorrhoea can be burning and replace menses. Strong sexual desire which increases during pregnancy and breastfeeding. *Skin*: Wounds bleed excessively. They may heal and then break out and bleed again. *Sleeping*: Generally on the right side. The person is better from taking naps and from sleeping. Sleepy during the day, restless at night. Vivid dreams.

Modalities: Symptoms get worse from lying on the left side or on the painful side, from slight causes, from cold or damp or changes in the weather, and from mental exertion. They improve from eating, sleeping, massage, sitting, cold food, washing the face with cold water and lying on the right side.

Phytolacca (Poke Root) *Phytolacca*

See Poke Root.

Pilewort (Lesser Celandine) *Ranunculus ficaria*

As the name suggests, this herb can be used for piles or varicose veins. It can be used internally, but it is probably best to make a decoction and use it externally, either as an enema or as a lotion, or combine in an ointment.

SUGGESTED DOSAGE Make an infusion if the leaves are used, or a decoction for the root: use 30g (1 oz) per pint of boiling water.

Pine Oil *Pinus sylvestris*

The main action of Pine Oil is on the respiratory tract. It is a powerful antiseptic and decongestant. It strengthens the lungs and can be used to treat bronchial infections, e.g. colds, coughs and bronchitis. It will help clear mucus from the throat and catarrh from the sinuses. It will also relieve hayfever. The antiseptic properties of Pine work on urinary infections, e.g. cystitis, pyelitis, and can be used to treat NSU (Non-specific urethritis). Pine Oil will create a refreshing, easing bath for aches, pains and smelly feet! Use up to 4 drops in the bath, or 1–2 drops in a saucerful of base oil.

Plantain *Plantago major*

This herb contains Vitamins C and K and the minerals zinc and silica. It has a cooling, drying action and is right for all catarrhal conditions, especially of the lungs and gut, and where there is apathy and a lack of confidence. It is also a specific herb to be given for infection of the middle ear (otitis media) or glue ear. Plantain is a diuretic herb and is antiseptic to the urinary tract, making it good for cystitis. It has strong anti-bacterial properties so it is used for healing skin problems such as ulcers, cuts, stings, spots and, as an ointment, for piles. As with all herbs, the freshly gathered plant is always preferable, but this is markedly the case with Plantain.

SUGGESTED DOSAGE Use 1 tspful of herb to 1 cup of boiling water, or 1–2ml of tincture in water, and drink 3 times a day.

Poke Root *Phytolacca americana*

This is a plant known and used by both herbalists and homoeopaths. It was at one time widely used by Native Americans to treat fevers, aches and pains. Homoeopathically, the mental and emotional indications are not particularly marked, although there may be a reluctance or indifference towards work and a general sadness.

Physical symptoms: Phytolacca affects mainly the tonsils or mammary glands, and works on inflammation of bones and glands in general. It helps: pains that come and go suddenly or those that move from spot to spot; pains that are shooting or feel like electric shocks; weakness; feeling faint on rising. Pains feel worse on the right side. The body feels chilly but the head and face can feel hot. There may be thirst, with frequent yawning and a restlessness from pain. The person may wake feeling very weak. They feel tired and worn out and want to lie down. There can be aching all over the body, with a bruised feeling, and painful throat that is inflamed or swollen, dry, rough, bruised and smarting, as if a ball of red hot iron is lodged in the throat – it feels full and choking. There can be pain at the end of the tongue and pain in the ears when swallowing. There is a sensation of a lump when swallowing or when the head is turned to the left.

Mumps: Phytolacca is a useful homoeopathic remedy for mumps where there is inflammation of the submaxillary and parotid glands, especially when they are hard like stones and there is pain shooting into the ear when swallowing. These symptoms are made worse by cold and wet. *Women's complaints*: Especially in the area of the breasts – when they become sore and lumpy, particularly before or during the period. It can help where the lymph glands are enlarged in the armpits and when the pain shoots all over the body. It is good for nipples that have become very cracked and sore and sensitive during breastfeeding. The breasts feel better from firm pressure. It is a good remedy for mastitis, when the breast becomes hard, painful, purplish and very sensitive.

Phytolacca is a good remedy to try when Bryonia and Rhus Tox fail, for rheumatic pains and stiffness in the muscles: when the joints are swollen and hot and the pains are like electric shocks. It can help right-sided sciatica. *Modalities*: Symptoms get worse on exposure to damp, cold weather or a change of weather, on getting up, from motion, swallowing hot drinks, heat, menses and rain. They improve in dry weather, from rest, lying on the abdomen or on the left side.

USING THE HERB

As a herb, Poke Root stimulates the lymphatic system. It is a good herb for glandular fever or colds, or where there are accompanying swollen glands in the neck and armpits. It can also be given for the treatment of mastitis. Use Poke Root for respiratory complaints, especially chronic colds and where there is inflammation. Although Poke Root is a very good herb it must be given with caution. It is not advisable to use it as a general lymphatic cleanser. It is not a gentle herb, such as Cleavers, and should not be taken over a long period of time.

SUGGESTED DOSAGE Dilute 1ml of tincture in water and take 3 times a day, or decoct 25g (1oz) of root to 570ml (1 pint) of water and take a tbsp 3 times a day.

Prickly Ash   *Xanthoxylum americanum*

This herb is an excellent circulatory stimulant which helps all sorts of disorders. It increases circulation to the joints making it good for rheumatism and arthritis. Use during the daytime as it increases the flow of saliva, it also increases sweating so it helps colds and flu. It is used for colic, spasm and watery diarrhoea. This herb is suitable for people with low blood pressure; it must be avoided by those with high blood pressure.

SUGGESTED DOSAGE Decoct 30g (1oz) to 570ml (1 pint) of water and take 2 tbsp 3 times daily, or dilute ½ ml in water and take 3 times daily.

Psyllium Husks   *Plantago psyllium*

The outer husks or the seeds are used for their mucilagenous and, therefore, soothing qualities. They can absorb a lot of water and are used to increase the peristatic action of the gut. The swollen and mucousy bulk will stimulate the colon to contract. It is good as a gentle laxative during pregnancy, or for the occasional bout of constipation. Use also to help soothe inflamed gut conditions.

SUGGESTED DOSAGE One way to take this herb is to mix a tbsful of husks with water and swallow the mixture. It may, however, be easier to take by mixing a spoonful with honey and then drinking a glass of water immediately afterwards. Take once or twice a day. If it is only required once, then take it at night.

Pulsatilla *Anemone pulsatilla*

This is one of the major homoeopathic remedies, it is primarily appropriate for women and children. *Mental and emotional indications*: The general indications are marked by changeability and a softness which puts up no resistance to confrontation. These people will tend to shape themselves around what they think will please, so trying to work out a remedy for a person requiring Pulsatilla is often tricky. They have very little sense of self, with no opinion of their own. They are easily dominated, being timid, shy and often embarrassed. Their emotions are quickly aroused, they can go from tears to laughter very quickly. They weep reading and feel much better for it, they can easily feel very sorry for themselves and will tend to whine and grumble, but they improve greatly with consolation and feelings of compassion.

Those needing Pulsatilla usually have a strong sexual desire but sometimes they have a dread of the opposite sex. They may be sensuous and needy or overdependent, this can lead them into being possessive and becoming victims of their own jealous feelings. They can be very demanding but are not aggressive or malicious, although they can become easily offended, irritable, touchy or angry through their lack of self-confidence. It is often possible to trace their symptoms to a time when they felt abandoned and forsaken. They have a strong desire for company, and fears about being alone, death, the dark and insanity which get worse in the evening. In women, hysteria, sadness and depression get worse before their period. A Pulsatilla person will crave the open air and hate stuffiness and although they can be chilly, they are averse to heat. It is one of the main remedies for babies and children where cold drinks or ice-creams tend to upset the digestion.

Physical symptoms: The changeable temperament is matched by changing symptoms. Pains shift rapidly and are erratic. There is a thirstlessness with nearly all complaints. Headaches pulsate and are bursting. Nervousness from overwork is improved by walking in the open air. *Eyes*: Symptoms include a thick yellow-green, profuse, bland discharge. There is a tendency to develop conjuctivitis from a cold, also recurrent styes. *Ears*: Earaches occur after colds, there is yellow-green discharge from the ears. Impaired hearing with catarrh of the Eustachian tubes. Earache is worse at night, and causes the child to become weepy and clingy. *Nose*: Loss of smell with catarrh, nostrils blocked with yellowish, bland discharge. These symptoms are worse when lying down and better in the open air. *Mouth*: It is a common feature in many Pulsatilla cases to have a crack in the centre of the lower lip, and there is a great need to lick the lips. This is often accompanied by an offensive taste in the morning when waking. There may be toothache which gets better with cold water held in the mouth. There is a marked thirstlessness but with a dry mouth.

Digestion and Abdomen: Gastric disorders come on from rich, fatty foods such as pork, sausages, pastry and ice-cream. Nausea and heartburn are symptoms of Pulsatilla, and so is vomiting food that has been eaten hours before. Digestion is slow and the stomach feels weighed down with an 'all gone' sensation. The person feels hungry but they do not know what they want. The abdomen is distended, stools are changeable in appearance, and diarrhoea can occur after a fright during the night. Diarrhoea is watery, greenish-yellow and can also arise from eating fruit, ice-cream or cold food. There can be piles which tend to improve during the menses. Cystitis can occur if the person lies on their back, and there may be involuntary urination during sleep or in pregnancy.

Women's complaints: Symptoms include amenorrhoea which comes on after getting the feet wet and debility and anaemia at puberty. Pulsatilla will generally regulate or bring on periods. It is a good remedy for late, irregular, scanty periods, clotted, dark, thick blood, and where there are changeable, bearing-down pains or cutting, griping pains during periods. It can help bleeding between periods (metrorrhagia) and is good for PMT when the person is nervous, touchy, restless, weepy, depressed and has headaches and swollen, tender breasts. It is a frequently-used remedy for breast problems: mastitis, swollen or cracked nipples, swollen breasts during breastfeeding, for thin, watery milk, and when the mother gets weepy every time the baby is at the breast. It can be used if the milk continues after weaning. Use for leucorrhoea that is acrid and cream-like or milky and thin. There may also be polyps in the vagina. Pulsatilla can be given to help correct the position of the foetus in pregnancy, for false labour or where the labour contractions are ineffectual and spasmodic. This remedy includes stinging and painful varicose veins that are worse during pregnancy.

Sleep: This is the remedy for sleeplessness due to persistent thoughts, and feeling wide awake at night and then exhausted on waking in the morning. Often the person lies awake, then drops off to sleep and wakes again for a long time. *Respiratory symptoms*: Pulsatilla is good for coughs when they are dry at night and then loose in the daytime. The cough is exhausting and racking. It gets worse at night and causes the person to wake up and then feel they must sit up. Coughs get worse with exertion and heat. There can be yellowish-green expectoration. It is a good remedy for coughs that come on after measles.

Pulsatilla is indicated for pains in the extremities which rapidly shift about. Joints can be painful, red and swollen. *Children's illnesses*: It is a good remedy and often indicated for chickenpox, measles, etc. The child will become weepy, irritable and clingy during the illness. *Modalities*: Symptoms get worse in warmth, warm air, a warm bed, from wet feet, in the evening, from rich foods, ice-cream, eggs, at puberty, during pregnancy and before menses. They get better in cold, fresh, open air, from gentle motion, from an erect posture, after crying, from applying pressure and lying down with the head up.

USING THE HERB
The herb must be used after it has been dried; if it is used when it is fresh, it will cause blistering. Its herbal uses are similar to its homoeopathic uses, and relate to the same emotional states. It will help vague, fleeting pains in both the male and female reproductive areas. Pulsatilla can help nervous, liverish migraines and a sluggish digestion, and where there are particular problems in digesting fats. It is good for all fleeting pains of the gut, gall bladder problems and rheumatic pains. It can be used for leucorrhoea and all thick, yellow or greenish catarrhal conditions, especially in the upper respiratory tract, sinusitis or glue ear. Pulsatilla is antiseptic and also diaphoretic, helping to induce sweat and lower feverish conditions; this makes it particularly appropriate in treating conditions where mucus has settled in the chest.

SUGGESTED DOSAGE Use ½ tspful of dried herb to a cup of boiling water and drink 3 times a day, or use 1ml of tincture diluted in water 3 times a day.

Purple Coneflower *Echinacea augustifolia* or *Echinacea purpurea*

See Echinacea.

Pyrethrum *Anacydus pyrethrum*

This is a very harsh, bitter herb. It should really only be used externally. Use in the garden in a spray against insects or for indoor use against cat fleas, and so on.

SUGGESTED DOSAGE Pour 570ml (1 pint) of boiling water onto 30g (1oz) of herb, cover and leave to stand for at least 10 mins before straining.

Raspberry Leaf *Rubus idaeus*

It is the leaf that is generally used medicinally, but the fruit is nutritious and has a cooling action. Raspberry Leaf is good to include in mixtures. Use it during any fitness routine as it will help to tone slack muscles. It is an astringent herb and can be infused and used as a gargle for sore throats, or combined with Agrimony for laryngitis, hoarseness and loss of voice. It helps gum conditions and can be made into a mouthwash similar to Sage, although Sage may have more anti-bacterial properties. It is useful in pregnancy, especially if you are prone to gum disease. Take it in the first three months of pregnancy as a digestive, its calming action will help with morning sickness. As a uterine tonic, it will tone the uterine muscles and this will help labour: combine with Chamomile and Peppermint and take for the three months before the birth. During labour, drink Raspberry Leaf to help prevent haemorrhage, and then continue regular drinking for 2–3 weeks after the birth to encourage the muscles to contract and resume their normal shape.

SUGGESTED DOSAGE Take 1–5ml of tincture 3 times daily, or infuse 1 tspful of herb per cup of boiling water 1–3 times daily.

Red Clover   *Trifolium pratense*

This is an alterative herb. It helps purify the blood and it is especially useful for weeping skin conditions and psoriasis. It can help eczema in children. It is a good cleansing herb to take in the late spring and early summer, and it can be combined with Nettles, Heartsease, Cleavers and Lavender. As well as being good for the skin, it is an expectorant and cooling herb and has anti-spasmodic actions. This makes it appropriate for lung conditions and the treatment of coughs, bronchitis and whooping cough.

SUGGESTED DOSAGE Infuse 1–2 tspfuls of herb in a cup of boiling water and drink 3 times daily, or dilute 1ml tincture and take 3 times daily.

Red Sage *and* Sage   *Salvia officinalis*

The actions of Red Sage and Sage are very similar, they are both antiseptic and healing. They can be used effectively to treat any inflamed and septic mouth conditions. Combine with Marshmallow in an infusion as a gargle for mouth ulcers, or to treat sore throats, tonsillitis, laryngitis and gum conditions that are sore and bleeding, such as gingivitis. Both will promote the circulation to any area so they are warming herbs that can be used for debilitated, weak, and cold people, especially if the body temperature is low. Caution must be used as Red Sage and Sage are abortifacients and should not be taken during pregnancy. They can be taken after the birth to dry up milk production, and can be used as a douche for leucorrhoea – combine with Lavender and Chamomile. They are good for menopausal hot flushes as they generally reduce sweating. For this reason, it is not advisable to take either during a fever or flu and where there is a need to sweat. They also raise the blood pressure, so avoid giving where there is high blood pressure.

Both Sages are good lung tonics and strengthen the lungs. Use for emphysema, asthma and where there is coldness and weakness associated with respiratory problems. Since they are bitter and antiseptic herbs, they are excellent for the digestive tract, helping liver, bile and pancreatic functioning. They increase hydrochloric acid production which is needed to help break down the food in the stomach. As general, overall tonics, both are good for nervous debility, convalescence or where the digestion is upset; and because they are antiseptic they help stop putrefaction. Although Red Sage and Sage will increase the peristaltic action in a sluggish gut, they can be given to someone with diarrhoea, if this is due to a general weakness and debility. The infusion is astringent and can be used externally as a wash for open pores and spotty skin. It is also said to restore colour to grey hair.

SUGGESTED DOSAGE Take ½ tspful of herb in a cup of boiling water, or 10 drops of tincture in water, 3 times a day.

SAGE OIL   *Salvia officinalis*
The properties of Sage make this an oil that can be used either on its own or as part of a mixture in a base oil, as a very effective warming massage. Where it is given for nervous and physical debility it can be mixed with Lavender; where there are rheumatic aches combine with Juniper; in a foot rub combine with Peppermint. After a cold, exhausting day try a few drops of Sage and Ginger in the bath. Sage Oil is very versatile, but remember not to use it during pregnancy, in feverish conditions or where there is high blood pressure.

Rhubarb Root   *Rheum palmatum*

This is a bitter herb which has an astringent and gentle laxative action. It is good to give for Bacillary dysentery, it will initially increase the laxative action and then tone the bowel without causing constipation. In smaller doses, Rhubarb Root is good for dyspepsia and diarrhoea, especially in the elderly and convalescents. It is sometimes used as a red-gold dye for blond hair. The powdered root can be combined with equal parts of Chamomile flowers and neutral Henna to give this effect.

SUGGESTED DOSAGE Use 1 tspful of powdered herb infused in a cup of boiling water. Leave to stand for 10 mins before straining, then drink 3 times a day. Or take 1ml of tincture diluted in water 3 times a day. For Bacillary dysentery give 5ml of tincture every 3 hours, and for children give 3 doses of 1–2ml tincture diluted in water.

Rhus Tox *Rhus toxicodendron*

This is a homoeopathic remedy that affects the fibrous tissue and any rheumatic symptoms of the ligaments or joints. *Mental and emotional indications*: There can be mental restlessness, with a feeling of despondency, sadness, anxiety and depression which gets worse in the evening, also a tendency to weep without knowing why and a desire to be alone. There can also be a mild restlessness with stupor or mild delirium. In children, there can be rigidity and anxiety, while being in the cold and damp makes them feel mentally worse. They can be forgetful, and there is a fear of being poisoned and of drowning.

Physical symptoms: Pains are tearing, sticking and shooting, and they get worse at night. It is difficult to find a position to rest in. The key indication to this remedy is that the symptoms are worse from rest and at the start of movement. They improve with prolonged movement. It is excellent for sprained ankles and wrists, strained ligaments and tendons around the joints or strained and pulled muscles. Symptoms get worse in cold, wet and damp conditions, they improve from the heat. *Skin*: Dry, hot and itchy. A triangular red tip to the tongue is a key indicator for this remedy. Rhus Tox is good for eruptions of vesicles, as in chickenpox and shingles. Itching is not relieved by scratching. There can be moist eruptions which are worse on hairy parts. Swelling of the joints. Red, spotty, itchy skin rapidly progresses to vessication and swelling, and then into yellow pus and scabs with surrounding yellow skin, which looks red and angry (as in chickenpox). Eczema, particularly of the face, neck and genitals. Eruptions are dark red. Swollen glands particularly under the arms (see also Graphites). The eyelids are inflamed red, stiff and agglutinated.

Rhus Tox is a good remedy to use whenever there is pain and stiffness that compels movement; this brings relief until exhaustion forces rest. Rest then makes the symptoms start up again. It can be given for heart trouble due to over-exertion. A Rhus-Tox fever is very hot with a high temperature, even though the person feels cold and needs extra covers. There is restlessness and slight relief comes from shifting positions, but the person may be motionless from exhaustion. Headaches feel as if a board is strapped to the forehead. Dreams are often of work and things that need to be done. *Fibrous tissues*: This is the remedy when they are inflamed from over-exertion, ligaments feel strained. Symptoms include slipped discs, back pain, lumbago in the small of the back, pains from trying to get up and stiff neck and back pains that are worse from cold and better from warmth. *Digestion*: There is hunger without appetite, an empty sensation in the stomach but no desire for food. Drowsiness after eating. A craving for cold drinks and ices, but this will create nausea after eating.

Rhus Tox is a remedy that follows Arnica well (see pages 190–1 for the homoeopathic dosage). *Modalities*: Symptoms are worse from rest, at the beginning of movement, from over-exertion, in the damp, cold and wet. They improve with continued motion, with heat and hot baths, from rubbing and from changing position.

Rosemary *Rosmarinus officinalis*

This is a strongly refreshing herb, it increases the circulation to the brain and is good for uplifting depressed, cold states. It improves memory and concentration and helps induce a feeling of well-being. It is good for people who tend to get dizzy when they get up. It stimulates and nourishes the nervous system, and is excellent to put in a bath for dull tiredness in the mornings. It is warming and stimulating to the digestive tract and will increase the appetite and help flatulence. It soothes cramps. It is a tonic for elderly people and convalescents. It can also help if periods have stopped as a result of being cold, or if they are very painful. It is a suitable herb to take if you are too tired to go to sleep, when the nervous system is overwrought. It can be made into an infusion for a hair rinse using 30g (1oz) to 570ml (1 pint) of water, because it strengthens the hair and adds shine to dark hair. This herb is contra-indicated in pregnancy and in high blood pressure.

SUGGESTED DOSAGE Infuse ½ tspful in 1 cup of boiling water and drink 3 times daily, or take ½ml tincture diluted in water 3 times daily.

ROSEMARY OIL *Rosmarinus officinalis*
Like the herb this oil is stimulating and raises blood pressure. It is particularly good in a massage oil for poor circulation, and for a weak heart where there is low blood pressure, especially in nervous people. Combine with Lavender for nervous headaches, migraines or confusion. Use an inhalation for catarrh or to unblock sinuses. Being antiseptic and anti-spasmodic, Rosemary Oil can be massaged in the abdomen for painful digestion and spasms. It can be beneficial

317

for rheumatism and cold, congested areas that need unblocking, e.g. cellulite. It is also good to add a few drops to the bath for painful or delayed periods.

As an oil, Rosemary can be added to Coconut Oil as a scalp treatment for dandruff. For an antiseptic and parasiticide, combine with Lavender against lice or scabies. Use in a massage where there is tension and over-tiredness, e.g. for exam nerves where there is a need to be alert but calm. Here it may be combined with Neroli.

Roses

Red roses may be used as a herb. Although mostly known as an oil, the red rose is a valuable tonic for the heart and lungs. As a tea, the petals are more astringent than the oil and have a tonic effect on the gut and the liver. They have a diuretic action and are said to increase the appetite. They have a very soothing effect on the skin: combine in a tea with Marshmallow and Elderflower to help eczema. Where there are menstrual problems and night sweats, add Borage and Chickweed. Consider adding Rose petals where there is an emotional aspect to a problem, and feelings of holding back. Roses are always good to add to a mixture of herbs for the bath.

ROSE OIL *Rosa damascena*

This is a beautiful deep, rich oil which is steam-distilled in Morocco, Bulgaria or Turkey. Rose absolute is more readily available, and this is extracted by means of solvents. Whether an essential oil or an absolute, Rose Oil has a powerful fragrance that in itself feels restorative. It has been combined into lotions and oils for the skin since ancient times, because of its anti-inflammatory and antiseptic properties. It affects the liver function and helps bring about cleansing. It is good for tired, lifeless skin. It is a balancer, both for the skin and for the vascular system – it strengthens the veins. Use for varicose veins and broken capillaries. It will also have a balancing effect on the heart, especially where problems arise from an overwrought lifestyle and stress.

The toning effect that Rose Oil has makes it appropriate for digestive problems. It strengthens the stomach and is good for gastro-enteritis and ulcers or where there is nausea and vomiting; it will help restore the appetite and is mildly laxative on the restricted gut and colon. It will soothe and cleanse the effects of physical abuse, e.g. from alcohol, and abuse on an emotional level. It is a calming, regenerative oil. It is an excellent oil to include in a massage or bath for helping problems in the female reproductive system, such as PMT and irregular or suppressed periods, and it also is very good in a massage during the last few months of pregnancy or during postnatal depression. Rose is a wonderful oil to use if you are feeling vulnerable, tired with life or sad. Adding Rose Oil to any combination of oils will contribute a depth of richness of fragrance. In particular, try adding one drop to a saucerful of base oil with either Sandalwood, Lavender, Geranium, Melissa, Olibanum or Bergamot.

Rosewood Oil (Bois de Rose Oil) *Aniba Rosaeodora*

Rosewood is a spicy, woody, sweet-smelling oil that is calming, cooling and safe to use. It is very useful as a mild expectorant and for all conditions that are dry and hot, e.g. feverishness or dry coughs. Use for digestive headaches. It can be massaged in when colds, flu or viral infections are difficult to throw off. It combines well with Rose for treating inflamed or hot, dry skin conditions. Rosewood is a very pleasant, gentle oil to use, it can strengthen the emotions and is good to use in times of crisis. Use 3–4 drops in a little base-massage oil.

Ruta *Ruta graveolens*

This is a good homoeopathic remedy to follow on from Arnica. It can be given for injured or bruised bones, fibrous tissue, tendons, cartilage or periosteum (tissue covering the bone). This remedy is indicated where there is injury and sprain, particularly when it involves the periosteum and wrists and ankles. Pains are sore, aching and bruised, there is a feeling of restlessness. It is an ideal remedy for treating strains around joints. Use for persistent stiffness after a sprain or strain. Give Ruta when Rhus Tox fails to work. Limbs can feel heavy and weak, legs give way on getting up or going up the stairs. There are pains in the hips and bones of the legs. There is unsteadiness when walking, and extreme weakness of the legs after straining the back, weariness and feelings of intense weakness and despair. Affected parts become sore even in bed. There may be a general feeling of dissatisfaction and a fear of anything new.

Ruta is a good remedy for the eyes or eye-strain which is then followed by a headache. Eyes can be red, hot and painful after reading small print or reading in a dim light. This remedy helps weak eye muscles. It is indicated for 'housemaid's knee', 'tennis elbow' and rheumatism, especially if due to strain or over-exertion. It is particularly indicated when the bony parts are affected. Use for sciatica which is worse from lying down or in the evening and gets better during the day. Give Ruta for osteo-arthritis which comes on from an old sprained ankle or knee. Use for prolapse of the rectum which has occurred on stooping, after delivery or during a stool. Ruta helps to strengthen prolapsed muscles. *Modalities*: Symptoms get worse from lying, sitting, eye-strain, cold air, wind, damp, sprains and injury from over-exertion. They improve from warmth, rubbing and lying on the back.

Sabadilla *Sabadilla officinarum*

This is a homoeopathic remedy which is often used for hayfever, 'flu or conditions affecting the mucous membranes. *Mental and emotional indications*: These are not very marked; the main ones are fears, confusion and fixed ideas, which are often to do with the state of the body.

Physical symptoms: These are persistent, spasmodic sneezing, with itching or tickling in the nose. The nose may be blocked or dry or with a profuse nasal discharge. The person may rub or pick the nose. The eyes may be watery or red, with coryza (nasal discharge); they will water when sneezing, coughing, yawning or walking in the open air. A marked indication of this remedy is an acute sense of smell, and nasal discharge will get worse with the smell of flowers. The face is hot and red, it burns as if scalded, the lips feel hot. The soft palette of the mouth itches. A sensation of a lump in the throat makes the person swallow constantly. Sabadilla is a remedy for worms where the symptoms are a craving hunger for sweet food and a crawling, itching anus, alternating with itching in the nose and ears. Sexual desire may increase with worms. *Modalities*: Symptoms get worse from cold air, drinks, periodically and during a full and new moon. They improve in the open air or from heat, warm food and drink, eating and swallowing.

Sabina *Sabina*

This is an important homoeopathic remedy for bleeding in the uterus. This can be due to either loss of tone in the blood vessels or a miscarriage. *Mental and emotional indications*: These are not marked although there is an intolerance to music, which can lead to excessive nervousness. There may be uneasiness, restlessness and increased sexual desire.

Physical symptoms: The main area that this remedy covers is the female reproductive organs. Sabina is a good remedy for leucorrhoea which is thick, yellow, smells foul and replaces periods. It can be used for periods that are early, profuse, protracted, part fluid and part clotted, or where the flow comes in waves. It may be accompanied by labour-type pains, paroxysms or colicky pains that go from the sacrum to the pubes, or pains shooting up the vagina. Blood is hot and gushing. There may be bleeding between periods accompanied by sexual excitement. There is a tendency to miscarry, especially around the third month. It is good for haemorrhaging from the uterus which follows a miscarriage or premature labour. This gets worse from the slightest movement but gets better from walking. Use where there are intense afterbirth pains and a retained placenta. There may be itching in the genitals, increased sexual desire and itchy nipples. Sabina can be given during the menopause where there is excessive bleeding. *Modalities*: Symptoms get worse at night-time, from heat, during pregnancy, during menopause and on hearing music. They improve in the cold and open air.

Sage *Salvia officinalis*

See Red Sage and Sage.

Sage Oil *Salvia officinalis*

See Red Sage and Sage.

St John's Wort *Hypericum perforatum*

As the homoeopathic remedy Hypericum, this is excellent to give in the case of any injury to a part of the body which is rich in nerve endings, e.g. fingers, toes or spinal cord. It is very good where tissues are badly damaged. The key symptoms which indicate this remedy are excessive nerve pains that shoot upwards. This may also be accompanied by drowsiness. Use Hypericum for bee-stings when the pain shoots upwards. It is a remedy to give in cases of tetanus (see also Ledum) – use Hypericum particularly after the onset, when tetanus has developed. It can be very useful for post-operative pain, particularly after eye operations, e.g. on the retina, because this is rich in nerves. Hypericum can be used for spinal injury, particularly to the coccyx, where there is violent pain shooting up and down the spine, or where limbs are crushed – especially when fingers or toes are involved. Give for animal bites or punctures, where there is injury to the nerves. *Modalities*: Symptoms are worse from motion, fear, shock, touch, exertion, a change of weather, cold and damp. They are better from lying face down and bending backwards.

USING THE HERB

As a herb, St John's Wort can be used in an infusion, tincture or oil. It is given when the body needs revitalising – it is good for burnt-out and overspent people, or when a person is very low in energy. The leaves contain 1 per cent volatile oil, which is red, also tannins, Vitamin C, flavonoids (hyperocide), hypericine and a glycocide, hyperium. One of its main actions is as an antidepressant. It can help lift moods (thymoleptic), is a very good nerve tonic, and can be given for conditions accompanied by anxiety, depression or where there are feelings of lethargy and a sense of being fed up. It is good, therefore, to consider during menopause (where there is depression), neurasthenia, for headaches or where there is cramping in the gut, uterus or bladder. Use on a poor, sluggish digestion and if there is a sense of coldness about the person; also for dysmenorrhoea.

The herb can be taken where there is night-time enuresis, and it is also indicated for insomnia or sleepwalking when there is associated depression. Use to help poor memory or lack of clarity due to a sluggish or depressed mental state. Use also for hypertension. St John's Wort needs to be taken for around 4 weeks before there is any change in the condition. Consider adding Rosemary for a more speedy effect. This herb stimulates cell respiration; it soothes pain of exposed or pinched nerves as well as aiding healing. It is also anti-haemorrhagic and anti-bacterial. These properties make it good for the treatment of peptic ulcers, varicose veins, trigeminal neuralgia, sciatica, shingles and burns. St John's Wort is able to stimulate the circulation, particularly to the gut and head areas, and it has a beneficial, spasmolytic effect on the arteries. It is also diuretic, so it can be helpful where there is high blood pressure, arteriosclerosis or senile dementia.

SUGGESTED DOSAGE 2–5ml of tincture diluted in water 3 times a day, or make an infusion using 1 tspful of herb to 1 cup water and drink 3 times a day.

HYPERICUM OIL
Macerated Hypericum Oil can be made by covering the flowers and leaves of the fresh plant in vegetable oil (traditionally olive oil is used) and exposing to the sun for 6 weeks. This oil can be used for external use, but make certain that the plant material is always covered by the oil, otherwise it will go mouldy.

Sandalwood Oil   *Santalum album*

This is a wonderfully relaxing oil. It has antiseptic and anti-inflammatory properties. It is a specific for treating genito-urinary tract infections, including cystitis and NSU (Non-specific urethritis). Being a cooling oil, it has an effect on inflamed mucous membranes and lung tissue. It can be used to treat bronchitis, laryngitis and chronic respiratory-tract infections. It is also good for hot, digestive symptoms, e.g. dysentery. Sandalwood is traditionally used as an incense and has a calming effect on the brain, it can quieten a restless body and soothe the nervous system. It is reputed to be an aphrodisiac, particularly for men. It really helps dry, ageing skin and has been used in cosmetic preparations for centuries. It mixes well with citrus oils, Olibanum and Rose, etc. Use a few drops either in the bath, or 2–3 in a saucerful of base-massage oil.

Sarsaparilla   *Smilax ornata*

This is a herb which is mainly used by men as it has a testosteronal activity and can be used for impotence and infertility. In the past, it was used to treat venereal diseases, but nowadays it is used mainly for cystitis and swollen glands. It is good for rheumatism and arthritis. It is an alterative and is a good blood cleansing herb, especially when combined with Burdock. Use for psoriasis and dry, scaly or itchy skin conditions or skin ulcers. Due to the testosterone in the herb it is best avoided by hirsute women. It is a bitter herb and will only be effective in medicinal doses.

SUGGESTED DOSAGE Use 1–2ml of tincture diluted in water 3 times daily, or 1–2 tspfuls of herb decocted per cup of water.

Saw Palmetto   *Sarenoa serrulata*

This is a very good tonic, especially for the reproductive system, because it helps to regulate the functioning of the organs of both sexes. It will also promote the proper functioning of the mammary glands and although it will not assist milk production, it will facilitate the process. It could be especially beneficial where there is scar tissue from breast reduction or where there are fibromas or breast cysts. Because this herb regulates the reproductive system, it may be of particular help to men as it helps to make healthy sperm, and therefore raises the sperm count. It has been used to treat infertility and is reputedly an aphrodisiac because of its tonic qualities.

SUGGESTED DOSAGE 3–5 berries can be eaten per day, or take 1ml of tincture, diluted in water, per day.

Scullcap   *Scutellaria lateriflora*

This is one of the main nerve-sedating herbs, but it also has a strengthening effect on the nerves. It is good to use in all conditions of agitation, restlessness, etc., such as St Vitus' dance, epilepsy and hysteria. Combine with Balm for anxiety which leads to insomnia. Combine with Crampbark and Valerian for physical spasms. Scullcap is similar in action to Passiflora for an over-excited mind, but it has a more active effect on the physical nervous system. It can be used during pregnancy for restlessness in bed and to calm a restless foetus.

SUGGESTED DOSAGE Preferably use in tincture 1–2ml diluted in water 3 times daily, or infuse 1–2 tspfuls of the herb in a cup of boiling water and drink 3 times a day.

Senna *Cassia angustifolia (Cassia senna)*

See Buckthorn.

Sepia *Sepia*

This is one of the main homoeopathic remedies, traditionally used for the martyred, toiling woman. It is made from the inky substance ejected by cuttlefish as a defence mechanism, and was used as a pigment in paints. It was discovered by Hahnemann (the eighteenth-century creator of homoeopathy) while he watched his friend paint pictures and lick his paintbrush. (See pages 189–91 on Homoeopathic remedies.) *Mental and emotional indications*: The overwhelming aspect of this remedy is being worn out – pressure a Sepia person and they will become irritable. They want to be left alone, they are indifferent to life and work and are easily offended, leading to anger and irritability. They appear to be sagging on all levels, including their spirits. Sepia is marked by sadness, there will be a tendency to cry when listening to music or when the person talks about their symptoms. They are averse to company but also dread being alone (see also Lycopodium). There is anxiety and confusion and a poor memory; also a sullenness which makes relationships with other people difficult. They are hardworking and refuse to give in but are worn out and turn on friends, often spitefully. The sense of sadness can alternate with indifference and resentment. Sepia is a remedy for people who force themselves to continue through a sense of responsibility, but find no joy in living or have no energy left.

Physical symptoms: Sepia is marked by dragging-down sensations and a gnawing, weak, hollow feeling. There may be a brown mark across the nose (an indication that the liver is overloaded), and venous congestion leading to protruding veins. Sepia is to do with slow circulation and stagnation – all organs sag. There can be a pot belly, varicose veins, piles, prolapse of the uterus and vagina. There are heavy bearing-down feelings in the pelvic organs and a sensation that they will drop out – this can create a desire to cross the legs. There can be sensations of a lump in the colon, in the throat or moving lumps in the stomach. All these symptoms are improved by exertion. Despite the worn out emphasis of this remedy, the person who fits the Sepia picture loves dancing and exercising. The Sepia person can think and talk about sex but have little or no capacity for involvement, or there may be a real indifference to

325

sex. The vagina may become very dry. Sepia is an excellent remedy for menopausal problems, especially hot flushes and loss of hair, if there is the accompanying Sepia picture.

Women's complaints: Sepia is known as one of the main hormonal homoeopathic remedies (see also Lachesis). It is very good to give for nausea or morning sickness which comes on at the sight and smell of food; also for thrush and leucorrhoea which are yellowish. Sepia 30C can be given for threatened miscarriage or where there is a tendency to miscarry between months 5 and 7 of the pregnancy. Use for period problems, periods which are early, late or absent, bleeding in the middle of the cycle and then periods which are heavy and clotted. Headaches may occur at the time of periods, either before or during, and they can be accompanied by nausea. They are usually left-sided and the eyelids feel droopy and heavy, the person is sensitive to a heavy, warm atmosphere.

Sepia includes catarrhal complaints, especially those of a chronic nature and where cheesy lumps are coughed up. It is also good for fungal complaints such as athlete's foot and ringworm. Constipation is of the type where stools stay in the rectum, often as small balls which can create a sensation of having a ball in the anus; these sensations are relieved by passing a stool. These constipation symptoms can come on during pregnancy. Urine can be red with sandy sediment. There can be cutting pains in the bladder before urination, which can be involuntary, especially upon coughing, laughing and sneezing. The Sepia person is prone to having droopy, lifeless hair, with sensitive roots. They are very chilly people, sensitive to the cold and they chill easily. *Modalities*: Symptoms get worse with the cold and cold air, before periods, during pregnancy, with intercourse or sexual excess. They improve with warmth, exercise and exertion.

Shepherd's Purse *Capsella bursa-pastoris*

This herb can be combined in mixtures and taken as a replacement for tea, as it is very helpful for stomach ulcers. It is particularly appropriate for very liverish women or those who habitually drink alcohol. It can be taken over a period of time to relieve heavy periods. It acts as a mild diuretic so it is useful where there is bloating. It helps leucorrhoea which is yellow and smelly. Shepherd's Purse can be used to relieve hot, burning cystitis where only a few drops of urine are passed. Also, it is good for hot, burning diarrhoea when the anus feels burning. Being an astringent, cooling herb it can be combined in a mixture for the treatment of varicose veins. It will help to tone the lining of the veins. Consider combining with Beth Root to take in the third stage of labour to help prevent or treat postpartum haemorrhage.

SUGGESTED DOSAGE For regular treatment, infuse 1 tspful of herb in a cup of boiling water, or 1ml of tincture diluted in water. Take either 3 times daily. During a period where there is heavy flooding, take 1–5ml of tincture diluted in water and repeat every 1–2 hours until the excessive bleeding stops.

Silica *Silicea terra*

This is a tissue salt associated with the astrological sign of Sagittarius. It is also a major homoeopathic remedy and is suited to complaints that develop slowly. *Mental and emotional indications*: The Silica person lacks stamina. There is a yielding submissiveness arising from a lack of energy to hold onto their own point of view. They will not oppose anybody else, even if they think them to be wrong. They tend to be refined, intelligent, easy going, mild and reserved, although they make friends and talk about themselves easily. They are not demanding of other people's time or impatient. They do not waste time on trivia. Children will take a reprimand to heart – they do not forget it and their behaviour is easily suppressed. They can grow up with fixed ideas. Silica is a good remedy to give for anticipatory fears, e.g. exams, public speaking, etc. The Silica person can be afraid of failing. They do well in whatever they undertake, but they get worn out, especially from a large amount of mental work. They can be obstinate and passively control others, and can be irritable to cover their underlying timidity. As children, they may learn to read and write slowly and have difficulty in understanding, they lack grit and are oversensitive to noise, touch or light and criticism. They avoid arguments.

    Physical symptoms: The children are thin and puny, often with weak ankles and a lack of stamina. They have large heads and a distended belly. The head and face sweat, rather than the whole body. Symptoms often develop in cold, damp weather, although they may improve in cold, dry weather. Silica will hasten the formation of abscesses and boils. It will help eliminate foreign bodies, such as splinters, warts, pimples, pustules and suppurating cavities. It should be taken for complaints that are caused by suppressed

327

discharges, particularly suppressed sweat. In this case, Silica can lead to thick catarrhal discharges. *Head*: Symptoms include chronic, sick headaches, with nausea and vomiting. The headache starts in the morning at the back of the head and by midday it is on the forehead. Headaches rise from the nape of the neck to one eye, especially the right eye. There are weekly headaches which are worse at night from light, noise, cold air and studying. They get better with heat, from pressure and from wrapping the head. There are profuse headsweats with headaches. *Skin*: Moist and scaly, and it has eruptions. Glands around the neck tend to enlarge with a cold. Glands become enlarged and hardened.

Eyes: May have blocked tear ducts, ulcers on the cornea and styes. Ears have an offensive thick, yellow discharge. There may be middle-ear infections, and catarrh of the Eustachian tube, with deafness. There may be hard, crusty scabs in the nose, catarrh and a loss of taste and smell. *Teeth*: This is the remedy when teeth tend to break and crumble. There is a loss of enamel, and mouth abscesses in gums which feel better from warmth. Also enlarged tonsils and chronic sore throats with enlarged glands. *Stomach*: Hiccups, nausea, vomiting, aversion to warm food; they can also have a dislike for meat and like cold things such as ice-cream and iced water. Symptoms are aggravated by milk. *Abdomen*: Constipation, caused by inactivity of rectum, the stool is partly expelled then recedes, faeces remain a long time in rectum. This is worse before and during periods.

Women's complaints: Symptoms include cysts in the vagina, fistula openings and abscesses along the vulva, if they heal they leave hard nodules. Silica is distinguished by offensive, cheesy-smelling discharges, and bloody discharges during periods. Periods come on from excitement or when breastfeeding. There can be profuse milky leucorrhoea and hard lumps in the breast. Also, breast abscesses and a tendency to miscarry or experience difficulties during pregnancy. *Coughs*: Dry, tickly with hoarseness, worse from cold and better for warm drinks. Green expectoration during the daytime. Colds go to the chest. If the picture fits, Silica is a good remedy for asthma, bronchitis and later stages of pneumonia. Silica is inimicable with Mercury. For treating an abscess, give Merc Sol, followed by Hepar Sulph, before Silica or Sulphur. *Modalities*: Symptoms get worse in the cold, with cold air, draughts and damp, suppressed sweat, mental exertion, pressure, nervous excitement, light, noise, full moon and alcohol. They improve with warmth, wrapping up the head, in the summer, in wet, humid weather and with profuse urination.

Slippery Elm   *Ulmus fulva*

The powdered bark of this tree is used mainly for its mucilaginous qualities. It forms a thick coating for the whole of the gut. It is also nutritious and can be mixed with milk for convalescents. It is good to give where there is any inflammation of the gut. Give for heartburn or hiatus hernia. As Slippery Elm forms a lining over the wall of the stomach, it helps soothe ulcers that are irritated by stomach acids. It is better than anti-acids as these actually stop the acids entering the stomach, which in turn impairs digestion. It is also excellent where there is inflammation of the bowel, e.g. colitis. Slippery Elm can be used externally in a poultice as it is very absorbing. Combine with Marshmallow for its anti-inflammatory properties.

SUGGESTED DOSAGE Use 1–2 tspfuls to make a dilution that you find desirable: take as a thick gel or in a drink with water or milk. Or, take a couple of tablets with water 3 times a day.

Speedwell   *Veronica officinalis*

This herb is used to help all liver conditions. It has a cooling and strengthening effect. It is good for liverish headaches where there is pain on top of the head, behind the eyes and in the forehead, that are both mild or pounding. It is a useful herb to take when you feel frustrated and irritable and unrested even after a night's sleep. It can be used for the sort of cough that makes you hold your ribs; here combine with Agrimony. Speedwell calms the heart when it is affected by the liver. It can also help balance blood pressure and is especially appropriate to give to help lower blood pressure in red-faced, angry people: combine with Hawthorn for this.

SUGGESTED DOSAGE Infuse 1 tspful of the herb to a cup of boiling water and drink 3 times daily, or dilute 1ml of tincture in water and drink 3 times daily.

Spongia   *Spongia tosta*

This homoeopathic remedy is good for coughs that take several days to develop, and where there is a rough sensation in the throat, with dryness in the nose and throat accompanied by sneezing. It can go on to develop into a dry, hoarse and barking cough. It can be a really good remedy to give children with croup. They can have a suffocating cough which will wake them, and they will be fearful, anxious and tearful. The cough will be tight, hollow, barking or crowing, and get worse after midnight. If Aconite is given for the cough earlier in the evening, and there is temporary improvement but it reoccurs in the early hours, then try Spongia. If the cough returns at around 5p.m. or the next day, try Hepar Sulph.

Spongia is good to use when breathing sounds as though it is through a sponge. It can also feel like this. There can be burning in the throat which gets worse at night. The cough does not sound bad during the day but by midnight it can sound barking and crowing. It is good for dry coughs that get worse on successive nights. Mucus can develop after several days, with a feeling of fullness in the chest; expectoration is usually easy. *Modalities*: Sore throat symptoms which get worse from eating sweet things or warm drinks. The throat is sensitive to touch.

Squaw Vine   *Mitchella repens*

This herb is an excellent tonic for the whole body, especially the uterus, and for preparing the body for childbirth. It is good to combine with Raspberry Leaf. Take for the first 3 months of pregnancy, especially if you are prone to miscarriage, and then in the last 3 months to generally tone up the uterus before labour. It is appropriate for debilitated women and so it is good to continue taking it after the birth as it causes rapid involution of the womb, and will also help to calm after-pains. Squaw Vine is generally classed as an emmenogogue (see Black Cohosh) in the sense that it is a uterine tonic and is good for painful, heavy periods, bloating and PMT. It also acts as a gentle diuretic and could help with toxaemia by assisting the kidneys. It is generally used for oedema, most appropriately for older women who suffer from swollen ankles and menstrual symptoms. It can also be used for colitis and problems with a sluggish gut.

SUGGESTED DOSAGE Use 5–10ml of tincture diluted in water and take 3 times daily, or 1–2 tspfuls of root to a cup, decocted, and take 3 times daily.

Staphisagria   *Delphinium staphisagria*

This is a major homoeopathic remedy. It deals with the suppression of emotions and any resulting physical symptoms. *Mental and emotional indications*: This type of person is reactive. They can become speechless through intense feelings. They will control their emotions but then go to pieces afterwards. They may suppress their anger for a while, then when it starts to come out they will tremble with it, making them unable to work or sleep. This is not a remedy for the aggressive type: there's a sweetness, sensitivity and refinement about these people, but there is grief in the background and often broken relationships. This is a divorce remedy. This patient will not want to cause any bother but if given time she will open up. They are too receptive, there's weakness on the emotional level. They want to please everyone, in particular those they love: they will not answer back or retaliate. When a woman gets beaten up by her partner, she feels worthless and there first to serve them. She feels overwhelmed by timidity, and intense feelings are easily aroused but not expressed. These people can have a very strong imagination. It is predominantly a remedy for women, but it is also good for children who have this remedy picture, and may have suffered from being afraid of parents that fight. They are developed sexually and frequently masturbate (this also applies to adults). This type of person is prone to fantasies, often sexual, which they can talk about but are unlikely to act on.

This remedy, if it is appropriate, will help make the person assertive. Generally they are inhibited by their fear of hurting others and have a very low self-esteem. Even if they have an outburst of anger, it will not be aimed at anyone for fear of causing pain. In a Staphisagria woman, the suppression of anger caused by a relationship may lead to breast lumps, fibroids and tumours. Later, she may become indifferent and adopt an uncaring attitude on a sexual level as well, even though a Staphisagria type is generally highly sexed. When they are hurt they withdraw and feel lonely and talk to themselves, although they want company and seek to be accepted. They are morbidly sensitive and very easily embarrassed. They are sensitive on all levels. Any situation that is invasive will have a major effect – such as the first time they have intercourse or a surgical operation. They may say that they have never fully recovered. Violation is a key word for this remedy. This is a remedy to consider giving after someone has been raped, mugged or assaulted. They will feel angry but powerless about the event. It is a remedy for victims, e.g. children who have been bullied at school.

Physical symptoms: These get worse from smoking. *Head*: Headaches feel as if the forehead is about to split open and this gets worse with movement and stooping. It feels as if the brain is bruised. It improves with yawning. It can feel as if there's a ball of lead in the forehead. There is vertigo which is worse from walking and turning rapidly. Also, a tingling, tickling scalp, dandruff and head lice. *Eyes*: Symptoms include recurring styes, nodosities on eyelids, heat and dryness in the eyeballs, bletharitis and sore, red, crusty eyelids. *Ears*: Deafness in children accompanied by enlarged tonsils. *Mouth*: The teeth are sensitive to touch, they can be black brittle and decayed. These people cannot bear having fillings and their gums bleed easily.

Stomach: Symptoms include the desire for milk, bread and soups; they like liquid foods, wine, brandy and tobacco. Use for severe pains after abdominal operations, hiccups, nausea that is worse in the morning and feelings of extreme hunger even when the stomach is full. *Abdomen*: Sensations of weakness and bearing down in the abdomen. The flatus smells of rotten eggs. Give after abdominal operations that are slow to heal or remain painful. *Cough*: Worse from vexation, cleaning teeth, indignation and tobacco smoke. Croupy cough in winter. *Skin*: There are warts which tingle like insects under the skin. Take for incised wounds causing great pain and for sciatica that comes on in the summer.

Urinary symptoms: Cystitis that occurs after intercourse; an urgent desire to urinate, pain after urination, pains after difficult labour. *Women's complaints*: Symptoms include extreme sensitivity of genitals, nyphomania, sexual fantasies, mind dwells on sex, inflammation of ovaries and feelings of burning and stinging. Periods are irregular, late, profuse or scanty. There can be amenorrhoea arising from anger or indignation. Can be given after a caesarean or an episiotomy where the scar is slow to heal and the area remains tender.

The Staphisagria type will find it difficult to sleep because their minded is crowded with ideas, they are wakeful at night with erotic dreams, and sleepy by day. Yawning and stretching will bring tears to their eyes. *Modalities*: Symptoms get worse from quarrelling, grief, indignation, humiliation, masturbation, sexual excess, tobacco, laceration and intercourse. They improve after breakfast, from warmth, with intercourse and rest at night.

Stone Root *Collinsonia canadensis*

This herb, as the name suggests, has several properties which help to break up stones. These will then ease their passage away from the kidneys and gall bladder. It will help relax spasms in the ureters and gall bladder, and has an astringent and tonic effect on the veins, making it helpful in treating piles and varicose veins. Stone Root is also a diuretic and will help to flush out the urinary system. Here are three herbal combinations which may be helpful as a guide to treatment: for kidney stones use equal amounts of Stone Root, Parsley Piert, Pellitory-of-the-wall, Marshmallow Leaf and Couchgrass; for gallstones use equal amounts of Stone Root, Fumitory, Fringetree Bark, Dandelion Root and Boldo; for piles use equal quantities of Stone Root, Witchazel Leaf, Plantain, Marshmallow Leaf and Marigold.

SUGGESTED DOSAGE For all these mixtures infuse 1 tspful per cup of boiling water and drink 3 times a day. Using the Stone Root separately use 30g (1oz) to 570ml (1 pint) of boiling water and drink a cup 3 times a day; with a tincture, use 2ml diluted in water and drink 3 times a day.

Sulphur *Sulphur*

This homoeopathic remedy covers more symptoms and is probably more often prescribed than any other. It is said to restore life to the spirit. It helps awaken the person to their purpose, putting them on the right path. *Mental and emotional indications*: Sulphur is an excellent remedy for those who are under-functioning, ineffective and generally not getting themselves together. They tend to be unkempt and scruffy and have a disregard for their personal appearance and cleanliness. They smell, sometimes even after bathing (which they do not like doing). They may be great philosophers and inventors, and are unconventional, independent, inquisitive, rebellious and argumentative. They can be selfish, egocentric and self-satisfied, they tend to be self-deceptive and are prone to mental and physical inertia. They are day-dreamers with poor memories and concentration. A picture of a typical Sulphur person is of someone who is working on a thesis or project: they will start off on one thing and then pursue another idea, and then another, and the thesis will remain incomplete. They can be irritable, impatient, critical, nagging, discontented and dissatisfied, and obstinate, sad or depressed.

Physical symptoms: A sulphur-type has a high-coloured face, red lips, red borders to eyelids, red ears and often stoops. They tend to feel hot easily. They are worse from standing and prefer to sit or lie down. Faintness or weak spells may be accompanied by great sleepiness. Sulphur is a good remedy to use where complaints get better then there are relapses again and again. Generally there is a tendency to congestion, burning, throbbing and flushes of heat. Mucous discharges are acrid, bloody, offensive and itchy. The top of the head feels hot, and feet feel cold. *Head*: Symptoms include headaches accompanied by nausea and vomiting, there are often headaches on Sundays (or days off) and with periods. The nose may feel burning, produce a discharge which gets worse outside and tends to be blocked indoors. There is frequent sneezing, and they may be very sensitive to smell, although unaware of their own, and feel nauseous about their own discharges. *Coughs*: These tickle the larynx, they are violent and worse lying on the back or at night. There is rattling of mucus and heat in the chest, and greenish expectoration. Sulphur is often very helpful for pneumonia or bronchitis which tend to linger and are difficult to throw off. It can also help asthma and hayfever.

Stomach: The appetite is either small or very large (Sulphur-type people can be greedy). They tend to drink more than they eat, and like sweets, raw foods, beer, fat and spicy and unusual foods. There can be sudden hunger at 11 a.m. accompanied by weakness, and an 'all-gone' sensation in the stomach. Headaches come on if they do not eat. There is vomiting and nausea during pregnancy. *Abdomen:* There is diarrhoea which is offensive, watery and involuntary and worse in the early morning. Often they wake early morning (6 a.m.) and need a bowel movement. Diarrhoea alternates with constipation, when the stool is hard, large and difficult to pass. The anus is red and itchy, there may be worms, and internal and external piles which are sore, bleeding, burning, itching, and worse during pregnancy (also compare Hamamelis and Calc Fluor). *Women's complaints*: The vulva and vagina burn, itch and are sore. Sulphur is a good remedy for thrush. Use for leucorrhoea which is yellow, burning and excoriating. Periods may be irregular, late, scanty, acrid, offensive and dark, there may be blackish blood which can bring about soreness or amenorrhoea. Also cracked nipples, which feel sore and burning; an offensive perspiration on the genitals.

Sleep: There is a need to keep the feet out of bed as the soles burn. Sleep is unrefreshing; these people can be sleepy during the day but wakeful at night, they have vivid dreams, talk, jerk and twitch during sleep and wake between 3–5 a.m., unable to go back to sleep. *Skin*: Symptoms include dry, scaly, rough, raw, itchy eruptions. There is plenty of itching and it is enjoyable to scratch, although the skin condition gets worse afterwards and may bleed. Skin burns after scratching and is made worse from wearing wool. It is unhealthy, slow to heal, worse from washing, wind and air. Sulphur is a very useful remedy to give for skin eruptions that have been suppressed, such as boils or crops of eruptions all over the body. One eruption is followed by another. There can be eczema which alternates with asthma. With skin complaints, it is better to give Sulphur in a low potency as it may aggravate the condition in high potency. *Modalities*: Symptoms get worse from suppressions (e.g. anti-perspirants, medicated ointments, drugs, etc.), bathing, heat, over-exertion, being in bed at 11 a.m., standing and periodically. They improve in the open air, from sweating, motion and dry, warm weather.

Sweet Orange Oil *Citrus auranticum*

See Grapefruit Oil.

Symphytum *Symphytum officinale*

See Comfrey.

Tarantula *Tarantula hispania*

A traditional method of overcoming this spider's bite was to dance all night, presumably in a state of mania. *Mental and emotional indications*: The indications for this homoeopathic remedy include great changes in temperament. The person is lively, restless and must keep moving, although this may make them feel worse. They are very sensitive to music and get excited, wanting to jump up and dance. This type of person is highly strung and can become hysterical; they are uninhibited, very sensitive to touch and cold, often preoccupied with sex and their nerve endings are very sensitive. They can have orgasms without any feeling of relief and there is frequent desire for genital excitement (consider also Platina), which can be followed by irritability and then depression. They have a poor memory and can be cunning and underhand. The mind is not strong, they are unscrupulous and unpredictable, with no control over their emotions. They may fake illness when they want something or tend towards kleptomania. When a Tarantula type is in an emotional state they tremble and can become physically violent to others as well as themselves. They suffer from delusions. Laughter can swing into depression.

Physical symptoms: One of the main uses for this remedy is for treating sepsis, even quite severe cases, in the form of: malignant ulcers, boils, gangrene, carbuncles. The remedy helps to evacuate pus rapidly. The tissue is bluish purple or red, skin is septic with burning, stinging pains. This condition can look similar to the Arsenicum or Lachesis pictures – if these two remedies do not work it may be worth trying Tarantula. Pains cause twitching and jerking. The spine can be very sensitive to touch and can cause pain in the chest and heart regions; there is extreme sensitivity in the tips of the fingers with a need to rub them.

Women's complaints: Periods can be early and profuse, accompanied by an increase of sexual desire and irritability. There may be a sensation of something being alive in the womb – this comes on particularly after a sleep and during the time of the period. It is a remedy for hysterical pregnancies. The ovaries can feel very sensitive. There is violent itching of the genitals; and this sensation can travel right up the vagina. There may be burning pains in the uterus. There is an increased dryness around the time of the period, especially in the throat, mouth and tongue.

There are different kinds of pains but a feeling of burning is most common, especially in the rectum, on the palms of the hands, soles of the feet and in the uterus. Neuralgia is like thousands of needles, especially in the head. These people like having the head rubbed and their hair brushed. There may be an intense thirst for cold water and an empty, all-gone feeling, with burning in the stomach. There can be coughs and respiratory symptoms included in this remedy's picture, these are generally better with smoking. *Modalities*: Symptoms get worse with movement, touching affected parts, at night, from bright colours, the cold and damp, with noise, from music and from intercourse. Symptoms also get periodically worse once a year. They improve with rubbing, sweating, in the open air, with bright colours, music and smoking.

Tea Tree Oil *Melaleuca alternifolia*

This is related to Eucalyptus, and is used primarily for its notable germicidal properties. It is highly antiseptic and can combat many different kinds of bacterial infections, including streptococcal and staphylococcal infections. Tea Tree has been shown to have significant anti-viral properties. It is excellent to use for respiratory infections, including colds and flu. One of the most important areas of use is on the genito-urinary tract. It is effective in the treatment of both acute and chronic cystitis, as well as being helpful for thrush, NSU (Non-specific urethritis), genital herpes and warts, and pruritus trichomoniasis. Diluted properly it is safe to use in vaginal douches (see page 183).

It is a very good oil for skin problems: apply locally to treat athlete's foot and ringworm. It also has mild analgesic and anti-inflammatory properties which help to bring relief to corns, callouses, warts, verrucas, wounds, cuts and burns. It can be included in a mouth wash for bad breath, mouth ulcers and gum infections. Use Tea Tree Oil as a first-aid remedy, apply locally undiluted or mixed with a base oil for respiratory complaints. Use up to 10 drops in hot water for an inhalation, or up to 20 drops in a hot bath.

Thyme *Thymus vulgaris*

Thyme herb contains approximately 1 per cent volatile oil. The main constituents of this are carvacrol which can irritate the skin and mucous membranes, and thymol, which is highly antiseptic, gentle on the skin and acts on the lungs and the digestive and urinary tracts. The herb also contains tannins, saponins and bitters. This herb has three main actions. In the respiratory system, it has an anti-spasmodic effect on the lungs, as well as being an expectorant; it can therefore help any respiratory infection where there are spasms, e.g. asthma, bronchitis, TB and emphysema. It will particularly help where there is tiredness and debility associated with the respiratory infection. Combine Thyme with Liquorice and Honey to use as cough mixture.

As an antiseptic herb, Thyme is very good for digestion that is slow and needs stimulating. It acts as a good general tonic to the system and can be taken for indigestion, inflammation or infection in the digestive tract. It is good for diarrhoea. Thyme is also anti-fungal, anti-bacterial and anti-viral. It can be used as a wash for ringworm.

Combine with Scullcap for scabies. It probably works against head and body lice. Make an infusion and use as a rinse after treatment or normal washing. It is traditionally used to add shine and strength to the hair.

SUGGESTED DOSAGE Use ½ tspful of herb to a cup of boiling water, or 10–20 drops of tincture diluted in water, 3 times a day.

THYME OIL   *Thymus vulgaris*
Care needs to be taken when using this oil: it is very strong and can burn or irritate the skin if it is not diluted sufficiently. It is, however, very effective in inhalations for chest infections, or to combine with a few drops of Rosemary in the bath. It is probably best to dilute the Thyme Oil in a base oil before adding to the bath as a globule of oil on the surface of the water may well sting badly on sensitive areas. It will be very warming and invigorating in winter, or when you feel sluggish and cold. Thyme Oil, diluted well, can also be used as a skin antiseptic for treating boils and sores. Use for treating athlete's foot. Research is being carried out on this oil because there is a great deal of interest in its anti-viral properties. It also appears to strengthen the immune system by stimulating the production of white blood cells.

Turmeric   *Curcuma zedoaria*

This herb has a strong action on the liver, it helps stimulate the flow of bile from the liver (cholugogue) and thereby helps with cleansing through elimination. It is good to use for jaundice and all liver disease, particularly during or following hepatitis, when the body is still very run down. Combine with Dandelion or Meadowsweet to counter acidity, or Marshmallow and Liquorice to help protect the lining of the gut. Tumeric will help increase the appetite but must be used with caution as it can irritate the mucous membranes. It is contra-indicated where there is hyperacidity or an irritable stomach.

SUGGESTED DOSAGE Take ½ tspful of the herb to a cup of boiling water 3 times a day, or use ½-1ml of tincture diluted in water 3 times daily.

Uva Ursi *Arctostaphylos uva ursi*

This herb is used as an urinary antiseptic. It has demulcent, astringent and diuretic properties. It is especially good for chronic urinary tract infections as it helps to restore tone in the urinary passage, and it is also good for both dissolving and helping the passage of stones and gravel. For stubborn infections, try combining with Couchgrass and Lavender. Uva Ursi is contra-indicated in pregnancy.

SUGGESTED DOSAGE Infuse 30g (1oz) of herb in 570ml (1 pint) water for 20 mins and drink a cupful 3 times a day, or take 1–2ml of tincture diluted in water 3 times daily.

Valerian *Valerian officinalis*

This strong-smelling herb is useful to relieve conditions which have been induced by anxiety and nervous tension. It has a calming effect on the heart and can be used for high blood pressure, a fast pulse, palpitations or angina. For these complaints it may be appropriate to combine with Hawthorn and Motherwort. Where a nervous disorder has led to hyperacidity and then to peptic ulcers combine Valerian with Meadowsweet. When it results in constipation combine with Crampbark. Valerian is a popular herb for insomnia; it can certainly be effective if the cause is anxiety, painful periods or fears, e.g. exam nerves. It is not an antidepressant and it is probably better to avoid using Valerian if there is any tendency to feel depressed. Too much Valerian can cause headaches.

SUGGESTED DOSAGED Use 10 drops of tincture diluted in water and take 3 times a day, or decoct ½ tspful of herb with a cup of boiling water and take 3 times a day.

Vervain *Verbena officinalis*

This herb contains bitter glycocides, volatile oil, mucilage, tannins and iron. It is good for anxiety and is often given for anxious states during pregnancy, because of the iron content. It reputedly increases milk production in nursing mothers. Vervain works on the liver and is calming to use in jaundice and for an inflamed gall bladder. It has diaphoretic qualities which make it useful to include in a tea for colds and flu. Generally it will aid digestion, soothe palpitations and help with insomnia and depression.

SUGGESTED DOSAGE Infuse 1 tspful of the herb in a cup of boiling water and drink 3 times daily, or dilute 1–2ml of tincture in water and drink 3 times daily.

Vitex (Chaste Berry) *Vitex agnus castus*

This herb has an effect on the pituitary gland and is said to have a progesteronal action, making it suitable to include in most initial prescriptions for the treatment of female disorders. It may be suitable for any cyclical problems, e.g. epilepsy, spots, period pains, etc. It has been used for men as an an aphrodisiac, and to dampen the male sex-drive – hence its other name, 'Monk's Pepper'. For women, Vitex acts more as a regulator and is said to have anti-bacterial effects on *Bacillus* and *Staph aureus* (the bacterium that cause yellow pus), it could be useful in chronic low-grade infections of the genital tract, e.g. for a problem that was treated in the past but has never quite cleared and maybe has a remaining discharge.

Vitex inhibits the release of the follicle-stimulating hormone (FSH) and it increases the leuteinising hormone (LH) production, therefore increasing the ratio of progesterone to oestrogen. Progesterone inhibits the spasm of smooth muscle and in this way prepares the uterus for pregnancy in that it can hold a baby. This action suggests that it could be a useful herb to give to women who tend to miscarry in the first few weeks of pregnancy.

Vitex can be a significant help with menopausal complaints; it can make a woman feel better by helping to keep her hormones in balance. It will have an effect on mood swings, hot flushes and night sweats, although it may not help dryness in the vagina. Clinical trials have shown that it can help breastfeeding women and with postnatal depression. It is also appropriate for pre-menstrual disorders because of its effect on depression, mood swings, bloating, swollen breasts and a swollen abdomen. Some women can get very severe cramps which are said to be due to a sudden drop in progesterone levels and Vitex normalises this level at the onset of the period by making the drop less sudden, and therefore the cramps less severe. Although Vitex is not an anti-spasmodic or analgesic herb in itself, it can definitely soothe period pains.

It is thought that it is most useful to use this herb, either on its own or in combination, for 3 cycles or months. It starts to work during the first cycle, regulates during the second cycle and establishes the new pattern in the third cycle. If the conditions improve then you could try not taking Vitex for a while, but generally it is better to continue taking it for some time as it is completely safe and has no side-effects.

Take this remedy when you come off the pill to help re-establish your own pituitary function, for example if you do not have a period straight away or if old complaints reassert themselves, e.g. with dysmenorrhoea. Generally we feel that if you are on the pill or HRT (Hormone Replacement Therapy) it is probably not worth taking this herb because it works by affecting hormone levels. Vitex encourages the pituitary to function properly whereas the pill or HRT will inhibit its function.

SUGGESTED DOSAGE Take 1ml (25 drops) of tincture per day, or infuse 1 tspful of herb in a cup and take 1–3 times per day.

Watercress *Nasturtium officinale*

Watercress is very rich in minerals and vitamins. It is used as a blood cleanser and nutrient. This makes it excellent to use as a spring tonic, for weak people, those with colds, anaemia and during convalescence. It will help to increase the appetite and aid digestion. Use to reduce swelling in the lymph glands and for spotty skin. It can be used as a hair tonic as well – it is said to help prevent hair from falling out. It is best to eat the fresh leaves or use recently dried ones, as properties fade with long storage.

SUGGESTED DOSAGE Eat a bunch of watercress a day, or infuse 2 tspfuls of dried herb to 1 cup of water 3 times daily.

White Deadnettle *Lamium album*

Traditionally an astringent herb known as Archangel, the white variety was used for white or general leucorrhoea, the yellow for yellow discharges and the red for haemorrhages. It is generally used for vaginal infections nowadays. With its astringent and

341

anti-spasmodic properties, it will affect the female organs because it balances the system. It is good for tired and debilitated women. White Deadnettle is very good to use in douches, especially combined with Lavender.

SUGGESTED DOSAGE Use 1ml tincture (25 drops) in water 3 times daily, or infuse 1 tspful of herb in a cup of boiling water 3 times daily. For a douche make a weak infusion with 1 tspful of herb to 570ml (1 pint) of water; strain very carefully before using.

White Horehound   *Marrubium vulgar*

This herb is mainly used for the lungs, its actions are anti-spasmodic and expectorant. It allows the bronchioles to relax and this makes it useful for asthma and whooping cough. It is good in conditions where there are spasms and excess fluid, e.g. bronchitis. White Horehound is a bitter tonic, it aids weak digestion and it is particularly helpful for chronic digestive problems. It can be used externally as a wash to promote healing in wounds.

SUGGESTED DOSAGE Infuse ½ tspful of herb to 1 cup of boiling water and take 3 times daily, or 10–20 drops tincture diluted in water 3 times daily.

White Willow   *Salix alba*

White Willow is the herb where salicylic acid was first isolated, Meadowsweet also contains it. This herb can be used in similar ways to Meadowsweet, but it is not such a specific for ulcers and is used more generally for fevers, pains, headaches and especially for rheumatism. It is also good for gut pains and diarrhoea.

SUGGESTED DOSAGE Infuse 1–2 tspfuls in a cup of boiling water and leave to stand for the full benefit. This can be drunk 3 times a day. In a tincture, 1–2ml can be diluted in water and taken 3 times daily.

Wild Cherry Bark   *Prunus serotina*

This herb can sedate the cough reflex, so it is chiefly used for dry, irritable coughs, smokers' cough or nervous and whooping coughs. When using this herb, care must be taken to also treat the underlying chest infection, as it tends to suppress expectoration. Wild Cherry is a bitter and a digestive stimulant, use for people with sluggish digestions.

SUGGESTED DOSAGE Use 1–2ml of tincture diluted in water, or 1–2 tspfuls of herb decocted in a cup of water. Take 3 times daily. Cherry juice is known to be specifically good for gout, drink 140ml (¼ pint) per day, or you could eat 450g (1lb) of cherries a day and decrease the amount slowly over several weeks.

Wild Indigo   *Baptisia tinctoria*

This herb is said to be an immune stimulant with a special effect on the upper respiratory tract. This makes it a useful herb to take for the treatment of sore throats, catarrh, swollen glands, coughs and colds, especially if there are accompanying headaches. The main use of Wild Indigo is for flu that is concentrated in the upper respiratory area: the head being the focus of discomfort. Take with caution as it can cause nausea. It can also be included in a mixture for ulcers and abscesses or used for gingivitis. It can be made into a decoction or used as a douche for leucorrhoea.

SUGGESTED DOSAGE 1 tspful of the root needs to be decocted with a cup of water that is brought to the boil and simmered, take a tblsful 3 times a day. Use ½–1ml of tincture and take 3 times daily.

Wild Yam   *Dioscorea villosa*

This is a good uterine tonic, and is taken for infertility as it relaxes the whole generative system and increases the production of female hormones. It is also said to promote male fertility by increasing the sperm count. Wild Yam can be given to treat the nausea of pregnancy. As an anti-spasmodic herb it will calm the nerves and help when there is a threat of miscarriage. It is a herb that can be taken throughout pregnancy and during labour to soothe the pain. It is good for pains that occur after giving birth, and it can be taken to increase milk production. Generally, Wild Yam is a helpful herb for ovarian and uterine pains and for pain during ovulation. It has a relaxing effect on the bile duct and gall bladder. It is good to use for bilious colic. Being an anti-inflammatory herb, it can be used for rheumatic pains and abdominal cramps.

SUGGESTED DOSAGE Because this herb is very hard, decoct 30g (1oz) to 570ml (1 pint) of water, and take 1 tbsp in a wine-glass of water 3 times a day. It is probably easier to take the tincture: dilute 1–2ml in water and take 3 times a day.

Witchazel   *Hamamelis virginiana*

As a homoeopathic remedy, Hamamelis acts mainly on the veins, making it a very useful treatment for varicose veins, piles and haemorrhages. Symptoms covered by this remedy are a bruised soreness of the affected part, with congestion and a bursting sensation. It can be used for nosebleeds, especially those that last a long time with blood that does not easily clot (this is more often seen in children). Also, piles which occur in pregnancy or childbirth and where there is a feeling of fullness and the pains are prickly and stinging and varicose veins which are painful and sore, again with the prickling stinging pains, and can be hard, swollen and knotty. Hamamelis also covers varicose veins in the vulva which occur during pregnancy. This remedy can be taken internally (see pages 190–1 on dosage) or by applying the tincture externally, as with the herb.

USING THE HERB
Herbalists use either witchazel leaves or roots and the main use is to soothe swellings, reduce inflammations and to stop bleeding. Its main action is on the blood vessels which it helps to contract. Witchazel can be taken internally for haemorrhages of the gut, and externally in a wash or tincture, for bruises, sprains and strains, cuts, bleeding varicose veins and piles. Use a well-strained infusion as an eyewash to soothe tired, red eyes; or mix 1 part witchazel to 20 parts of sterile, purified water for an eyebath. Witchazel is popular to use as a face cleanser or wash. It is refreshing and pleasant and may well help broken capillaries in

the face; it also has astringent properties to help greasy or open-pored skin.

Woodruff *Asperula odorata*

This is a herb that is good for the congested liver where there is constipation and irritability. It calms the nervous system, especially when the digestion is affected and where there is insomnia. Use when it is difficult to get to sleep or when you wake up very easily and cannot get back to sleep. Woodruff is a herb that seems more aromatic when dry, and can be used either on its own or with Lavender as an insect repellant.

SUGGESTED DOSAGE Use 1 tspful of herb to a cup of boiling water and take 3 times daily, or 1ml of tincture diluted in water 3 times daily.

Wormwood *Artemisia absinthum*

The main action of this herb is on the nervous system and the digestive tract. It is very good for weak, convalescing people, it increases the appetite and it can be useful for anorexics. It aids digestion and stimulates the liver and gall bladder. Wormwood is a very strong herb, a little added to a mixture will help to combine the rest of the herbs. If a herb is clearly indicated, and is being taken over a long period of time but then appears to stop working, add a little Wormwood as this can be very effective.

Caution must be taken with Wormwood as it contains thujone which is an abortifacient. It must not be used during pregnancy as it will harm the baby, and in large quantities it is known to cause nerve deterioration, then epilepsy and brain damage. The liqueur, absinthe, contains Wormwood and has been banned in some countries for this reason.

SUGGESTED DOSAGE It is advisable to only take 5ml per week. Use 5 drops of tincture in water 3 times a day, or infuse 30g (1oz) of herb in 570ml (1 pint) of water and only take 1–2 tspfuls 3 times a day.

Yarrow   *Achillea millefolium*

This herb was once used as a 'heal-all'. The essential oil contains chamazulene, as does Chamomile, and it has many of the same properties as Chamomile but is less relaxing, and has a more powerful effect on the lungs. It is an important diaphoretic herb, which makes it very good for fevers and colds: an excellent combination is Yarrow, Elderflower and Peppermint. By selectively stimulating and relaxing aspects of the digestive system, Yarrow improves both digestion and absorption; it contains iso-valerianic acid (as in Valerian) and this relaxes the gut. It also restores tone to the bowel and helps to heal gastric ulcers.

Yarrow tones blood vessels and has the effect of lowering blood pressure, especially when it is raised due to tension. It is therefore very good to give to someone with high blood pressure caused by stress. Put it into a mixture for piles and varicose veins. It is very appropriate for old people where the veins are very noticeable on their hands and feet. Combine with Hawthorn and take for a long period, such as 6 months. It can also help to heal wounds by clotting the blood and preventing haemorrhages, so that it can be used internally, as in bleeding ulcers or where blood occurs when coughing. It is also said to cause *and* cure nosebleeds.

Yarrow regulates periods especially if they have stopped through being cold; and it helps relieve pelvic cramps. It is a mild emmenogogue but it is generally quite safe to take in pregnancy.

SUGGESTED DOSAGE Use ½–1 tspful per cup of boiling water, or 1–2ml of tincture in water 3 times a day.

Yellow Dock Root   *Rumex crispus*

This is a nutritious herb for poor liver functioning which results in hepatitic congestion. It helps to increase bile flow. It also acts as a laxative, helping constipation and where there are chronic, itchy skin conditions, such as psoriasis, acne and eczema; it is an excellent herb for pustular or oozing skin. It can be used externally for ringworm or scabies. For scabies, combine with Scullcap as this seems to alter the pH balance of the skin. Yellow Dock is generally a good blood cleansing herb. It can be used during pregnancy and where there is constipation, anaemia or bad skin.

SUGGESTED DOSAGE Decoct 30g (1oz) to 570ml (1 pint) of water and take 1 tbsp 3 times a day, or take ½–2ml of tincture in water 3 times a day.

Ylang Ylang Oil *Cananga odorata*

This is a very sedating oil, it is excellent to use a few drops in the bath when returning home from a tense, overwrought day, or after shock or fear. It will calm high blood pressure, is good for red-faced people and where there is rapid breathing. Ylang Ylang has a very powerful, sweet fragrance, produced from the yellow flowers of the *Cananga odorata* trees, which are found in Indonesia. It is an oil that can be substituted for Jasmine as it is said to have similar, aphrodisiac qualities. It blends well with Rosewood or citrus oils. Only 1–2 drops are needed in a saucerful of base oil.

Lifestyle

Introduction to Healing Ourselves

To enjoy good health we need to look after the spiritual, mental and emotional aspects of our lives as well as our physical health. The flow of energy between these different aspects of our self integrates and keeps us whole; disharmony in any one of these areas will push all the others out of balance.

Daily stresses and life events tend to throw us into a state of imbalance. And if we become stuck for too long in this imbalance then we have dis-ease. Our ability to adapt and deal creatively with life's up and downs will determine the mental and physical processes that we experience as good health. We all have an innate desire to create the conditions for balance within ourselves, and in our environment, and it is the aim of the various systems of natural healing to help us achieve this.

Our potential for good health is based on the unique mixture of our parents' genes (inherited factors), the physical and mental environment in which we were nurtured, and our individual ability to deal with all these factors. We need to strike a balance between accepting the basics of who we are, e.g. as woman/man, black/white, able-bodied/handicapped, and recognising that there are also huge areas of choice about what we can do with our lives. One of the most debilitating states of mind, and the cause of many people's depression, is to feel that there are no options to choose from. It is important to remember that there are always options, even if these are only a question of our attitude towards problems.

Knowing that we always have choices means that we also need to make decisions, and this is not always easy. As our lives have become more complex in the modern world, our choices have also multiplied. We have to make decisions continually about such things as how, when and what to eat, where to live, what to spend our money on, what paid work to pursue, whether or not or when to have children, and what kind of relationships to have. In the past, and now in less developed societies, many of these choices were restricted by environmental or social factors.

When making a decision, we can be positive by choosing the option that best supports the whole. We, in the industrialised West, have shown little concern with this kind of decision-making, and our damaged physical environment exemplifies the danger of choosing on the basis of short-term gain and exploitation. Not all societies have been so reckless. The Native American tribes, for example, placed great importance on living in harmony with their environment, and made decisions as a group aimed at maintaining its integrity and not depleting resources.

On a personal level, the principle of decision making is the same: we cannot choose personal gain or individual happiness at the expense of anything or anyone else, and at the same time sustain integrity in our life. Every time that we make a decision, we can think of what best supports the whole. When we go shopping we can choose products that are environmentally sound, we can use unleaded petrol, we can encourage free-range farming methods by buying these products. We can work in jobs that we feel are contributing something to society as well as paying our wages.

The principles of natural medicine are based on the same idea: that we have to treat the individual as a whole and not just as a set of physical symptoms. The aims of natural medicine are to create better conditions for health to exist within the person, and to encourage them to throw off disease on every level. The disadvantage of much orthodox modern medicine is that it tends to remove a particular physical symptom without dealing with why the symptom developed in the first place. This approach not only leads to the suppression and distortion of symptoms, but has also led to the use of drugs which, whilst being powerful in removing one illness, cause side-effects that damage other parts of the person.

Again, the same principle applies to our emotional life: the best way of dealing with a problem is by choosing the option which best supports the whole. If we suppress our negative emotions or fail to acknowledge the aspects of ourself that we don't like, we will never come to terms with our whole self, and we will never be able to use the whole of our potential and energy. It is only by accepting our negative emotions that we can change, and use the energy that is released. This may mean taking what feel like risks at the time, but will quickly add to our experience and enrich our lives. There are many very moving, and inspiring, accounts of women who have suffered, for example the death of a child through a particular disease or drug abuse, who don't dwell on their anger and grief, but use the experience to help others by setting up support groups and so on.

In this section we set out an approach to health and the enjoyment of life in the fullest sense. We examine the different aspects that make up our life experience, and show how, by seeing ourselves as part of an interconnected whole, we can both enrich our individual lives, and create a better world for us all to live in.

Our Spiritual Selves

In this section we are going to explore what it means to be healthy in our spiritual lives, and what we can do to improve things when we feel dissatisfied. As women, it is especially important to have a positive spiritual outlook because this will determine to a great extent our ability to be creative, our feelings of self-worth and the value that we put on our life experience. This, in turn, will be passed on to our children, and to all the people with whom we interact.

It is our spiritual self that links us to everything beyond the personal self; it gives us awareness of and contact with the interconnectedness of life. When we acknowledge that we are part of an interconnected whole, we realise that we cannot exploit any one person, group of people or any resource at all, without damaging the balance of the whole, and in effect damaging ourselves.

Our western society, with its emphasis on exploitation of resources, and material gain, has created a society in which it is very difficult to feel profoundly connected to other people and to the planet as a whole. The promotion of modern science as the answer to all our problems, both philosophical and practical, has meant that we have lost the ability to be in touch with the overview, because science always tends to focus on material gain, technological advance and the importance of research, whatever the cost to the whole. What this has led to on a physical level, is a widespread depletion of resources, and pollution on a scale that now threatens our very survival. On a spiritual level it has led to very many people suffering from a sense of alienation and lack of purpose.

Thankfully there is now an upsurge of awareness that we are all linked to each other, and to the planet as a whole. Writers such as Fritjof Capra in *The Tao of Physics*, and Gary Zukav in *The Dancing Wu Li Masters*, have combined philosophical understanding with an interpretation of modern physics, to illustrate that life is not made up from bits of inert substance that can be dissected up and examined out of context, but rather it is a flow of interweaving energy that creates a whole. There is a reawakened interest in the principle named after the earth goddess Gaia: that our earth is a living, evolving entity that has a life cycle and life processes like any other organism, but on a planetary scale.

The Green Movement in politics and business has grown out of the awareness that our materialistic society has been depleting finite resources, and polluting our environment, to the degree that our planet is now showing symptoms of disease. Many rivers can no longer sustain life, and global warming is threatening established weather patterns. These are just two examples of what it means for a planet to become diseased.

What can we do about this? One important thing that we can be aware of is that, as consumers, we have an effect on the sort of goods that are produced. We can therefore contribute towards a more politically and ecologically-sound lifestyle. For example, we can use unleaded petrol in our cars, we can buy environmentally-friendly washing powder, we can recycle paper and glass, and we can avoid dealing with companies that exploit the Third World. Separately, all these things seem trivial, but they are examples of how we can make choices in our everyday lives that are in accordance with our overall ethical aims, and that if enough of us support these issues we can bring about considerable changes. It is becoming increasingly important that we educate ourselves about environmental and ecological matters because of the increasing hype that surrounds 'green' issues. More and more companies are claiming that their products are ecologically sound. We need to be able to base our choices on knowledge rather than on ignorance and fear.

If we want to take our commitment for change further, we can join one of the groups that are campaigning for environmental issues, such as Greenpeace or Friends of the Earth (see page 399 for addresses). We can develop our awareness of political issues by reading informative newspapers and books. But most importantly, we can realise that each of us can make a difference: we can change our own lives and have an effect in the world. If every individual acted out of an awareness of the interconnectedness of all things, then we would all feel motivated to improve the society in which we live, and ecological sustainability would be a natural part of planning any project. The sense of empowerment that this attitude creates further reinforces our ability to feel and be creative and purposeful in our lives, which is the other function of our spiritual selves.

Being in contact with our spiritual self enables us to have an awareness beyond the mundane activities of life, and to gain insight into the larger issues of our existence: it is a source that provides us with our sense of purpose, and our innate desire to be creative. The spiritual aspect of our selves needs looking after just as much as the physical body does. We need to create time in our lives to cultivate the contact and expression of our spiritual self. It is only by continually making the commitment to allow the spiritual impulse into our lives, that our daily experience is enriched with a true feeling of purpose.

The cultivation of the spiritual aspect of our lives involves the process that is known as 'becoming conscious'. This means thinking about what we do and how we live, examining all our old patterns and habits and beginning to experience life as a process of insight, inspiration and purposefulness. This may seem like a huge step to take. It need not be. We can only start from where we are, and even very small changes in our behaviour and attitudes can begin to break up the habits and personally-imposed restrictions that we all allow ourselves to fall into.

If you would like to try and set the process of breaking through some old patterns and restrictions in motion, and therefore clear a space to let some fresh insights and creative energy into your life, here are some suggestions:

- try sleeping in a different position to your usual one
- give up a personal habit that has annoyed you for years
- eat completely differently for a while (e.g. try the cleansing diet at the back of this book)
- make a conscious effort to do routine things a different way each day (e.g. put your socks on in a different order or get out of bed on the other side)
- try concentrating totally on the task that you are doing at every moment of the day, and do them all with enthusiasm
- try to start the day with a clear mind, and whenever you start thinking of something, think it right through to its conclusion
- when you meet with criticism or accusation, instead of trying to justify yourself, try to find out what gave rise to it and the point of view behind it (whether you agree with it or not)
- try not to make an excuse of any kind for anything

- take every opportunity to understand someone from another culture that seems foreign and strange to you
- practise making a conscious effort to contact your inner source each night before going to sleep.

Try each one of these exercises for a couple of weeks, and then try another one. The idea is to just watch how you react to trying something different – don't worry if it isn't easy or if you forget for a while, just observe that and have another go.

The results often appear to be truly miraculous, but as any therapist or counsellor interested in spiritual development knows, whenever a person makes a commitment to becoming more conscious, tremendous energy is released into her life, and suddenly she realises what to do next in order to make progress. Really all that is necessary to bring ourselves more into contact with ourselves as spiritual beings, is to commit ourselves to change and growth. Be committed to being true to your perceived purpose at any time, to what is best for your own growth, and also to what is necessary for the development of anyone else with whom you come into contact.

It is an unfortunate reflection of our society that so many people complain of feeling purposeless, or that although they feel there may be some greater purpose for their life, they don't have a sense of what it is. Finding a purpose – your purpose – is not so much about searching around for what you think fits your expectations, but more a question of identifying where you are now, and what your potential is. Lack of purpose is really alienation from society, and from anything bigger than yourself; so it is also necessary to acknowledge that you, whilst being an individual, are also part of the interweaving patterns of life, and that your contribution is as important as anyone else's.

Questions like 'Who am I really?' or 'What should I be doing?' can only be answered by accepting who you are and what you are doing right now. It can feel very painful and restricting to accept that we have to start with what we are now, as opposed with what we would like to be, but from that point of acceptance we can acknowledge our strengths and our weaknesses, and then what we can change in our lives.

If you do feel totally in the dark about your purpose in life, it can be helpful to review your life up until the present time. Take time, this process can take several days. It is important not to become too attached to any one issue, nor to apportion any blame to yourself or anyone else, just look at your life as if it is on a television screen in front of you. At the end of the review, consider what the things are that have given you most satisfaction, such as caring for others, gardening, writing, teaching, being creative or physical exercise. It may be something that you have not done for a long time, if your life has gone off in other directions. But if you do realise there are some things that you find particularly satisfying, then project your review into the future and imagine ways in which you can develop this potential. Commit yourself to finding more time and chances to express these in your life, and be especially open to any chance or occasion that may arise to facilitate your chosen direction.

Another way to get in touch with a sense of purpose in your life is to spend some time doing the above exercises to free up your habitual way of doing things. We have to make room for new experiences, and our habits, resistances and excuses for not trying something 100 per cent can block the flow of energy from our spiritual contact. The most important thing is to consciously commit yourself to cultivating a sense of purpose in your life, to be prepared to let go of how you think things should be, and to be open to change and any new opportunities when they present themselves.

You will know when you are in touch with your inner purpose because you will feel very empowered. It is the same feeling as being in the right place at the right time. When a person is acting out their purpose great things become possible, because tremendous energy flows along the channel that is created by being in line with our inner source.

It is important to remember that a particular role is only an expression of the purpose. The role itself, whether that of a plumber, doctor, mother, teacher, cleaner or poet, is unimportant unless it expresses your purpose at the time. We may need to do many different things at different times in our lives in order to stay in touch with our purpose. It is doing what seems appropriate at the time that is important.

Being in contact with your purpose is the same as being in touch with your source of energy and inspiration, or your spiritual self. This is also the source of what is called impersonal or unconditional love. Nearly all of us will recognise the experience of feeling in contact with something greater than ourselves at some time in our lives, and the aim of cultivating our spiritual life is to have constant access to this source of energy, to get it flowing through every aspect of our lives. It is this love that creates an empathy and sense of contact between people, and it brings the gift of enjoyment and well-being into our existence.

People that radiate this kind of energy come across as powerful and expansive. It is as if you can sense the love that is emanating from them. Such people are often far from 'perfect', in the sense of conforming to the ideal that society expects, and they may have some obvious shortcomings, but nevertheless other people will always be attracted to being around them because of their tremendous energy.

Many women and men feel at their most connected and powerful when they 'fall in love'. The outpouring of energy towards another person leads us to an experience of love filling our lives and often this creates a feeling of benignness and well-wishing on the whole world. This is a sense that could be seen as sharing some of the qualities of a profound spiritual experience. However, what we actually do is project all of our energy and emotion onto another person, who has become an 'object' of our desire. When that initial stage of infatuation passes, we return to whatever state we were in before, and do not really learn or build in any lasting qualities as a result.

The highest expression of love is of service. This concept can be hard to understand, but it means responding to your own needs, and the needs, but not necessarily the wants, of others. It implies caring about everything without expecting results, committing yourself to your purpose without becoming goal-oriented. This aspect of service is also known as unconditional love. This is not something that we can really try and achieve, but it is an ideal that we can hold in our minds and try and return to whenever we realise that we have been acting out of our own selfish wants or desires.

An experience that can both connect us with a sense of our inner energy, and also create the feeling of profound contact with another person, is the experience of sex. Sex can be a celebration of the link between spirit (our inner source) and matter (our body), an expression of our creative impulse and a profound exchange of energy with another person. However, our ability to 'make love' is going to be limited by any expectations or judgements, and by inhibitions on any level. Sex is an expression of where we are at, and it will reflect our limitations and unconscious habits, as well as our ability to express love and enjoyment.

When we consider commonly accepted attitudes to sex, we have another example of how we have become exploitative and self-oriented as a society. Whenever we use something for our own pleasure we denigrate it and objectify it. Women in particular have been seen as objects of sexual gratification that men have rights

359

over. When sex becomes free of rights and obligations, and instead is valued as an exchange of intimacy and tenderness with another unique and vulnerable human being, then we can enjoy sex more fully as an expression of energy and life.

What else can we do to help us find our source of consciousness? There are many techniques that have evolved over the centuries to help us get in contact with our spiritual selves. All of these require freeing ourselves to some degree from our habitual way of responding to things, and our unconscious patterns, as we have discussed. They also require us to reach beyond the rational, concrete part of our brain, to the more abstract, intuitive mind, and then even beyond that. This is the aim of many self-development and meditation groups.

Meditation is a tool that can enable us to calm the chattering of our brain, and create a contact with the part of our mind that uses symbols and images, and is beyond the rational and mundane. It can help us to restore our contact with ourselves, and with our real needs, so that we are motivated from inside. In this way we can have an effect on our lives and our environment, instead of being motivated only by what happens to us from the outside, and always being affected by our environment.

We have used the following meditation techniques, and if you would like to try them, then do have a go. There are lots of different kinds of meditation using a variety of techniques, although the purpose is generally the same: to open us up to an experience of ourselves that is beyond that of the petty personality. If you want to find out about some different kinds of meditation turn to page 401 at the back of this book.

In common with most forms of meditation, we first suggest that you sit in a comfortable position, with your spine straight, and allow yourself to become relaxed. Then breathe regularly and evenly, so that the length of the breath in is equal to the length of the breath out. Concentrating on breathing can always seem a little strange at first, but it helps to achieve a state of balance. When you get more used to it, you can try to lengthen the length of the breath in and out a little, and a deeper sense of relaxation will follow.

The next stage in this meditation routine is to bring your awareness to a focus in the centre of the forehead. In traditional terms this centre is called the 'third eye', but it is generally known as the seat of consciousness. From this centre you should be able to view things in a more detached manner. When you have become familiar with focusing your awareness on the centre of the brow, you can return there when you need to see an overview of a situation, or when you want to function on a level beyond that of the petty personality.

When you feel that you are focused in the brow-centre, use your imagination to create a circle of light travelling anti-clockwise around your head. This circle of light is a technique of the western meditation tradition, and it is the same idea as a halo, or an aura. If other people are present you can also include them in the circle of light and it will create an area of positive energy. It is also possible to imagine someone who is ill or suffering inside the circle of light, but it is important to wish nothing specific on them, just direct a sense of well-being towards them.

If you have managed to maintain these exercises, you can establish your consciousness in your spinal column by imagining that it is full of light. The lighted spine can represent your base, or your home, and you can return to this image as a way of centring yourself, or contacting your inner source.

If you want to take your meditation a step further, then you can visualise a globe of light above your head, like a sun, and bring a ray of the light down and in through the brow centre, and then down your spine. When your spine is filled with this light, you can radiate it out through every pore of your body, and fill your atmosphere with light and positive energy. When you breathe in bring down the light, and when you breathe out radiate the energy out. If at any time you feel your mind or your concentration wandering, then just bring your awareness back into the brow-centre, and start again with the basic exercises of relaxing your body and balancing your breath.

This bit of the meditation – bringing down light – is very useful for those people who need to feel inspired, and want to create a flow of positive energy in their life. For those of us who have a problem concentrating, and are prone to feeling 'spaced out', then a more useful technique can be to do the exercises including relaxing, balancing the breath, focusing in the forehead and creating a circle of light around you, but then visualise sending down roots deep into the earth, like a tree. You can then bring energy up from the earth, and up through your feet into the rest of your body. This energy can then be radiated out into your atmosphere, and it will have a more 'earthing' effect for you.

You can meditate daily, weekly or just whenever you feel like it. The meditation is not really an end in itself – its purpose is to help us to contact our source of energy, and to get that positive energy flowing into every area of our life.

Another technique that can be used to open our lives up to the spiritual is ritual. There are as many variations of ritual as there are mystical philosophies and religions, but the intention is generally the same: to create a link between the spiritual and the physical. Another useful aspect of ritual is that we can use it as a set period of time in which to practise being 100 per cent conscious during every action. This can thus help us to develop an increased awareness and sense of purpose.

Some people feel very uncomfortable about ritual in general, or about ritual that is not done for them by a religious 'expert', but any action that has a symbolic as well as a literal meaning is actually a ritual. For example, decorating a fir tree at Christmas is a ritual, so is putting candles on a birthday cake or and placing a wreath on a grave. In fact, other functions of ritual are that it can help us to develop an appreciation for the use of symbols, and it can also enrich our understanding of our cultural heritage.

There is a tradition of using ritual in the West that is based on the four elements. This can be done by dividing an area up into four quarters, and choosing which element to place in which quarter. Here is one suggestion:

North – Water

West – Earth   East – Air

South – Fire

Within this space you can creat a context for any activity that you consider to be sacred. For instance, it can be used for healing, meditating or creating something very special. You can divide up a room in this way, or a table top, or part of a garden, or just an imaginary space. If you want to choose symbolic objects that represent the elements to you, then you can place them in the appropriate quarter. The space that you have created can be purified by sprinkling it with water, and consecrated by the burning of incense. Candles can be lit in the centre as a focus of energy and light.

To help you develop the potential of ritual, you can take any object, word or idea and consider what it means to you, both literally and symbolically. Take the example of water from the suggested layout above: water can be used as an element that represents clarity, purity, reflection and tranquillity. It is often associated with the emotions, it is generally seen as a feminine element and it is connected to the moon through the ebb and flow of the oceans.

Further illustrations can be drawn from the example above to help develop an understanding of the other elements. Air is a symbol of truth, inspiration and communication, it is associated with spring in the cycle of the year. Fire gives us courage, enthusiasm, warmth, love and is associated with midday and midsummer. Earth offers solidity, stability and endurance. From earth, we can learn about our relationship with the material world, it represents the time of the harvest. To gain a more personal understanding of these elements, and how you relate to them in your daily life, you will have to reflect on them yourself.

Everything in nature can be looked at ritually. The cycle of the seasons can be considered symbolically as well as literally. Try asking yourself what winter means to you, and then spring, summer and autumn. Consider the cycle of day and night, and what your associations are with night, sunrise, midday and evening. We can begin to see why night and winter and death have been associated with each other through the ages. Likewise why spring, sunrise, the east and new life or rebirth, are connected to each other. Some of the rituals that exist in our culture may then have more meaning for you. We can see, for example, why easter eggs are given in the spring, the symbolic time of new life.

By building up our associations with the symbols that we use in ritual, we can become more conscious of our relationship with them in our everyday lives. The relationship that you have to water in a ritual, the associations that you make and the ease with which you are able to establish a contact with it, are all reflections of the role of water in your life. For example, if you find it difficult to imagine and establish a sense of contact with water during a ritual, it may be that you find it difficult to express your emotions, or to feel relaxed and able to flow in your everyday life. Ritual enables us to go inside our own psyche, it helps us to understand our relationship with the world.

By means of a conclusion to this section, we would like to emphasise that we feel that cultivating contact with and expression of our spiritual selves is a very important part of developing a sense of well-being and purpose in our lives as a whole. The actual nature of this contact, and the way that we choose to manifest it in our lives is entirely up to each one of us, and we can only offer some very broad guidelines and simple exercises in a book of this kind.

The important thing to remember is that it is bringing the spiritual impulse into our everyday life that will create health and well-being in ourselves. There is for example, very little point in just going to church once a week, without the feeling of inner purpose enriching our day-by-day life experience.

When we become more confident about our contact with the spiritual part of ourselves, we find that we have more resilience to help us overcome some of the traumas and painful experiences of life. If we feel connected to our own sense of being we can draw on it as on a source in times of need. If we feel that there is more to our life than a physical body then we become less afraid of death. If we feel that we are ultimately connected to everybody and everything else, then we will truly want what is best for the development of the world as a whole, even if that means re-evaluating what we think we want for ourselves.

Our Mental and Emotional Selves

We are going to explore what it means to enjoy ourselves in our mental and emotional life, and what we can do to improve things when we recognise that changes need to be made. The theme that we will develop is that of encouraging a healthy and well-balanced mental and emotional life by being prepared to accept and learn from the whole of an experience. This means accepting the 'good' and the 'bad', the plus and the minus, the pain and the pleasure, of all our experiences.

Firstly we will look at how 'accepting the whole' operates in our relationships with other people, because enjoying the relationships in our life is so important to our mental and emotional well-being. For example, you cannot enjoy a meaningful relationship with someone unless you acknowledge that there are things about them that you feel good about, and things about them that you find more difficult to accept; and that you will have some good times together, but also some painful and challenging times.

Every relationship with another person enriches our life, and provides a unique opportunity for us to learn and grow. We are born to certain parents, and into a certain family, at a particular point in time. These family relationships, and all the others that we go on to form, provide precisely the interaction and contact that we need in order to develop as individuals.

What is the advantage of viewing relationships as learning experiences? We need to know that we are in a relationship because we have a mutual need for that particular interaction. Once we realise this, we can both appreciate it more, and be more willing to make changes when those needs are no longer satisfied. Also, we never need to fear letting go of a relationship that we have outgrown, because we will always form others that are more appropriate to our current learning needs.

If you and your partner decide to commit yourselves to a relationship together, then you are in fact creating a third entity – a sort of pool to which you both contribute and draw out. This pool is a resource for both of you, and one that builds up over time and experiences shared together. You will develop a sense of care, respect and tolerance for the relationship itself, and it will become trusted as a source of nourishment. The partners within a relationship such as this can carry on their development as individuals, and are respected as individuals by the other partner.

However, so many relationships start out well but become stuck in a destructive process. Both parties then become judgemental, blaming and petty. If this situation is prolonged then the couple tend to support each other in their failings and weaknesses, with neither person being free to transform and grow. At the worst this leads to frustration, violence and a diseased state of mind and body. It is very unfortunate that there can be considerable pressure from society to stay in a marriage-type relationship, and that we can be made to feel a failure when such a relationship has to end.

We feel that it may be far better to consider ending a relationship where the needs of either partner are not being satisfied, and honour the rights of both individuals to change, rather than remain in an unsatisfying life. When the purpose of a relationship has ended, no matter how much effort is put in, the potential of both individuals will be unfulfilled because the relationship itself will be restrictive, rather than a source for expansion and growth.

How can we sort ourselves out and enjoy our lives to the full? How can we enjoy being ourselves, and enjoy our friendships and our relationships? This really means how do we stay healthy? We need to appreciate our life as a process of transformation and growth. We need to allow ourselves to experience our dark side as well as our light side, to experience that aspect which we believe to be bad and wrong, that which we go to great lengths to conceal from others. We will not be able to change and grow unless we truly know ourselves, including our negative thoughts and emotions.

If we only allow ourselves to appear to be a 'nice' person or a 'good' person, and hide away the fact that we also have 'horrid' thoughts and 'bad' feelings, then we will carry what we are trying to hide around inside ourselves. We will come to feel guilty, fearful and self-critical, and lose our sense of self-worth. It is only by re-learning to acknowledge and accept the 'bad' as well as the 'good' in ourselves that we can come to know who we really are.

We can begin to live as a whole person fulfilling our potential only when we accept ourselves. This does not mean that we can go around projecting our bad temper, frustrations, and so on, onto other people, but we also don't have to appear nice at the expense of our health and growth. Take a risk and express some of that concealed 'bad' behaviour. You can still be sensitive to what seems appropriate and what doesn't, and to other people's reactions. You may be surprised to that other people find your hidden 'vices' perfectly acceptable.

We have grown up learning how to hide the bits of ourselves that are not approved of from a very early age. Babies quickly adopt strategies of behaviour as part of the process of learning how to survive in their environment. These behavioural tendencies are at first copied from one of her or his parents, or another available role model, and are then developed and moulded according to the feedback that the infant receives. We experience this process in action whenever we recognise that a child 'takes after' one of his or her parents.

As well as the contribution of the parents to the personality of the child, there is also the contribution from the society and the culture that the child is part of; there is the environment and the personal experiences that the child is exposed to; and there is also the innate ability and the individual characteristics of the child. It is the unique combination of these factors that will determine the habits that we develop as an individual.

What exactly do we mean by habits? We mean the unconscious responses that we make to particular situations. These unconscious responses are the result of past experiences, for example if we respond in a certain way to a particular situation and we meet with a reasonable degree of success, then when a similar situation arises in the future the habitual response will be to behave in the same way again. If an infant cries when she is hungry, and as a result her mother feeds her, then she will come to associate crying with being fed. If a child initially expresses her anger and frustration visibly, but is forcibly made to be quiet and not express it by a parent, or at school, it is probable that this child will come to habitually suppress her anger.

These successful strategies become programmed-in as our methods of survival and control using the best options that we have available at the time. Our personality is built up largely from the complex pattern created by the interface between this programmed behaviour, and the experiences that we are subject to. The problem is that the programming remains even when the circumstances change, and we are left stuck with a limited number of options as to how we perceive and respond to a situation. If I am an introverted young person, afraid of expressing an opinion because my parents always put my opinions down, then even when I no longer live with my parents, I am still likely to have a problem being assertive and expressing myself.

Because the experience and feedback that each individual is exposed to is completely individual, the exact pattern of behavioural habits that develops is unique to each person. These habitual responses not only affect our behaviour, but also our emotions and thoughts. If I believe it when I am told at school that I have an awful singing voice, then I will probably avoid situations where I have to sing, and I will also feel inhibited and lack confidence about my ability to sing. Thus habits can lead to inhibition, self-criticism, an absence of self-worth and the tendency to suppression.

Habitual behaviour also limits our ability to change as well as our creative potential. For example, much habitual behaviour is part of a pattern of fear: fear of change, of disapproval, of being criticised, or of not being loved. These habits lead to a defensiveness that prevents us from participating fully in an experience, and can also prevent us from being prepared to take the risks necessary to make a change in our lives. If I avoid asking for help when I do not understand something in a class I am attending, because I am afraid of being thought stupid, then I am unlikely to learn as much as I could, and I am also unlikely to really enjoy the class. Similarly, if I turn down a new job because I am afraid of taking a risk and making a change, then I have rejected the opportunity for growth and new experience in that area of my life.

We learn not to risk ourselves, and we learn not to be ourselves. It is this that prevents us changing our lives and from really communicating. Supporting another person in their habits, for example by allowing them to become dependent on you, is the worst thing that you can do for them. It kills their opportunity for change and growth.

When we allow our unconscious habits to repeat themselves again and again, the suppression involved is like a record getting stuck in a groove. A deeper and deeper rut is created, and it becomes more and more difficult to change the habit. Habitual behaviour comes to affect our relationships with other people, how we feel about ourselves, and all our activities. In fact it is this process of becoming stuck in habitual ways of being that creates disease. An example is someone who has got into the habit of continually worrying about work. This person will become tense and obsessive, they will alienate their family, they may become too anxious to sleep, and typically they will begin to suffer from a 'nervous' digestion, which leads to a stomach ulcer, or to develop high blood pressure.

So, how can we change habitual behaviour? Firstly, we have to realise that this will be an ongoing process; it is part of the process of becoming conscious that we described in the Spiritual section. It is not that we suddenly stop acting out of our unconscious habits, but that we try to become more aware of when we are responding habitually, and that we continually reaffirm our commitment for change and growth.

The exercises given in the Spiritual section (see pages 356–7) to loosen up some of our habitual ways of doing things are appropriate here. If you feel that you really don't know where to start, there are many psychotherapists and group dynamic processes available today that aim to unravel some of the complex patterns of threads that make up our habitual behaviour (see pages 398–9 for some suggestions).

A general guide to giving up a particular habit is that first we must acknowledge it, and then we must let it go. Acknowledging a habit means becoming aware that we have responded to a situation in an unconscious way. Watch yourself react. When something seems to go wrong, ask yourself why it went that way. Don't blame something or somebody else, instead check whether or not your response was appropriate to the situation. If it wasn't, consider where your reaction came from, and how could it be different next time?

The motive for giving up many of our habits emerges when we realise that the pain caused by the habit is actually greater than the pain caused by giving it up. It is always difficult to give up a habit because our unconscious operates by adopting behavioural habits for survival, and so there will always be an initial resistance to change while we are retraining the unconscious to adopt a new pattern. This is why it is often the best strategy to replace an old habit with a more positive, new one. For example, if you are someone who always walks out of the room in the middle of an argument, practice instead letting go of your pride and trying to see the other person's point of view. Putting your energy into trying something new has a very different effect from suppressing an emotion: it opens the door for change, rather than closing it. You know when you have done something differently because there is a sense of freedom and excitement accompanying the action.

Another reason why it is difficult to change a habit is because the habit originated to satisfy a need and we will still have to deal with the need. If I decide to give up smoking, I will only be successful if I am confident that the benefits from giving it up outweigh the advantages or 'pay-off' of smoking. The advantages of smoking, like with many habits, are complex and subtle. There is a physical addiction to nicotine, but we know that removing the nicotine will not actually cause us any physical harm, merely some initial readjustment. What I really have to confront when I give up smoking is the removal of an emotional prop for controlling vulnerability, and deflecting a sense of exposure. If I am conscious of the need behind the habit (in this case the need to hide my vulnerability), then I can at least be patient with myself if there is an emotional backlash when I try and change. In fact, trying to give up a habit is a very good way of getting to know more about yourself, and your needs and props, even if you resume the habit in the end.

So far we have dealt with how habits affect the individual. We can also see that groups and societies operate habitually. These habits need to be reviewed and changed when the damage they cause outweighs any advantages. A society where the purpose was to establish material growth and technological advance, has created tremendous progress in scientific knowledge and communications. However, the habitual abuse of natural resources, so often accepted as being necessary for material growth, has resulted in widespread despoilation and pollution of the land. This has now become so damaging that we need to change our approach to materialism in order to survive. We need to build in new habits that are based on an appreciation of the balance between giving and taking. We need to become conscious of the results of our actions, and be prepared to put something back in return for what we use.

How can we make these very necessary changes as a society? We can only transform a society if enough individuals recognise the need to change their personal wants and desires, and their attitude to the earth and her resources. Government legislation is necessary to enforce restrictions on the discharge of pollutants and the exploitation of natural resources. But the legislation will only come about if it is demanded by determined individuals. Business practices will only change if individual customers demand that changes are made in what they want to purchase. Every individual needs to reassess their material needs and their contribution to society, in order to make change happen on a global scale.

Be wary of stereotyping people. Every time that we have an expectation about the way a certain group of people do something or feel about something or are capable of achieving something, we have limited their potential. If girls are not expected to be good at science in school, we create a reality by not encouraging them and teaching them adequately. We need to be aware of how these habitual attitudes towards people limit and damage both individuals and society as a whole. There are terrible restrictions on freedom and growth in a society that is essentially racist, sexist, classist or ageist. In fact, whenever we hear or use a word with 'ist' or 'ism' at the end we need to beware of prejudiced or judgemental attitudes.

The way that a society creates the different roles of men and women is of the most significant contributions to habitual behaviour. Gender expectations and obligations significantly form the unconscious habits of individuals, and by return, build up more entrenched attitudes and expectations for future generations to adopt. Although the Women's Movement has done much to break down the habits and pressures of a male-dominated society, there is still a long way to go before both women and men are free from the limitations of stereotyped attitudes. How often do you excuse your behaviour because you are a woman?

A baby is genderised immediately from birth. The infant is reacted to differently if she is a girl or if he is a boy. Boys are expected to be aware that they are different from girls at a very early age, and that they are better at doing some things, and not so good at others. They learn quickly that they are supposed to be physically adept, and they are encouraged to play with constructional toys. They are also expected to be more competitive than girls, and they are more likely to be encouraged to go off and explore their environment. Boys are not usually expected to read very early, or to talk a lot.

As a boy grows up there is often considerable pressure on him to become successful in the world. He is generally encouraged to become achievement-oriented and ambitious. Boys are approved of if they 'go for what they can get', they are taught to pursue what interests them, and to be brave and withstand hurt. They are told not to cry, and they are not generally encouraged to be sensitive or considerate and caring to others.

As adolescents, boys are teasingly encouraged to 'prove themselves', and be good at conquering women. This attitude leads to the idea that girls are something to be possessed and taken. This unconscious process of turning girls into objects in the minds of men, creates the conditions for men to commit rape. Women have become something for men to possess. This is true with any form of pornography and sexual harassment.

How can we improve the way we bring up young men? Adolescents need clear definitions from their parents about what is right, because adolescents will, and have the right to, challenge every assumption and every dictate from authority. Honest communication and tolerance is extremely important to allow an adolescent to become an independent adult. It is important to remember that we do not own our children, and that they have the right to live their own lives. It can be very difficult to be a constant source of loving support and tolerance without making it conditional.

Aggression in a developing male is seen as 'natural'. Violent behaviour is the outcome of frustration and a breakdown in communication. Control through fear will never create a healthy society, in the same way that suppression of an illness by drugs will never create a well person. Police and prisons are symptoms of social failure. Everybody, but especially the developing youngster, needs to know what is or is not acceptable behaviour within the family, and in society. They must learn that 'discipline' is something that comes from inside the individual. Imposed discipline can never be an adequate substitute for discipline from within.

Adolescent boys have to work out their relationships with teachers, friends, parents and society. Behind all this is the working out of their role as a man. The traditional role of man is seen as the one who goes out to hunt for food to bring back for the dependent women and children. We suggest that a more empowering way of understanding this symbolic image for the man (and woman), is that of the hunter who uses his spear with choice.

In Native American society, where men and women were not in such an exploitative relationship to each other, or to the earth, as we have become, they appreciated how important it was to select the right moment to throw the spear. The hunter took only what was necessary for survival, and only that which was the most appropriate to take – the weakest of the species, so that the strongest would be left to reproduce and support its survival. Wielding his power as an expression of purpose and with consideration as to the result of his action, the role of man gains clarity, direction and the active expression of purpose. The spear is a symbol of the way man consciously exercises choice to achieve his purpose.

We can empower ourselves by having this same attitude of choosing when and how to act in our everyday use of resources. We can do this by not buying more food than we need; by supporting public transport; by using money rather than accumulating it. Native Americans never killed more animals than they were going to eat in a given period of time. This is a long way from our attitudes of accumulation and acquisition today. Try asking yourself the following questions:

- Do you enjoy work?
- Do you work just for the money?
- Do you really need the money?
- What do you need the money for?
- Do you need the money to support a particular way of life?
- Do you really enjoy your way of life?
- Does your work contribute to your sense of purpose?
- Does your job contribute to the community?
- Do you enjoy the companionship of where you work?
- Do you feel obliged to work to satisfy somebody else?
- Could you risk the disapproval if you were not the main provider/breadwinner?
- Are you still trying to fulfil your parents' or society's expectations for success?
- What does success mean to you?
- What does power mean to you?
- To what degree is material gain your purpose?

So many of us work in jobs whose contribution to our own purpose and to the well-being of society is detrimental. We feel strongly that everybody should question the integrity of the work that they do. Some of us have very little choice about our work because we do need to support our families. If you are stuck in an unsatisfying job then to some extent society is at fault because it pushes people towards material obligations and provides too few mobility opportunities. However, the more we are all aware of a need for change, the more likely is the possibility of it happening.

There is a 'grey area' of jobs that are justified by society because they are 'beneficial', that we feel are questionable in the light of our view that we should all strive for the well-being of the whole, and not for the benefit of one section or part. Much scientific research falls into this category. Animal experimentation exploits the animal kingdom for the so-called benefit of humans. Moreover, animal experiments continue despite evidence that there are frequently alternatives to using animals, and also that animals are often not an exact enough substitute for the research to be of real value to humans.

It is worth remembering that 49 per cent of our genes are made up of opposite sex. We are taught esoterically and psychologically that we are feminine and masculine on different levels. This means that we need to look at both the masculine and feminine parts of ourselves.

Girls are genderised from birth just as much as boys are. It appears that even the youngest of girls will play differently to their male counterparts. Girls tend to be less interested in constructional games, and more readily involved in social and communication-oriented games. They become interested in looking pretty with the minimum of encouragement, or even at times with active discouragement. It is very difficult to identify what causes these differences in behaviour between girls and boys: it may be due to inheritance, biological make-up, parents, society, or a combination of all these factors.

A girl's development is further determined by the educational process. Girls are treated very differently from boys at school, however careful and informed the school attempts to be. They are generally considered to be easier to deal with in the classroom, they tend to apply themselves more, and they learn quickly that they get approval by being 'good'. Girls tend to mature more quickly than boys, and are usually more advanced at reading and writing than boys of the same age.

In recent years schools have generally made more effort to offer equal opportunities to both sexes. Reading material for early readers has been reviewed to remove some of the more explicitly-sexist ideas. Teachers play a crucial role in society: they are the spearheads of change. Unfortunately, the power for making changes in education has been placed in the hands of politicians, whose decisions are based on votes and not vision. Teachers need to be leaders within the community; their contribution towards creating our future through education is of vital importance. Children need teachers who are committed, and have a sense of purpose. We need to create the conditions within our education system that allow teachers to inspire children, or at least pass on the willingness to learn.

Young people are subjected to a huge amount of advertising as they grow up. The media persists in perpetuating the stereotype of young women as pretty and desirable objects. A girl's sense of self-worth becomes dependent on her attractiveness, and how she fits into the standards of society. The adolescent girl is desperately trying to fit in, to make herself acceptable to her peers and attractive to the opposite sex.

Adolescent girls need a lot of reassurance that they are all right, and that they are loved because they are who they are, and not just because they are seen to be attractive. It is helpful to encourage girls to be self-reliant, and not to be dependent on others for approval. Teach them practical things, for example, how to repair plugs, bicycles and so on, to do things around the house like putting up shelves, as well as how to make clothes, grow things and cook. They need to learn how to be independent human beings, and not vulnerable and dependent within their own environment.

Self-discipline needs to be encouraged in girls as in boys. This is not always considered to be important, and as a result girls can become gullible, lack discrimination and attract abuse.

Girls pick up the need to be protective from their mothers. They often enjoy caring for and nuturing animals and babies when they are still very young. This is a very fine quality, but it can develop into a tendency to overprotect and stifle other people. If mothers overprotect their sons, then the boys will grow up with a lack of independence and an inability to be creative. If mothers overprotect their daughters then girls also become overprotective and unable to let things go their own way. This is the mechanism by which girls can become emotionally manipulative and security-seeking.

Women seem to become over-materialistic and competitive out of a desire for control too often. Why do we need to control? Why do we need to stand out as special people, as 'prima donnas', queen bees or even martyrs? Because it gives us a sense of power, a feeling of being more significant than we suspect we really are. What we need to develop is a sense of our true power as women: we need to find an inner sense of worth based on our appreciation of our own strengths.

Whenever we resign ourselves to our weaknesses, or refuse to acknowledge our failings, we collude with all that is second rate in society. We accept poor quality food, we put up with the appalling services public places provide for our children. Whenever a woman tries to prove her worth through her attractiveness she is putting down her real inner worth.

For a woman to function effectively and positively in our society, it is important not to lose touch with the positive qualities of being a woman. A positive archetype that we can draw on for inspiration is that of the Goddess. The energy of the Goddess is the earth itself, in all its abundance. The Goddess is in touch with the processes of life and death: she is the healer, the seer, the inspirer, the sister, the lover and the mother.

Too often women lack a sense of purpose. We easily confuse this with what society approves of in us, that is by being responsive and submissive. The Goddess image allows us to sense our power and our purpose, without losing touch of our femininity. If we have a sense of our inner worth, we do not need to rely on that which is external to prove our value. We need to trust the process of growth and renewal in ourselves and in the earth. The Goddess is the earth, from her and through her all life is sustained.

Our Physical Selves

In this section we are going to look at how we can look after our body so that we are able to resist disease and enjoy ourselves. Health has become a complex issue in recent years. Although better nutrition and hygiene has improved our health enormously in some ways, a new and different pattern of chronic and stress-related disease is being established.

The main factors that contribute to how susceptible we are to disease today are inherited factors, individual habits, environmental stresses (including pollution), medication and diet. Our ability to be healthy depends on whether we can steer a reasonable path through these factors. We have to acknowledge that there are today a great deal more choices involved in our daily life, for example as to what we eat, how hard we work, etc., and that the choices we make influence our health.

We can all think of people who appeared not to look after themselves well, probably smoking or drinking heavily, and who thrived into a perfectly healthy old age. This kind of constitution is not so common any more. Increasingly we do need to look after ourselves in order to stay healthy. Pollution, over-medication, refined diets and stressful lifestyles, have all placed a strain on our ability to eliminate toxins, adapt to our environment and remain healthy.

Maintaining our good health requires a degree of balance in our diet and the exercise and rest that we take, and we will look at all these factors in detail in this section. If we already have a specific health problem, we need to consider consulting a therapist of some kind, as well as reassessing our lifestyle and the factors in it which may have contributed to the problem.

Choosing a particular form of therapy or a therapist can be difficult just because of the wide range that are available. Probably the best way to choose is to go for one which feels to be the most appropriate for you at this moment in time. Becoming healthy is a process and this process may involve seeing more than one therapist, as well as making a variety of changes in your lifestyle. The important thing is to make a start now, and not worry if the therapy that you choose does not seem to be absolutely ideal for you, or that your therapist does not have all the answers. If you discover later that a different therapy feels better for your needs then change, although you need to give any therapy long enough to have a fair chance of working (a year or more may be necessary).

Why choose wholistic medicine rather than orthodox medicine? The aim of wholistic medicine is to understand the process of disease, and how these processes have led to a particular set of disease symptoms for an individual. Unlike orthodox medicine, the treatment will be directed at changing the disease process, and not just removing the symptoms that are the end result. This is known as curing the tendency to disease, rather than suppressing the symptoms.

We described in the Mental and Emotional section (see pages 365–76) how an individual's habits can lead to disease developing in the physical body. By habit we mean any behaviour, response or attitude that prevents us from being in touch with, and expressing, our inner purpose. Curing disease requires changing the habits, which may be mental, emotional or physical. Only when the habits have been changed is the body able to come back into a state of health and maintain it. Wholistic medicine is one of the tools that we have available to help us become more aware of our habits, and to change them. At the same time, natural remedies will encourage the body to throw off, or eliminate, the symptoms of the disease.

Disease can be seen as an opportunity for growth, not by accepting the disease itself but by accepting that the process is our own, and that it is within our potential to change it. Our disease is our link with our past – we can look back at the development of the disease and see where the wrong choices were made. This can be very empowering, not if we blame anything or anyone else (or ourselves) for our disease, but if we recognise that we can make changes in our own life, and that these changes will affect our own health and well-being. Blaming anyone else, or ourselves, for our disease will create anger and resentment or guilt, which only serves to add to our ill-health and further prevent our growth.

The starting point, or the 'soil', for our health is our genetic inheritance. Not only can specific physical diseases be inherited, but also our susceptibility to types of disease, and our general constitution. Orthodox medicine has never been very good at explaining or understanding how the more subtle processes of inheritance work. Traditional Chinese medicine and homoeopathy have made greater contributions to our understanding of how inherited tendencies affect our health.

In Chinese medicine, it is the state of the flow of body energies in the man and the woman that contribute to the health of the child. A man with a healthy and vital flow of energy will produce healthy sperm; and a woman with a healthy flow of energy will provide the right environment for a foetus to develop in the womb. In homoeopathy, the theory of 'miasms' explains how subtle characteristics are passed down in families, and the same disease tendency will crop up in different members of the same family, although the actual symptoms may differ from person to person. For example, it may be one particular miasm in the family that contributes to asthma developing in one child and eczema and hayfever developing in another child in the same family. Constitutional homoeopathic treatment aims to minimise the impact of these disease-inflicting miasms.

Food and Diet

As well as our inheritance, our health will be determined by our diet, our environment, and our lifestyle. Food is one of the basic necessities for life, but this basic need becomes overladen with personal and social habits and values.

Many of our eating habits stem from sharing meal-times together. Children learn social and cultural values during meal-times, as well as getting nourishment. This early socialisation contributes to the eating habits that we develop when we are older. It is generally the mother who is mainly responsible for giving children their food. Children need to be encouraged by their mothers to be aware of food as the produce of the earth. We all need to be aware that we are fortunate to have enough to eat. Wasting food is a profound waste of resources.

Food should be appreciated, shared and enjoyed. As mothers we must be careful not to make our children feel guilty if they do not want what we think they should have. At the same time, children need to be offered nutritious food, and they need regular meals. It is a good idea to educate children about basic nutrition at home, and involve them in the preparation and cooking of food, so that they can grow up with good habits.

There is a huge amount of advertising of food products, and this is aimed at trying to prove that one brand is better than another. The food we buy is also subject to class, racial and lifestyle factors. Diet needs to be tailored to suit individual needs and tastes within broad nutritional guidelines. We do not know the full effects living on a diet of TV dinners and refined foods have on our health because they have not been around for long enough. However, there are indications that the health of ourselves, and of our children, is being seriously undermined by a modern diet of processed and refined foods.

In the past we have been willing to let the 'experts' decide what is good food for us and our children. Now we are becoming more aware about some of the implications of the type of food we eat, and we are starting to question those 'experts'. After 1945 great emphasis was placed on consuming sufficient milk, butter and meat. Recently there is concern over the level of heart disease connected with a western diet that is high in animal fats. Children frequently suffer from allergies connected to the additives in our food.

In order to fulfil our food requirements factory farming has been developed. There have been some alarming incidents in recent years to indicate that we need to reassess our attitude to producing food. Battery-farmed chickens have led to outbreaks of Salmonella. Feeding cows on an unnatural diet of meat products has led to the development of BSE (Bovine Spongiform Encephalopathy) or 'mad cow disease'. The over-use of nitrates in agricultural practices has led to the pollution of our water. There are many other examples of how short-term, profit-motivated ideas have led the developed world to seriously disrupt the balance of agriculture.

There is now a shift underway towards eating more of a wholefood-oriented diet, and towards producing organically-grown vegetables and free-range animal products. Children themselves are often very concerned about the welfare of the animals in factory farming, and are making choices about the food they are prepared to eat. However, this recent development only applies to the western world. We still supply chemicals for intensive production of foods in underdeveloped countries. Refined foods are still very popular in less developed countries, partly as a sign of wealth, and also because food companies have looked for new markets as their domestic ones have shrunk. We need to reassess our food production practices on a global scale.

What kind of food should we eat? Basically, food retains more of its nutritional value the closer it is to its original state. Food needs to be as fresh and as unprocessed and unrefined as possible. We need, where possible, to eat the whole of the product, as with brown rice or wholemeal flour.

Food is an area where we can all have a great effect on what is produced by exercising our choice about what we buy. Women, as the main purchasers of the family's food, have encouraged supermarkets to offer more products that are additive and colouring-free by choosing brands and foods without additives and colourings. The food industry will respond to our demands if we make them known. Make a point of asking for what you want to buy, not just accepting what the retailer has decided you can have.

Refined foods are often low in vitamins, and to compensate for this, some foods actually have vitamins added back in. This is a total waste of resources. The fact that intensive agricultural methods have caused a decline in the natural vitamins and minerals in our food has led some nutritionists to favour taking food supplements. There is no substitute for good, fresh food, and if we take steps to have a varied and balanced diet, with a high proportion of organically-produced foodstuffs, then food supplements should not be necessary.

Food supplements are manufactured using complex technological processes, and the full implications of taking synthetic vitamins are not fully understood. Vitamin and mineral supplements are also usually supplied in very large doses, much larger than we would ingest at any one time from eating a well-balanced meal. Another issue involved with taking synthetic vitamins is that the only companies who have the capital to set up the expensive technology to manufacture them are the major drug companies, and so we are supporting them by buying vitamin pills.

If you would like to know more about what foods to eat in order to benefit from natural sources of particular vitamins or minerals, then consult the Food Charts on pages 392–4.

We may soon be expected to accept irradiated food as an alternative to genuinely fresh food. This is another process where we will only discover the long-term effects when it is too late: because we will have already suffered any detrimental effects to our health before they are acknowledged and the practice changed. What we must do in this case is make our opinions known, and refuse to accept irradiated food if it concerns you.

If you are aware that you have not had a very good diet for some years, or that your diet is contributing to a particular disease, you should consider consulting a dietary therapist or naturopath for specific advice. The naturopathic approach to health is that we need to be able to clear out impurities or toxins in our system, rather than letting them build up and contribute to disease. If we are reasonably healthy we should be able to eliminate a small amount of additives and toxins through our bowels, bladder and skin. However, if the level of toxins in our diet is too high, or if our eliminative processes are blocked or underfunctioning, then symptoms of disease will result.

A detoxifying or cleansing diet can be a good way to clear out the system – and a good start to making improvements in your diet if you feel that to be necessary. Either consult a naturopath or dietary therapist who will guide you through a cleansing regime, or follow the cleansing diet on page 395. A traditional time to do a cleansing diet is in the spring, so that we can clear out the effects of stodgy winter foods, and prepare ourselves for the new yearly cycle.

Another area related to food that has become a big issue in our society is that of body weight. We live in a society where women are expected to be nymph-like creatures, and so many of us are unhappy if this is not what our bodies are like. For some women trying to lose weight is a constant struggle and cause of anxiety; some other women give up completely under the pressure, and do become obese. Neither is a very satisfactory way of being.

For some time it has been known that calorie-counting diets are rarely an effective way of losing weight and maintaining the lower weight. Calorie counting requires an attitude of self-denial and an artificial, obsessive approach to food. We need to get back in touch with what foods suit us as individual people, given our particular tastes and our lifestyle.

What is basically wrong with our attitude to weight is that being overweight has become confused with being unfit. We often use being overweight as an excuse for not making the attempt to be fit. We can become fit by concentrating on improving the quality of the food that we eat, and by taking regular exercise. It is much more sensible and enjoyable to set your purpose at being fit, than to try to live up to an image of what you would like to look like.

In addition to eating a diet based on fresh and unrefined wholefoods there are a few other general guidelines that we recommend if you are considering making improvements to your eating habits. Eat a wide variety of foodstuffs that supply a balanced range of nutrients. Eat regular meals – say three times a day. Do not eat just before going to bed. Eat for the purpose of being healthy, and active, and to get energy, and not for other reasons. Talk to other women about your food concerns. Join a fitness centre or exercise class. Work on being positive and improving your general self-esteem, rather than just concentrating on what you look like.

Our society has attached an exaggerated importance to certain foods. These foods are often the ones that are likely to make us put on weight, for example chocolate, cream or sweets. These luxury foods have become readily available and commonplace, whereas once they were genuinely treats for special occasions. If we say no to these foods we can become caught up in feelings of self-denial that we may feel the need to rebel against.

The fact that so many women have eating disorders, and have even become closet eaters, or anorexic, is a fundamental sign of how mixed up we are as a society about eating and weight. These kind of problems will require an in-depth assessment and investigation of the patterns behind the self-denial, and poor self-esteem, that are causing the eating disorder. A visit to a counsellor, psychotherapist or other professional therapist will be necessary to treat these more serious eating disorders.

Exercise

In order to take regular exercise we have to decide that it is an important part of our daily life. Also, we have to have developed enough self-esteem to recognise that our personal needs are important, and that one of those needs is to keep fit.

Creating the leisure time to take exercise can be a real problem for many women. If you work, and have children, then it is always difficult to find time for yourself. It is best to set aside a small amount of time on a regular basis – an amount that you know is realistic. There are many good exercise books and videos to help you create your own exercise routine for yourself and stick to it. It can be fun to encourage a friend to take up an exercise with you so that you can swim, jog or create a dance routine together.

There are many benefits to taking exercise, but generally it improves your level of energy by stimulating your vitality. Exercising also assists the elimination of toxins by increasing lymphatic drainage. It tones the circulation, and improves muscle tone. Regular exercise is particularly important in women, as over a period of years exercising encourages bone growth and helps to prevent osteoporosis.

Some forms of exercise are costly, so if you are hard up you need to find ways of exercising that do not involve joining an expensive fitness club or paying for classes or equipment, and so on. Contact your local council for information about subsidised sports centres. Adult Education Institutes often offer subsidised fitness classes, or contact your local women's support group.

It is worth remembering that you can take every opportunity in your daily life to exercise and use muscles. Try running up and down stairs, and walking up escalators. If you travel to work on a bus or tube, get off a stop early and walk the last bit. If you live in the city, try to set aside one day each week to go to the countryside for a walk, and if you have children take them with you.

As we get older it tends to become even more of an effort to make sure that we get enough exercise to stay supple and fit. If we feel tired and without energy, then we may be unfit, and probably lack self-esteem about our physical body. What we need is to do more exercise, but because we feel tired anyway we do less, and a vicious cycle needs to be broken. Concentrate on pleasurable exercises like walking, swimming or gardening. It is keeping moving that is important.

Getting older does require us to find different ways of enjoying life. We need to recognise that we are more than just a physical body, without neglecting our fitness. Later in life it is possible to do the things that you never had the time for during a career and looking after children. Take up those activities that you used to be interested in again, or do the things you always wanted to do. Involve yourself in the surrounding community. Try checking out your local libraries, Adult Education Institute or local council for appropriate activities. Now is the time to cultivate a special interest.

Sleep and Rest

It has been said that our bodies can only repair themselves during the hours that we are asleep. We need sleep for good physical and psychological health, although the amount of sleep needed varies considerably from person to person, and at different times of our life.

Newborn babies spend the majority of their time asleep, and within a few months usually become used to more regular sleeping patterns, averaging about twelve hours a day. It is very important for all children to get enough sleep to sustain their intensive growing. Most children will need about ten hours of sleep until their teens. Severely disturbed sleep in children is often caused by hyperactivity.

There are many theories as to why hyperactivity occurs, and we suggest that you consult one of the hyperactive children support groups to investigate this problem further (see on page 400).

Sleep can become out of balance in either extreme, and may be an indication of being out of balance in other ways also. If you desire to sleep constantly, and for long periods of time, it may be that you are unwell, in which case it is normal to want to sleep more in order for the body to repair itself. If this tendency is prolonged, then you may need to find out if you are trying to avoid your daily life, and consider seeking professional advice.

If you have trouble going to sleep, then you need to assess your ability to 'let go' generally. Look at the section on Insomnia on page 105. Try to avoid stimulants such as coffee and smoking all day (not just in the evening), and make building in the time for relaxation a priority. Taking daily exercise in the fresh air can help you to sleep through the night.

Another reason that we need to sleep is to allow ourselves to dream. Dreaming complements the active, outgoing part of our life, and is the reflective, more passive balance to it. Problems that have been left unresolved by our rational, conscious minds can be explored through our dreams.

We can work with our dreams to come to a better understanding of ourselves. Try writing down your dreams in a special notebook kept by the side of your bed. Recording your dreams will often increase your ability to remember them. It is worth remembering that your reaction to your dream can be as significant as the dream itself, and when you record your dream you can convey how you felt about it also. If you want to examine your dreams with someone else, then there are various forms of therapy that work with dreams; consult your natural healing centre and ask about their psychotherapists, or if they run dream workshops.

Sex

Our sexual expression is an expression on one particuar level of who we are. Our sexual relationships will reflect how we relate to our bodies, and how we relate to our parents, as well as how we relate to other men and women.

Sex for procreation is natural. This is a basic urge. Sex for pleasure is a human capability, and there are a lot of opinions around, just as there always have been, about what is and is not 'right' in terms of sex. All religions have guidelines and restrictions about our sex life. Unfortunately, rigid guidelines and opinions will always lead to feelings of guilt in those people who do not easily conform to the proscribed attitudes. There is more sexual freedom in our society in recent years, although we still have to deal with many social expectations and opinions.

We can only experience a sense of sexual well-being if we feel good about our particular sexual needs. This does not mean devaluing sex. But we need to develop sex as an expression of love and tenderness, without necessarily excluding any particular sexual orientation.

Sexual intimacy gives us an opportunity to explore our inner selves, and our mutual vulnerability with another person. Sex is a time when we can experience a sense of closeness with another human being. The important thing is to respect your own body, and your partner's, during sex. There are no easy solutions to the power-based struggles that often develop between sexual partners, but it is worth bearing mind that a sexual relationship offers great opportunities for self-learning and growth.

Our level of interest in sex does not make us more or less of a woman or man. We must guard against making assumptions about other people. When we question why some people are more interested in sex than others, we must be wary of accepting that there is a 'normal' level of sexual behaviour.

Sex education in schools varies widely, but however good this education may be it can only be secondary to the openness that parents should have with their children. We should be well enough informed to answer anatomical questions, and we should be close enough as a family so that the growing-up process is simply part of everyday living together. Questions regarding birth control, menstruation, and so on, can all be dealt with as they arise.

Essentially sex, like eating, sleeping and exercise, is part of living. Be aware of what you do and its effects, and allow yourself to enjoy it because you are alive.

Appendices

Natural Remedies First Aid Kit

Ointments

ARNICA: For bruising, sprains, strains and so on. Apply externally to the injured part. Do not use on broken skin.

HYPERCAL: A general purpose antiseptic and healing ointment for use on abrasions, cuts, spots and insect bites, etc.

Tinctures

EUPHRASIA: A soothing and anti-inflammatory lotion made from the herb eyebright. Dilute in cool, boiled water and use as an eyewash for eye infections, sore eyes, etc. Seek medical advice if you suspect there are any particles of grit or whatever left in the eye.

HYPERCAL: An antiseptic and healing lotion. Apply neat for small cuts, bites, spots, etc. To clean wounds, dilute a few drops of the tincture in a little cool, boiled water and gently bathe the area with a piece of cotton wool dipped in the solution.

Essential Oils

LAVENDER: Antiseptic and anti-inflammatory. Pour neat onto minor burns and scalds. Hold near the nose and inhale the vapours if feeling faint.

Healing Herbs of Dr Bach

FIRST-AID REMEDY: For shock, fear and panic. Take a few drops straight in the mouth as often as required. Alternatively, add a few drops to half a cup of water and sip as often as required. If the patient is unconscious, or cannot swallow, moisten any pulse point, eg. temple or wrist, with a few drops of the remedy.

Homoeopathic Remedies

Keep these remedies in a box and store in a dark, cool place away from strong smells. If you are taking homoeopathic remedies abroad with you, ask for them not to be X-rayed at airports, as this will reduce their efficiency.

The remedies listed below are for first aid and acute situations only. If symptoms are severe, or persist, professional advice must be sought.

For first aid and acute use, remedies in the 6th potency should be taken, one dose every two hours until there is some improvement, then dosage should be less frequent. Remedies in the 30th potency should be repeated only once or twice, preferably at eight-hour intervals. For further indications look the remedies up in the Materia Medica section of this book.

ACONITE 6: First stages of fever and inflammation; after-effects of exposure to a cold wind; earache; hoarse, dry cough; after-effects of shock or fright.

ARNICA 30: A very useful first-aid remedy to take after any accident or injury. Helps to reduce bruising, prevent haemorrhage, and ameliorate shock; concussion; over-exertion.

ARSENICUM 30: Food poisoning. After-effects of bad food or drink with diarrhoea and vomiting; great weariness; anxiety and restlessness. Acute asthmatic and allergy attacks marked by anxiety. Worse at night.

BELLADONNA 30: Fevers with a high temperature. Patient is hot, red and may be delirious. Sunstroke. Throbbing, hammering headache. Inflammation where the affected part looks red and has a violent, throbbing pain.

FERRUM PHOS 6X: For the beginning stages of a cold or sore throat; hoarseness; nosebleeds. Externally this remedy may be used by crushing a tablet and sprinkling the powder onto a wound to stop the bleeding and help prevent infection.

GELSEMIUM 30: Influenza with an aching body, heavy headache, shivering. Trembling and diarrhoea before an ordeal, or following a shock.

HYPERICUM 30: Injury to parts rich in nerves such as fingers or spine. Any injury marked by severe pain. Lacerated wounds; punctured wounds such as from a nail, needle or splinter.

LEDUM 30: Wasp, bee or other insect bites or stings. Animal, bites, such as dog bites, where there is bruising surrounding the wound. Black eyes, any injury with a lot of bruising, with swelling and puffiness. Prophylactic for tetanus.

NUX VOMICA 6: After-effects of over-indulgence in food, drink or stimulants (hangover). Irritability, nausea and headache. Any stomach disorder where there is nausea that is greatly relieved by vomiting.

RHUS TOX 6: Sprains and strains following an injury or over-exertion. The painful or injured part stiffens up during rest, and is ameliorated by gentle motion. Colds or flu following exposure to cold, wet weather.

Food Charts

Chart 1: Good Sources of Vitamins

VITAMIN A: Fish-liver oils, liver, butter, egg yolk, cheese, herring, mackerel, carrots, dried apricots, kale, parsley, spinach, pumpkin, peas.

VITAMIN B1 – THIAMIN: Brewer's yeast, yeast extract, rice, wheatgerm, soya beans, sunflower seeds, broad beans, rye, lentils, chickpeas.

VITAMIN B2 – RIBOFLAVIN: Yeast extract, brewer's yeast, liver, soya beans, wheatgerm, eggs, yoghurt, almonds, mushrooms, millet, kelp, broad beans, sesame seeds, mung beans.

VITAMIN B3 – NIACIN: Brewer's yeast, meat, liver, mackerel, brown rice, cod, peanuts, kelp, pulses, almonds, dates, millet.

VITAMIN B5 – PANTOTHENIC ACID: Brewer's yeast, liver, wheatbran, egg, lentils, cashew nuts, almonds, soya beans, brown rice, peas.

VITAMIN B6: Brewer's yeast, liver, mackerel, avocado, banana, walnuts, yoghurt, millet, rye, sunflower seeds, sesame seeds.

VITAMIN B12: Liver, fish, meat, free-range eggs, cheese, yoghurt, milk. Rarely found in cereals, fruit or vegetables, although there is a small amount in cauliflower, comfrey and alfalfa.

VITAMIN C: Blackcurrants, parsley, broccoli, green pepper, straw-berries, cabbage, oranges, guava, cauliflower, watercress. You should eat vegetables raw to obtain maximum levels of Vitamin C, and all foodstuffs should be fresh.

VITAMIN D: Sunshine, oily fish, egg yolk, sunflower seeds, alfalfa.

VITAMIN E: Wheatgerm oil and other cold-pressed vegetable oils, sesame seeds, tahini, almonds, wheatgerm, millet, Brazil nuts, peanuts.

VITAMIN K: Fresh leafy green vegetables, green and red peppers.

FOLIC ACID: Brewer's yeast, liver, green vegetables, eggs, lentils, milk.

Chart 2: Good Sources of Minerals

CALCIUM: Dairy products, watercress, wheatflour, cabbage, eggs, brown rice, fish, meat, sesame seeds, nuts, chickpeas, kelp, parsley, broad beans.

PHOSPHORUS: Cheese, lentils, wholemeal bread, eggs, meat, fish, brown rice, sunflower seeds, barley, kelp, sesame seeds, almonds, rye, millet.

POTASSIUM: Brewer's yeast, dates, mushrooms, cabbage, meat, bananas, watercress, tomatoes, yoghurt, wholemeal bread, kelp, soya beans, dandelion.

FLUORINE: Tea, oats, rice, watercress, most fresh vegetables, goats' milk.

MAGNESIUM: Brazil nuts, soya beans, wholemeal flour, chocolate, lentils, parsley, kelp, almonds, sesame seeds, spinach.

IRON: Liver, cocoa, treacle, parsley, lentils, dulse, kelp, sesame seeds, haricot beans, wholemeal bread, eggs, watercress, dried fruit.

MANGANESE: Tea, whole cereals, beans and peas, nuts, pineapple, grapes, beetroot, watercress, kale.

ZINC: Meat, oysters, cheese, lentils, most nuts, sunflower seeds, sesame seeds, rye, olives, haricot beans, eggs.

IODINE: Iodised salt, white fish, yoghurt, kelp, eggs, almonds, wholemeal bread, spinach, strawberries, turnip, okra.

Cleansing Diet

This cleansing diet is a 10-day programme which is suitable if you are basically healthy but want to clear your system out. If you have a particular health problem, you should have a consultation with a dietary therapist or naturopath before going on a special diet.

It is particularly beneficial to do a cleansing diet in the spring and/or autumn.

DAY 1: Fruit for breakfast, lunch and in the evening. Choose one fruit for each meal from the following: apples, pears or grapes. Eat as much fruit as you like at one sitting. Drink lots of mineral water throughout the day.

DAY 2, 3, 4, 5, AND 6: Fruit for breakfast. Choose one fruit each day from: apples, pears, grapes, tomatoes, kiwi fruit and grapefruit.

Raw vegetables for lunch. Make a mixture of at least five salad vegetables: mix roots (carrots, grated beetroot, and so on), sprouts and leafy vegetables.

In the evening eat cooked vegetables. Make a soup by boiling a mixture of at least five vegetables, preferably including onions. Do not add any salt or seasoning.

DAY 7, 8, AND 9: Breakfast – as Day 2.

Lunch – as Day 2, but in addition eat two slices of dry Ryvita crispbread biscuits.

Evening – as Day 2.

DAY 10: Breakfast – as Day 2.

Lunch – as Day 5.

Evening – as Day 2, but in addition eat a baked potato with a small knob of butter.

Notes

Drink lots of mineral water every day.

If you prefer, you may add a small amount of dressing to the raw-vegetable lunch, made from virgin olive oil and a little fresh lemon juice only.

If you feel weak and very hungry between meal times, drink a cup of barley water made as follows: boil pot barley in lots of water until the water begins to turn pink and the barley is soft. Keep adding water if it gets low. When done, strain off the water and discard the barley. Add a little fresh lemon juice and a teaspoon of honey to each cupful. You can take this drink in a flask if you need to keep going at work.

Eat as much organically-produced fruit and vegetables as possible.

It is not unusual to get symptoms such as headaches, tiredness or skin eruptions during a cleansing diet. This is an indication that toxins are being released from the tissues and into the bloodstream before they are eliminated. If you drink enough water these symptoms should not be severe, and they usually disappear before you have finished the diet.

Important things to avoid altogether throughout the diet are: tea, coffee, smoking, salt, pepper, drugs (whether recreational or prescribed), alcohol and late nights.

Don't binge the day after you finish the diet. You will regret it. Readjust to the new range of tastes and foods available to you slowly.

Useful Contacts and Addresses

To find a practitioner of natural medicine write to the appropriate organisation listed below, seek a personal recommendation from a friend or acquaintance, or look up your nearest natural health centre by looking under 'Clinics' in the local telephone directory.

In Britain, the Institute for Complementary Medicine publishes a yearbook which is a directory of practices, colleges, therapies and information. Write to:
The Institute for Complementary Medicine
21 Portland Place, London W1N 3AF.

ABORTION ADVICE
Pregnancy Advisory Service
11–13 Charlotte Street, London W1 (0171–637 8962).

ACUPUNCTURE
The Council for Acupuncture
Suite One, 19 Cavendish Square, London W1M 9AD (0171–409 1440). Will supply a joint register of practitioners from the main acupuncture societies.

AIDS
National Aids Helpline
Freephone: 0800 567 123.
Positively Women
0171–490 5515.

AROMATHERAPY
International Federation of Aromatherapists
Department of Continuing Education, Royal Masonic Hospital, Ravenscourt Park, London W6 0TN. Send sae for information.

BATES METHOD
Eyesight training to overcome eye and vision problems naturally.
Bates Association
Peter Mansfield, Friars Court, 11 Tarmount Land, Shoreham-by-Sea, W. Sussex BN43 6RQ (01273 452623).

BREASTFEEDING
La Leche League
BM3424 London WC1V 6XX (0171–404 5011).

CHILDBIRTH
Active Birth Centre
55 Dartmouth Park Road, London NW5 1FL (0171–267 3006).
Association of Radical Midwives
62 Greetby Hill, Ormskirk, Lancashire L39 2DT.
Independent Midwives' Association
65 Mount Nod Road, London SW16 2LP.
National Childbirth Trust
Alexandra House, Oldham Terrace, London W3 6NH
(0181–992 8637).
The Maternity Alliance
59–61 Camden High Street, London NW1 7JL (0171–388 6337).

CHIROPRACTIC
British Chiropractic Association
Premier House, 10 Greycoat Place, London SW1P 1SB (0171–222
8866). Send sae for register.
The Institute of Pure Chiropractic
PO Box 127, Oxford OX1 1HH (01865 246687). Send sae for list
of practitioners.

COUNSELLING AND PSYCHOTHERAPY
Association of Child Psychotherapists
54 Gayton Road, London NW3 (0171–794 8881).
British Association for Counselling
37a Sheep Street, Rugby, Warwickshire CV21 3BX
(01788 78328/9).
Provides list of local counsellors and general information.
Institute of Dream Analysis
8 Willow Road, London NW3 (0171–794 8717).
The Institute of Family Therapy
43 New Cavendish Street, London W1 (0171–935 1651).
The Institute of Group Analysis

1 Daleham Gardens, London NW3 (0171–431 2693).
Relate (National Marriage Guidance Council)
Herbert Gray College, Little Church Street, Rugby CV21 3AP
(01788 73241).
Women's Therapy Centre
6 Manor Gardens, London N7 6LA (0171–263 6200).
Westminster Pastoral Foundation
23 Kensington Square, London W8 5HN (0171–937 6956).

CRANIAL OSTEOPATHY
Craniosacral Therapy Association
3 Sandgrove Cottages, Horsley, Nailsworth, Glos GL6 0PS.

DRUGS
Drug Advisory Centre
9 Brockley Cross, London SE4 (0181–692 4975).
Drugwatch
157 Waterloo Road, London SE1 8XF.
The Drug and Alcohol Service
Woodlands Colindale Hospital, Colindale Avenue, London NW9
(0181–905 9955).

ENVIRONMENTAL ISSUES
Friends of the Earth
56–8 Alma Street, Luton, Beds. LU1 2TH.
Greenpeace
30/31 Islington Green, London N1 8XE.
Women's Environmental Network
287 City Road, London EC1V 1LA (0171–490 2511).

ETHICAL BANKING
Mercury Provident plc
Orlingbury House, Lewes Road, Forest Row, Sussex RH18 5AA
(0134282 3739). Encourages depositors to take responsibility for
the way in which their savings are invested.

FLOWER REMEDIES – DR BACH
Bach Flower Centre
Mount Vernon, Sotwell, Wallingford, Oxfordshire OX10 0PZ
(01491 39489).
The Healing Herbs of Dr Bach
PO Box 65, Hereford HR2 0UW (01873 890218). Make and
supply the 38 Flower Remedies, and offer courses and training.

FOOD
The Soil Association
86 Colston Street, Bristol BS21 5BB (0117 9290661). Publish
regional booklets listing local suppliers of organic foods.
Parents for Safe Food
Britannia House, 1–11 Glenthorne Road, London W6 0LS
(0181–748 9898). Supply information about food safety issues.

HERBALISM
National Institute of Medical Herbalists
9 Palace Gate, Exeter, Devon EX1 1JA (01392 426022). Send
large sae for list of members.
The General Council and Register of Consultant Herbalists
Grosvenor House, 40 Seaway, Middleton-on-Sea, Sussex PO22
7SA (01243 586012). Send sae for list.

HOMOEOPATHY
Society of Homoeopaths
2 Artizan Road, Northampton NN1 4HU (01604 21400). Send
sae for regional list of registered homoeopaths.
British Homoeopathic Association
27a Devonshire Street, London W1N 1RJ (0171–935 2163).

HYPERACTIVITY
Hyperactive Children's Support Group
59 Meadowside, Angmering, Sussex. Publish diet sheet and general
advice.

MISCARRIAGE
Miscarriage Association
18 Stonybrook Close, West Bretton, Wakefield, West Yorks WF4
4TP (01924 830515).

NATUROPATHY
General Council and Register of Naturopaths
6 Netherhall Gardens, London NW3 5RR (0171–435 8728). Send
large sae for register of members.
Incorporated Society of Registered Naturopaths
1 Albemarle Road, The Mount, York YO2 1EN. Send sae for details
of your nearest practitioner.

ONE PARENT FAMILIES
Gingerbread
35 Wellington Street, London WC2 7BN (0171–240 0953).

OSTEOPATHY
British and European Osteopathic Association
6 Adelaide Road, Teddington, Middlesex TW11 0AY (0181–977
8532). Send sae for register of members.
General Council and Register of Osteopaths
(01734 576585). Register of members available.
London School of Osteopathy
110 Lower Richmond Road, London SW15 (0181–785 2267).
Send large sae for register of members.

PERSONAL DEVELOPMENT
Neal's Yard Agency
14 Neal's Yard, London WC2H 9DP (0171–379 0141). Free
advice on workshops, holidays and courses. Will also help you to
find a counsellor or psychotherapist.

REFLEXOLOGY
Association of Reflexologists
110 John Silkin Lane, SE8 5BE. Send sae for register of members.

SHIATSU
The Shiatsu Society
14 Oakdene Road, Redhill, Surrey RH1 6BT.

SPIRITUAL HEALING
National Federation of Spiritual Healers
Church Street, Sunbury-on-Thames, Middlesex TW16 6RG
(01932 783164).

SUPPLIERS
All the products mentioned in this book are available from branches
of Neal's Yard Remedies. A mail order service is also available. For
details telephone 0181–379 0705.
Neal's Yard Remedies
15 Neal's Yard, Covent Garden, London WC2 (0171–379 7222).

Chelsea Farmers Market, Sydney Street, London SW3 6NR
(0171–351 6380).
68 Chalk Farm Road, London NW1 8AN (0171–284 2039).
2A Kensington Gardens, Brighton BN1 4AL (01273 601464).
126 Whiteladies Road, Clifton, Bristol BS8 2RP (0117 9466034).
26 Lower Goat Lane, Norwich NR2 1EL (01603 766681).
5 Golden Cross Walk, Cornmarket Street, Oxford OX1 3EU
(01865 245436).
Little Priory, Fore Street, Totnes, Devon TQ9 5HJ
(01803 864640).

WOMEN'S ISSUES
National Women's Aid Federation
(Battered Women's Refuges)
374 Grays Inn Road, London WC1 (0171–837 9316).
Women Against Rape
71 Tonbridge Street, London WC1 (0171–837 7509).
Women Into Business
46 Westminster Palace Gardens, London SW1 (0171–976 7263).
Women's Environmental Network
287 City Road, London EC1 (0171–490 2511).
Women's Health and Reproductive Rights Information Centre
52 Featherstone Street, London EC1 (0171–251 6332).
Women's Therapy Centre
6 Manor Gardens, London N7 (0171–263 6200).

In Australia

Association of Massage Therapists
18a Spit Road, Mosman, NSW 2088 (969 8445).
Association of Remedial Masseurs
22 Stuart Street, Ryde, NSW 2112 (878 2159).
Australasian College of Natural Therapies
620 Harris Street, Ultimo, NSW 2007 (02 212 6699).
Australian Academy of Osteopathy
7th Floor, 235 Macquarie Street, Sydney, NSW 2000 (233 1655).
Australian Federation of Homoeopaths
21 Bulah Close, Berowra Heights, NSW 2082 (02 456 3602).
Australian Natural Therapists Association Ltd
PO Box 522, Sutherland, NSW 2232 (02 521 2063).

Australian Traditional Medicine Society
120 Blaxland Road, Ryde, NSW 2112 (808 2825).
National Herbalists Association of Australia
14/249 Kingsgrove Road, Kingsgrove, NSW 2208 (502 2938).

In the USA

ABORTION ADVICE
National Abortion Federation
1436 U Street, NW, Suite 103, Washington, DC 20009 (202 667 5881).

AIDS
National Resource Center on Women and AIDS
2000 P Street, NW, Suite 508, Washington DC 20036 (202 872 1770).

BREASTFEEDING
La Leche League International
9616 Minneapolis Avenue, PO Box 1209, Franklin Park, Il 60131–8209 (708 455 7730).

CHILDBIRTH
International Association for Childbirth at Home
PO Box 430, Glendale, CA 91209 (213 663 4996).

CHIROPRACTIC
American Chiropractic Association
1701 Clarendon Blvd, Arlington, VA 24203 (703 276 8800).

COUNSELLING
Association for the Development of
Social Therapy
c/o Barbara Silverman, 474 Third Street, Brooklyn, NY 11215 (718 499 3759).

DRUGS AND ALCOHOL
Alcoholics Anonymous World Services
PO Box 459, Grand Central Station, New York, NY 10163 (212 686 1100).

ENVIRONMENTAL ISSUES
Earth Island Institute
300 Broadway, Suite 28, San Francisco, CA 94133 (415 788 3666).

Greenpeace USA
1436 U Street, NW, Washington DC 20009 (202 462 1177).
World Women in Environment
1250 24th Street, NW, 4th floor, Washington DC 20037 (202 347 1514).

ETHICAL BANKING
Working Assets Money Fund (Socially Responsible Money Markets Fund)
230 California Street, San Francisco, CA 94111 (415 989 3200).

FLOWER REMEDIES – DR BACH
Dr Edward Bach Healing Society
644 Merrick Road, Lynbrook, NY 11563 (516 593 2206).

HERBALISM
Flower Essence Society
PO Box 1769, Nevada City, CA 95959 (916 265 9163).
California School of Herbal Studies
PO Box 39, Forestville, CA 95436 (707 887 7457).

HOMOEOPATHY
National Center for Homoeopathy
801 N Fairfax Street, Alexandria, VA 22314 (703 548 7790).

OSTEOPATHY
American Osteopathic Association
142 E Ontario Street, Chicago, IL 60611 (312 280 5800).

SPIRITUAL HEALING
Common Boundary Inc
7005 Florida Street, Chevy Chase, MD 20815 (301 652 9495).

WOMEN'S ISSUES
National Organization for Women
1000 16th Street, NW, Suite 700, Washington DC 20036 (202 331 0066).
National Association of Women's Centers
c/o Sylvia Kramer, Women's Action Alliance, 370 Lexington Avenue, Suite 603, New York, NY 10017 (212 532 8330).

Suggested Reading

GENERAL

Campbell, J., *An Open Life* (New York: Harper & Row, 1989).

Capra, F., *The Turning Point* (London: Wildwood House, 1982).

Carter, F., *The Education of Little Tree* (Albuquerque, USA: University of New Mexico Press, 1976).

Gawain, Shakti, *Creative Visualisation* (Mill Valley, CA, USA: Whatever Publishing, 1986).

Gawain, Shakti, *Living in the Light* (Mill Valley, CA, USA: Whatever Publishing).

Heindel, M., *The Vital Body* (London: Fowler, 1950).

Howe, Dr E. Graham, *The Mind of the Druid* (London: Skoob Books, 1989).

Lessing, D., *The Marriages Between Zones Three, Four and Five* (London: Granada, 1980).

McLuhan, T., ed., *Touch the Earth: A Self-Portrait of Indian Existence* (London: Abacus, 1973).

Pearson, C., *The Hero Within* (New York: Harper & Row, 1986).

Russell, P., *The Awakening Earth* (London: Arkana, 1982).

Starhawk, *Dreaming the Dark* (London: Mandala, 1990).

Stein, D., *The Women's Spirituality Book* (St Paul, Minnesota, USA: Llewellyn Publications, 1987).

Waring, M., *Counting For Nothing* (Wellington, New Zealand: Allen & Unwin, 1988).

Zukav, G., *The Dancing Wu Li Masters* (London: Fontana, 1979).

HEALTH – GENERAL

Chaitow, L., *Vaccination and Immunization: Dangers, Delusions and Alternatives* (Saffron Walden, England: C.W. Daniel, 1987).

Curtis, S., Fraser, R., & Kohler, I., *Neal's Yard Natural Remedies* (London: Arkana, 1988).

Dethlefsen, T., and Dahlke, R., *The Healing Power of Illness* (London: Element, 1990).

Scott, J., *Natural Medicine for Children* (London: Unwin Hyman, 1990).

Urs Koch, M., *The Whole Health Handbook* (London: Sidgwick & Jackson, 1981).

WOMEN'S HEALTH

Amner, C., *The A-Z of Women's Health* (London: Thorsons, 1983).

Campion, K., *A Woman's Herbal* (London: Century Hutchinson, 1987).

Drake, K., & J., *Natural Birth Control* (London: Thorsons, 1984).

Nissim, R., *Natural Healing in Gynecology* (London: Pandora, 1986).

Phillips, A., & Rakusen, J., *The New Our Bodies Ourselves* (London: Penguin, 1989).

PREGNANCY AND CHILDBIRTH

Balaskas, J., *Active Birth* (London: Unwin Paperbacks, 1983).

Balaskas, J., *Natural Pregnancy* (London: Sidgwick).

Gaskin, I., M., *Spiritual Midwifery* (Summertown, TN, USA: The Book Publishing Company, 1977).

Kitzinger, S., *Freedom and Choice in Childbirth* (London: Penguin, 1987).

Kitzinger, S., *Pregnancy and Childbirth* (London: Penguin, 1986).

HERBS

Grieve, M., *A Modern Herbal* (London: Penguin, 1931).

Hoffman, D., *The Herb User's Guide* (London: Thorsons, 1987).

Hoffman, D., *The Holistic Herbal* (Scotland: Findhorn Press, 1983).

Lust, J., *The Herb Book* (New York: Bantam, 1974).

McIntyre, M., *Herbal Medicine for Everyone* (London: Penguin, 1988).

McIntyre, A., *Herbs for Pregnancy and Childbirth* (London: Sheldon Press, 1988).

Mills, S., *The A-Z of Modern Herbalism* (London: Thorsons, 1985).

Tierra, M., *The Way of Herbs* (Santa Cruz, USA: Orenda/United Press, 1980).

HOMOEOPATHY

Castro, M., *The Complete Homoeopathy Handbook* (London: Macmillan, 1990).

Cummings, S., & Ullman, D., *Everybody's Guide to Homoepathic Medicines* (London: Gollancz, 1984).

Goodwin, J., *The Biochemic Handbook* (London: Thorsons, 1980).

Lockie, Dr. A., *The Family Guide to Homoeopathy* (London: Hamish Hamilton, 1989).

Phatak, S., *Materia Medica of Homoeopathic Medicines* (Delhi, India: IBPS, 1977).

Speight, P., *Before Calling the Doctor* (Saffron Walden, England: C.W. Daniel, 1976).

Vithoulkas, G., *Medicine of the New Man* (London: Thorsons, 1979).

AROMATHERAPY

Davis, P., *Aromatherapy: An A-Z* (Saffron Walden, England: C.W. Daniel, 1988).

Maury, M., *Marguerite Maury's Guide to Aromatherapy* (Saffron Walden, England: C.W. Daniel, 1989).

Price, S., *Practical Aromatherapy* (London: Thorsons, 1983).

Ryman, D., *The Aromatherapy Handbook* (Saffron Walden, England: C.W. Daniel, 1984).

Tisserand, M., *Aromatherapy for Women* (London: Thorsons, 1985).

Tisserand, R., *The Art of Aromatherapy* (Saffron Walden, England: C.W. Daniel, 1980).

Valnet, J., *The Practice of Aromatherapy* (Saffron Walden, England: C.W. Daniel, 1980).

Worwood, V., *The Fragrant Pharmacy* (London: Macmillan, 1990).

FLOWER REMEDIES – DR BACH

Bach, E., *Heal Thyself* (Saffron Walden, England: C.W. Daniel, 1931).

Bach, E., *Twelve Healers* (Saffron Walden, England: C.W. Daniel, 1933).

Barnard, J., *A Guide to the Bach Flower Remedies* (Saffron Walden, England: C.W. Daniel, 1979).

Chancellor, P., *Handbook of the Bach Flower Remedies* (Saffron Walden, England: C.W. Daniel, 1971).

Index

abortion, 117–18
abscess, 263, 327; mouth, 69; see also
  Infections
accidents, 7–14, 95, 206
Achillea millefolium see Yarrow
acne, 162–3, 213, 218, 223, 228, 246,
  255, 264, 271, 279, 287, 346
Aconite, 12, 33, 46, 48, 50, 51, 76, 78,
  103, 117, 156, 157, 159, 197–8, 204,
  253, 330, 390
Aconitum napellus see Aconite
addiction, 100–2, 362–4, 369–70
Aesculus hippocastanum see Horsechestnut
ageing, 384
Agnus castus see Vitex
Agrimonia eupatoria see Agrimony
Agrimony, 64, 198–9, 324
Agropyrum repens see Couchgrass
AIDS, 81–2, 129, 246, 248
Alchemilla vulgaris see Ladies' mantle
alcoholism, 100–2, 289, 299, 318, 326
alfalfa, 56, 60, 115, 144, 199
allergies, 82–4, 155, 157, 158, 165,
  167–8, 204, 296
Allium cepa, 156, 158, 199–200
Allium sativum see Garlic
Aloe vera, 9, 13, 200
alterative herbs, 179
Alumina, 66, 200–1
amniocentesis, 119–20
Anacydus pyrethrum see Pyrethrum
anaemia, 55–6, 199, 226, 237, 253, 296,
  301, 341
analgesic herbs, 179
Anenome pulsatilla see Pulsatilla
Anethum graveolens see Dill
Angelica archangelica see Angelica root
Angelica root, 35, 39, 101, 201–2
angina, 57, 266, 339
Aniseed, 23, 46, 51, 60, 69, 157, 202,
  230, 247, 249, 252
Aniseed oil, 202
anorexia nervosa, 264, 274, 345, 383, 300

Ant crude, 45, 202–3
Ant tart, 157, 203–4
anticipation, 205, 256
anti-inflammatory herbs, 179
Antimonium crudum see Ant crude
Antimonium tartaricum see Ant tart
antiseptic herbs, 179
antispasmodic herbs, 179
anxiety, 102–3, 205, 207, 209, 221, 257,
  267, 273, 278, 286, 297, 300, 305,
  322, 324, 339
aperient herbs, 180
aphrodisiac, 246, 270, 319, 323, 324,
  340, 347
Apis, 8, 51, 69, 74, 77, 84, 94, 147, 168,
  172, 189, 204–5
Apis mellifica see Apis
Apium graveolens see Celery seed
appetite loss, 229, 272, 274, 299, 345
Arctium lappa see Burdock
Arctostaphylos uva ursi see Ura ursi
Arg nit, 103, 205
Argentum nitricum see Arg nit
Ariba rosaeodova see Rosewood oil
Arnica, 8, 9, 10, 11, 12, 14, 35, 37, 38,
  68, 72, 94, 95, 105, 117, 118, 163,
  206, 245, 317, 319, 389, 390
Arnica montana see Arnica
Arsenicum album, 45, 67, 74, 76, 78, 84,
  103, 109, 156, 158, 164, 207, 297,
  336, 390
Artemisia absinthum see Wormwood
Artemisia maritima see Cina
artery diseases, 55, 56–7, 255, 281, 299,
  304, 322
arthritis, 93–5, 216, 218, 232, 254, 266,
  270, 296, 301, 309, 320, 323; see also
  Rheumatism; Rheumatoid arthritis
Asperula odorata see Woodruff
asthma, 83, 155–6, 157, 203, 241,
  249, 255, 269, 272, 273, 277, 279,
  281, 282, 287, 295, 304, 314, 334,
  337, 342

Witchazel, 8, 10, 12, 13, 45, 62, 68, 291, 333, **344**
Woodruff, **345**
worms, 71, 237, 256, 281, 320
Wormwood, 8, 71, 345
wounds, **13**, 213, 227, 242, 278, 279, 285, 291, 322, 332, 337, 346

Xanthoxylum americanum *see* Prickly Ash

Yarrow, 9, 50, 59, 62, 68, 76, 77, 83, 144, 157, 172, 173, 219, 248, 287, 304, **346**
Yellow dock root, 18, 56, 69, 86, 162, 166, **346**
Ylang ylang oil, 59, 60, 101, **347**

Zea mays *see* Cornsilk
Zingiber *see* Ginger

Natural Healing in Gynaecology

Rina Nissim

"*Natural Healing* compels us to care for our health in an intelligent and truly preventative manner. It provides a wealth of healing alternatives from eastern and western cultures and critiques the limits of conventional western medicine giving us the power of choice. Its friendly conversational style is a delight, as though a wise woman were guiding us through whatever problem we have and helping us figure out what to do. An unusual and invaluable resource indeed."
— *Boston Women's Health Collective*

Natural Healing in Gynaecology describes the use of herbs, trace-elements and diet in ensuring the proper functioning of the body and in the treatment of gynaecological disorders. It is intended as a tool for health care workers interested in natural healing and in alternatives to modern western medicine.

At the same time, as a product of the self-help movement, this manual is equally intended for women seeking to deepen their knowledge of their own bodies and their health care.

The Tentative Pregnancy

Barbara Katz Rothman

"Anyone who thinks that prenatal diagnosis is liberating for women should read this book."
— *Ruth Hubbard, Harvard University*

More and more women are having children when they are over thirty and amniocentesis, primarily used as a test for Down's Syndrome, is becoming a routine part of prenatal care.

In this groundbreaking book, Barbara Katz Rothman draws on the experience of over 120 women and a wealth of expert testimony to show how one simple procedure can radically alter the way we think about childbirth and becoming a parent. The results of amniocentesis, and the more recently developed chorion villus sampling, force us to confront agonising dilemmas. What do you do if there is a 'problem' with the foetus? What kind of support can you expect if you decide to raise a handicapped child? How can you come to terms with the termination of a wanted pregnancy?

Passionate, sympathetic and at times heartbreaking, Barbara Katz Rothman's book is a must for anyone thinking of having a child.

". . . makes women's experience of the technology visible for the first time . . . an immensely intelligent, sensitive and passionate book. No one can read it and remain unmoved."
— *Gena Corea*

Preventing Breast Cancer

The politics of an epidemic

Dr Cathy Read

Breast cancer is the most common cancer among women. It is predicted that across the world it will claim the lives of one million women annually by the turn of the century.

These deaths are preventable.

As Cathy Read argues in this powerful and provocative book, breast cancer is not the mysterious and unavoidable epidemic many would have us believe. Conventional medicine has failed to find a cure for breast cancer. This book addresses the root causes, which lie in our diet, environment and social structures. Breast cancer is not 'women's fault' — but it is not beyond our means to control it.

By laying bare the politics of an epidemic, *Preventing Breast Cancer* calls on everyone, women and health professionals alike, to stop the wringing of hands and unravel the real story behind breast cancer.

NATURAL HEALING IN GYNAECOLOGY	0 86358 069 6	£5.99 ☐
THE TENTATIVE PREGNANCY	0 04 440912 5	£8.99 ☐
PREVENTING BREAST CANCER	0 04 440909 5	£7.99 ☐
ALWAYS A WOMAN	0 7225 2643 1	£8.99 ☐
HERBAL THERAPY FOR WOMEN	0 7225 2722 5	£4.99 ☐

All these books are available from your local bookseller or can be ordered direct from the publishers.

To order direct just tick the titles you want and fill in the form below:

Name: _____

Address: _____

_____

_____ Postcode: _____

Send to: Thorsons Mail Order, Dept 3, HarperCollins*Publishers*, Westerhill Road, Bishopbriggs, Glasgow G64 2QT.
Please enclose a cheque or postal order or your authority to debit your Visa/Access account —

Credit card no: _____

Expiry date: _____

Signature: _____

— to the value of the cover price plus:
UK & BFPO: Add £1.00 for the first book and 25p for each additional book ordered.
Overseas orders including Eire: Please add £2.95 service charge.
Books will be sent by surface mail but quotes for airmail despatches will be given on request.

24 HOUR TELEPHONE ORDERING SERVICE FOR ACCESS/VISA CARDHOLDERS — TEL: 0141 772 2281.